T0318469

A Social History of Medicines in the Twentieth Century
To Be Taken Three Times a Day

A Social History of Medicines in the Twentieth Century
To Be Taken Three Times a Day

John K. Crellin

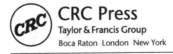

CRC Press
Taylor & Francis Group
Boca Raton London New York

CRC Press is an imprint of the
Taylor & Francis Group, an **informa** business

First published 2004 by The Haworth Press, Inc.

Published 2023 by Routledge
Taylor & Francis Group
6000 Broken Sound Parkway NW, Suite 300
Boca Raton, FL 33487-2742

Visit the Taylor & Francis Web site at
http://www.taylorandfrancis.com

and the CRC Press Web site at
http://www.crcpress.com

PUBLISHER'S NOTE
This book has been published solely for educational purposes and is not intended to substitute for the medical advice of a treating physician. Medicine is an ever-changing science. As new research and clinical experience broaden our knowledge, changes in treatment may be required. While many potential treatment options are made herein, some or all of the options may not be applicable to a particular individual. Therefore, the author, editor, and publisher do not accept responsibility in the event of negative consequences incurred as a result of the information presented in this book. We do not claim that this information is necessarily accurate by the rigid scientific and regulatory standards applied for medical treatment. **No warranty, expressed or implied, is furnished with respect to the material contained in this book. The reader is urged to consult with his/her personal physician with respect to the treatment of any medical condition.**

Cover design by Marylouise E. Doyle.

"To Anni Besant, Marie Stopes"—Reprinted from, *CMAJ* 1966, Volume 64, Page 1015 by permission of the publisher, © 1966 Canadian Medical Association.

Library of Congress Cataloging-in-Publication Data

Crellin, J. K.
  A social history of medicines in the twentieth century : to be taken three times a day / John K. Crellin.
       p. cm.
Includes bibliographical references and index.
    ISBN 0-7890-1844-6 (hard : alk. paper)—ISBN 0-7890-1845-4 (soft : alk. paper)
    1. Drugs—North America—History—20th century. 2. Drugs—Great Britain—History—20th century. 3. Drug utilization—North America—History—20th century. 4. Drug utilization—Great Britain—History—20th century.
    [DNLM: 1. Prescriptions, Drug—history—Canada. 2. Prescriptions, Drug—history—Great Britain. 3. Prescriptions, Drug—history—United States. 4. Drug Therapy—history—Canada. 5. Drug Therapy—history—Great Britain. 6. Drug Therapy—history—United States. 7. History of Medicine, 20th Cent.—Canada. 8. History of Medicine, 20th Cent.—Great Britain. 9. History of Medicine, 20th Cent.—United States. 10. Social Change—history—Canada. 11. Social Change—history—Great Britain. 12. Social Change—history—United States. QV 711 AA1 C915s 2004]
I. Title.

RM45. C74 2004
615' .1'0973—dc21
                                                                              2003012397

ISBN 13: 978-0-7890-1845-8 (pbk)

To JDC for healthy skepticism and a whole lot more.

ABOUT THE AUTHOR

Dr. John K. Crellin holds British qualifications in both medicine and pharmacy. He also holds a PhD in the history and philosophy of science. His principal interest is self-care, particularly the role of complementary medicine. Dr. Crellin has taught undergraduate, graduate, medical, and complementary/alternative medical students in the United Kingdom, the United States, and Canada. His present position is John Clinch Professor of the History of Medicine at Memorial University of Newfoundland; he gives frequent public and professional talks on complementary/alternative medicine.

Dr. Crellin's publications range widely on the history of medicine and pharmacy, as well as on herbal medicine and home medicine in general. His books include *Professionalism and Ethics in Complementary and Alternative Medicine* (Haworth, with F. Ania), *"By the Patient and not by the Book": Constancy and Change in Small Town Doctoring* (with P.I. Crellin); *Herbal Medicine Past and Present* (with J. Philpott); *Home Medicine: The Newfoundland Experience; Alternative Health Care in Canada: Nineteenth- and Twentieth-Century Perspectives* (co-edited with R. Andersen and J. Connor); and *Healthways: Newfoundland Elders, Their Lifestyles and Values* (with R.R. Andersen and B. O'Dwyer).

CONTENTS

Preface and Acknowledgments

A Social History of Medicines in the Twentieth Century: To Be Taken Three Times a Day is written for everyone who has wondered how they came to be taking one medicine rather than another, either as self-care or a doctor's prescription. This includes all those who are additionally involved in the complex business of prescribing, dispensing, advising on, and administering modern medicines. Today, expectations are that everyone takes an increasing responsibility for his or her health and is sufficiently knowledgeable about these medications. It is a time, too, when countless concerns exist regarding poor patient compliance with prescription medication directions. Before discussing this dilemma, the reader is taken through a complexity of issues to explore why, throughout the twentieth century, physicians and sick people on both sides of the Atlantic prescribed or chose a particular medicine—perhaps validated it—often when others felt it was of little or no value or remained uncertain of it.

Historical explorations can serve many purposes. One hope is that the perspectives in this book, dealing with everyday usage rather than discovery, will help readers to sharpen their thinking and ponder questions about how we reached a situation in which medicines have become so dominant, not only in public worries about rising health care costs, but also in the lives of countless individuals.

The writing of this book was prompted by a series of oral histories taken from retired pharmacists and the need to place the information in historical and social context. From there, in the absence of a general account of the everyday use of medicines in the twentieth century, it grew into the present work that examines medical, pharmaceutical, and sociocultural influences.

Particular thanks go to many people who, wittingly and often unwittingly, have helped in many ways. Living in England, the United States, and Newfoundland, Canada, over the years allowed me to imbibe understandings and perspectives from three countries. Education in both pharmacy and medicine at the University of London initiated my firsthand exploration of attitudes toward medicines in the

1960s and 1970s. In North Carolina, perspectives on everyday medical and pharmaceutical practice were gleaned from innumerable sources. Many informative hours during the 1980s were spent chatting with James Semans at Duke University Medical Center about the changing pulse of American medicine. Invaluable, too, was the pharmacy at Patterson's Mill Country Store in Durham, North Carolina, founded by Elsie and John Booker, as well as my involvement at the Country Doctor Museum in Bailey, North Carolina. Living in Newfoundland, part of Canada since only 1949, offers a variety of insights from the attitudes of a one-time British colony overtaken by the mainland.

Particular thanks go to the Newfoundland Pharmaceutical Association where Joan O'Mara (curator of the James J. O'Mara Pharmacy Museum) and Donald Rowe (secretary-registrar) have been totally supportive. A particular debt goes to those who gave oral history interviews during the 1990s. In addition, the number of people who helped with brief conversations and responses to questions is tremendous. Members of the Medical History Society in St. John's (sometimes described, not quite accurately, as the retired physicians' society), and, from time to time, many other physicians have been helpful over the years with reminiscences about medical practice and attitudes. Special thanks are noted in places for particular information, but here I want to express profound thanks to Ian Rusted, Nigel Rusted, John Martin, and Paddy Warwick. The Rusted brothers, who must never have thrown away a scrap of paper with potential historical value, are the sources of information many historians can only dream about.

Over the years, I have met with countless senior citizens when giving talks on home medicines in seniors' homes and complexes; no one has ever been shy to add perspective on the most popular medicines in everyday use and why he or she took them. On the level of a more formal study, I thank colleagues Raoul Andersen and Bernard O'Dwyer for our work on the Healthways project. When actually writing this book, whenever I wanted to check information, an e-mail to David Cowen invariably brought an immediate response. Thanks also to John Parascandola, John Swann, and Ernie Stieb. JDC, with a much sharper memory for events than my own and an invaluable questioning approach to almost everything, has challenged and sharpened many interpretations.

At Memorial University of Newfoundland, I am grateful to research assistance from students, especially Nancie Ridout and Margaret Ann Lee. The help of Rosalind Nichols has been inestimable in patiently arranging and rearranging the text as the overwhelming amount of twentieth-century material was sifted and, if appropriate, added to or discarded from the initial outline. Cheerfully, beyond the call of duty, she also dealt with the hiccoughs that arose in transferring the manuscript from WordPerfect to Word software.

The staff at The Haworth Press have been exceptional in copyediting and checking the manuscript. Special thanks to Peg Marr, Jennifer Durgan, and Ryan Crissy.

Chapter 1

The Big Canvas: Issues and Context

A desire to take medicine is, perhaps, the great feature which distinguishes man from other animals.

William Osler
"Recent Advances in Medicine"[1]

SOME KEY QUESTIONS

This book examines the social, medical, and pharmaceutical influences that shaped the everyday availability and usage of medicines in the twentieth century. The story is far more complicated than the triumphal parade of such new medicines as antitoxins, Salvarsan, insulin, and other hormones (e.g., adrenaline, thyroxine, testosterone, and estrogen), sulfonamides, antibiotics, antihistamines, antihypertensives, tranquilizers, antidepressives, immunosuppressives, and many others. Although the story of the introduction of these and other milestone developments has often been told, the countless sociocultural factors that shaped (and shape) their use by individuals have generally received much less attention.[2]

Exceptions do exist, especially in writings that focus on a single medicine or a class of medicines. Covering the second half of the twentieth century, for instance, Mickey Smith (1991) explores some relevant issues in his *A Social History of Minor Tranquilizers*. He looks at diverse factors encouraging and undermining the use of medicines and poses such questions as, Why do doctors overprescribe? What is the influence of the media? Did the availability of medicines actually create medical conditions (for instance, anxiety becoming a commonplace diagnosis)? And why do many medicines have a "life cycle" of overvaluation on their introduction, followed by misuse,

1

emerging problems, undervaluation and condemnation, and finally critical usage?[3] Another recent author, David Healy (1997), in *The Antidepressant Era,* raises some of the same questions as he tells a fascinating story of ambiguities, ideologies, and diverse interpretations of scientific and clinical data from the 1950s to the 1990s.[4] All such writings make clear not only the influences of society on usage, but also the specific impact of many medicines on society; some, such as Prozac, became "cultural events" and contributed to what is commonly viewed as the twentieth-century medicalization of society.[5]

Various issues considered in these and other writings are examined further in this book in order to illustrate the broad array of circumstances and attitudes that surround the choices, prescriptions, and use of medicines by physicians and patients. In the text a "Mr. Brown" or a "Ms. Smith" are mentioned from time to time as a reminder that this story of medicines is very much concerned with patients and that, given the wide range of attitudes individuals have toward medicines, the generic patient does not exist. One recurring question is, Why did certain medicines become or remain widely accepted and validated as useful by patients and physicians, even though serious doubts existed subsequently (if not at the time) about their effectiveness or safety? The question is particularly apt for the first half of the 1900s, which is often viewed as being "premodern" in the story of medicines. For the second half of the century, amid changing circumstances—from the establishment of double-blind clinical trials of medicines to the growing involvement of the powers of government and the pharmaceutical industry—the issue is not so much about doubts regarding effectiveness; it is more the extent to which prescription medicines were accepted given the worries over side effects, the challenges to the authority of physicians, the distrust of the pharmaceutical industry, and the concerns whether governments were protecting the public adequately.

In exploring validation, or otherwise, of medicines by the general public, various factors are looked at, aside from the severity of an ailment, that can affect or shape physician prescribing, purchase of over-the-counter medications, or the taking of a medicine. For instance, what were the public's general attitudes toward medicines, and in what ways did they change? How did patients respond to new choices of medicines? To what extent did the advertising of over-the-counter medicines encourage confidence in particular medicines and, perhaps, reinforce popular lay beliefs about health and disease? Why did over-the-counter medicines push aside homemade remedies? Did similarities between over-the-counter and prescription medicines help in validation? Did the authority of doctors and the mystique of the prescription foster lay confidence in "doctors'" medicines? What was the influence of pharmacy, especially community pharmacy, in shaping everyday attitudes to, and usage of, medicines? Did limiting public access to many medicines through legislative and professional controls encourage confidence in or fear of those medicines? How significant was the curtailment (often due to cost containment) of physicians' clinical freedom to prescribe certain medicines? Why did alternative medicine mushroom in the final decades of the twentieth century? And have changes in physician-patient relationships affected attitudes toward medicines?

To anchor the questions and discussions, I provide as much comment as possible on selected medications, for a social history of medicines without any details about the medicines would be like a leopard without spots. Indeed, the character and symbolism of a medicine can be significant factors in usage and validation (see Figure 1.1). One must remember that amid multiple factors affecting decision making—which wax and wane in significance over time—people with worries and health problems have always drawn on various beliefs and resources—some conventional, some not. They selectively draw from the constantly changing big picture of medicines and other treatments according to their particular beliefs, needs, and circumstances. Decisions are personal. Although these choices may reflect current fashions in medication, individual idiosyncrasies always exist.

SOCIAL VALIDATION OF MEDICINES

Why did certain medicines eventually become accepted even though they were viewed with suspicion at one time, and later were considered useless or even dangerous? Countless medicines in use prior to the modern era were widely castigated while still in their heyday; in 1936 they were seen as survivals of "tradition [and] credulity," due to the "disinclination to oppose 'the general consensus of opinion,' and

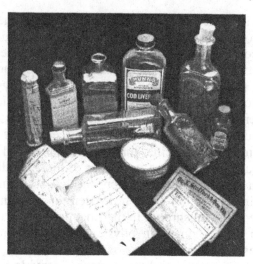

FIGURE 1.1. A medicines montage. Physicians' prescriptions and medicines (both dispensed and over the counter) are witnesses of their times. Like all artifacts, those shown here embody lives, parts of lives, and stories in one way or another. They embody a doctor's knowledge and idiosyncracies, the pharmacist's skills and art in dispensing patients' social circumstances, health beliefs, lifestyles, and medical problems. (*Source:* Author's collection.)

the neglect to use proper controls in making therapeutic tests on actual patients."[6] In more recent times, historians and others have been equally hard-hitting. Influential American physician/writer Lewis Thomas is not alone in saying that all treatments before his time—he qualified in 1937—were "the most frivolous and irresponsible kind of human experimentation."[7] Physician James McGrath wrote less bitingly in 1974 that

> looking back, it is hard to believe how limited was effective medical treatment in 1922. . . . At least ninety-eight percent of all medicines were worthless, as are the majority of those we swallow to-day, but to-day at least a substantial proportion of medicines are effective and useful.[8]

Such subjective views are bolstered by a study that examined therapies in use in 1927 and in 1975 for 362 medical conditions; it was concluded that the therapeutic value of 60 percent in 1927 and 22 percent in 1975 was "nil, harmful, useless, of questionable value, or merely symptomatic."[9]

The response in this book to charges of ineffectiveness is in line with historians who stress that, rather than being dismissive, we must try to understand how societies, or groups and individuals within those societies, came to see particular treatments to be at least useful.[10] Such social validation has always had a particularly important role, by which we mean that widespread (not necessarily universal) public acceptance of a particular remedy is dependent on more than just the authority of "scientific" evidence. The latter has been of constant influence, but interpretation of data has always been contingent on the thinking and social settings of the researcher and of other observers.[11] Although this was more obvious before the current era of clinical trials, consensus conferences, and evidence-based medicine, questions about interpretation and bias remain. During the first half of the twentieth century, the assessments of medical science that reached everyday medical practice depended very much on the authority of physician-leaders (the medical elite of "consultants" and "specialists"), their interpretations, textbooks, and reviews. Some promoted "rational" or science-based therapeutics, as did the American Medical Association's Council on Pharmacy and Chemistry from 1905 onward.[12] However, as will be discussed, throughout the twentieth century there was debate and often disagreement between science and experience, between the academic physician and the general practitioner.

Social acceptance of particular medicines by patients is undoubtedly a complex issue, as it is for physicians who, at one time or another, accepted widely used practices before they fell into disfavor. Striking, well-studied examples of socially validated treatments other than medicines include surgery for autointoxication and lobotomy for psychiatric disorders.[13] Patients' use of a medicine may rest on their beliefs (popular, religious, scientific, pseudoscientific, or a mix) about the cause or causes of disease; whether a diagnosis of a particular disease (or perhaps nondisease) is fashionable at the time;[14] attitudes toward the authority of physicians; opinions about medicines in general (were they safe or did they "act like toxins"?); the persuasiveness of testimonials for a medicine (perhaps from a friend, newspaper, support group, or health care practitioner); effectiveness of commercial promotion; and local health and social conditions.[15]

Such considerations undoubtedly embrace the views and practices of society in general, including broad national characteristics as emphasized in Lynn Payer's (1988) *Medicine and Culture: Varieties of Treatment in the United States, England, West Germany, and France.*[16] Intriguing differences are revealed in the use of prescription and over-the-counter drugs in the four countries; for instance, some "commonly prescribed drugs in France, drugs to dilate the cerebral blood vessels, are considered ineffective in England and America."[17] Various explanations have been put forward to account for national differences. One author seems to reflect stereotypical views when suggesting that the higher use of antihypertensive angiotensin converting enzyme (ACE) inhibitors in Italy compared with Britain was "perhaps due to the increased incidence of drug induced impotence with β-adrenergic blockers [that] is more unacceptable to Italians than British patients or their wives."[18]

Cultural characteristics may lead to prescriptions for inappropriate therapies in consequence of a person's physical responses (known as *somatization*) to psychological and social stress, a significant issue in increasingly multicultural societies. For example, late twentieth-century depression among Asian immigrants in the United Kingdom often presented as generalized weakness, bowel consciousness, exaggerated fear of heart attacks, and other symptomatology.[19]

REGIONALISM IN THE STORY OF MEDICINES

Historians, geographers, and others are always interested in regional distinctiveness in health care, particularly the impact of diseases. Significant nuances and exceptions to broad national/international generalizations are frequently highlighted, for instance, differing features between northern and southern states in the United States,[20] the endemic opium eating in the Fen district of Britain in the nineteenth century,[21] and the twentieth-century local popularity of headache remedies manufactured in North Carolina up to the 1950s.[22] In this book, Newfoundland serves as a sounding board and mirror, particularly for the earlier part of the social history of medicines. By contrast and comparison, particularly with the United States and Britain, Newfoundland's medical history is used to weave an account of overall trends and distinctive features in the use of medicines on both sides of the Atlantic. Although late-twentieth-century medicine is often seen as being globalized, the philosophies of everyday practice in Britain and the United States have often been noted as being different. For instance, the view that the clinical freedom of a doctor in the second half of the century was more constrained in the nationalized and bureaucratic health system of Britain than it was in the United States, where professional "free trade" and self-determination prevailed.[23] Newfoundland has been characterized, as has Canada as a whole, as holding many attitudes that fall midway between the attitudes of Britain and the United States, though this is not always so.

Newfoundland's story offers much more than just another local history. It is distinctive and in many ways unique because of its social history as a self-governing British colony and, from 1949, as a Canadian province.[24] Isolated in the turbulent North Atlantic, Newfoundland's attitudes toward medicines help to raise questions about attitudes elsewhere. In other countries the more subtle influences on the use of medicines may be hidden behind broad national or global trends. Although discussion of the social conditions is necessarily brief, it should alert the reader to the importance of recognizing that a person's sense of place is frequently relevant to understanding attitudes to and use of medicines, even aside from availability. The island's reliance on imported medicines is noteworthy—from Britain, the United States, and Canada—throughout its years of independence, and it prompts questions about the shaping of choices of medicines by entrepreneurial market forces. In 1905, readers of the British *Pharmaceutical Journal* were told that "British traders who only send representatives there once in about two years will do well to make a note of the fact that Canadian and American merchants send traveling agents to the colony twice in each year."[25]

Newfoundland acts as a sounding board in other ways. One example comes from U.S. reports on public health in the island prior to the establishment of U.S. military bases there during World War II. The disparaging nature of the reports raises questions of U.S. attitudes toward a "colony" in the context of policies to safeguard the health of 10,000 servicemen.[26] Yet whatever attitudes were expressed in reports, far-reaching social change in the island was brought about by the bases. Countless Newfoundland lives were altered by the availability of new jobs on the military bases or by marriage to a "Yankee." Physicians from both countries interacted, though this had been happening for some time with constant visits from U.S. physicians and medical students to the renowned Grenfell Mission, once described as "an American colony."[27] In addition, a constant stream of volunteers came to Newfoundland eager to gain experience in providing health care in a remote place.[28] These visitors, who often left a record of their stay, included U.S. medical students looking for medical experiences they could not get at home. A Johns Hopkins medical graduate, John Olds, practiced in a small Newfoundland community from 1930 to around 1980, and encouraged innumerable U.S. medical students and young physicians to work with him for short periods.[29]

Newfoundland, then, with its problematic social conditions, offers an ideal resource from which (1) to prompt questions about social factors affecting everyday use of medicines; (2) to use as a sounding board to raise questions about trends and practices in other countries; and (3) to consider general matters of interest such as the transmission of ideas and practices.

ORGANIZATION OF THE BOOK

The book first provides an introductory overview of selected medicines and of pharmacy in Newfoundland from the seventeenth to nineteenth centuries. It spotlights topics relevant to the early history of therapy throughout North America; for instance, how new local remedies were "discovered" in Britain's North American colonies, how some of these remedies—even of doubtful value—became socially validated, and on how the boundaries between self and professional care changed. Certain topics, too, have interesting parallels to the twentieth century, such as how self-care in the 1800s drew on new alternative medical practices, just as happened in the last decades of the twentieth century.

The detailed discussion on the twentieth century—the core of the book—looks at the period from 1900 to around 1950, and then the second half of the century. The latter is a dramatically different time from the first half in many ways, aside from the vastly different armamentarium of available medicines. The second half can be described not only as the prescription-only era but also as a time of particular attention to "drugs," in part because of the widening scope of illicit drug use.[30] The natural break in the story around 1950 allows comment on differences and on how relevant a characterization of the two time periods by medical historians is to the medicines story. The first half of the century is viewed widely as one of dominance of medical authority that owed much to a new public optimism that science (e.g., physiology, bacteriology/immunology, and pharmacology) was finding solutions to diagnostic and treatment problems. In contrast, the second half of the century is seen as a period of curtailment of medical authority through such challenges to the profession as patients' rights and widespread acceptance of alternative medicine. By 1982, Paul Starr writes at length that the autonomy and dominance of the medical profession is in jeopardy.[31]

Although the broad characterizations of historians are accepted in this book, the situation in Newfoundland prompts the general question: did the two halves of the twentieth century differ more in emphases than absolute differences? After all, there was, as will be seen, more than a little ambivalence toward the authority of physicians in the early decades. Moreover, just as the consumer culture was evident in the United States in the early decades of the century (preceding an organized consumer movement), it also reached, at least with respect to over-the-counter medicines, into the countless, small Newfoundland communities at the time.[32]

Throughout the book, I use the term *medicines* (or *medications* and *remedies*) rather than the commonly employed *drugs*. Amidst many often slippery definitions of *drugs* and *medicines* (e.g., a medicine is a licensed drug), I prefer *medicines* not only because it is more appropriate for the compounded preparations common to the first half of the 1900s but also because the term *drug* covers illicit substances and recreational usage of prescription-only products. It is of interest that the efforts of U.S. druggists in the 1920s to stem the growing popularity of such terms as *drug abuse* or *drug evil,* rather than *narcotic abuse* etc., ultimately failed.[33] Another term used throughout is *patients,* rather than, say, *consumers* or *clients,* which commonly appeared in the medical literature during the 1990s. I prefer the term *patients,* because it reflects the power imbalance that is still commonplace in the physician-patient relationship despite the changing nature of that relationship.

RURAL SCENES

Here, and in the next two sections, introductory comments on rural health care, public/community health, and colonial mind-sets focus primarily on the first half of the 1900s. These matters are chosen not only to compare situations and practices in Newfoundland with those in other countries but also to outline, on the big canvas of health care, some of the social circumstances that directly and indirectly shaped the availability and use of medicines.

The Newfoundland scene, in prompting questions about the quality of medical practice in small towns and rural areas, is a good jumping-off point to raise awareness of rural-urban differences that impinge on health care and the use of medicines elsewhere.[34] Except for its capital city, St. John's, the island in the pre-1950s not only conjures up analogous pictures of conditions in, for instance, the Appalachian region and many poor southern states in the United States, as well as the Highlands and Islands of Scotland, but also raises general questions about rural health care throughout Britain and the United States. It has, after all, been said that in Britain, between the two world wars, "comparative death rates showed that those who lived in urban areas were more likely to be offered . . . new treatments successfully than those who lived in the countryside."[35]

Difficult terrain and harsh weather challenged the provision of effective medical services to about half of Newfoundland citizens (of a population of around 350,000 in the 1930s), who lived in the 1,300 or so small communities (known locally as outports) scattered around the 6,000 miles of rugged coastline of an island slightly larger than Ireland. The general absence of roads until the 1960s (with transport by boat to most communities), the small population, the heavy reliance on the vagaries of the fishery, the frequent inaccessibility to conventional medical practitioners, and the limited cash economy all handicapped the provision of conventional health care. This is reflected in an interpretation made by the 1930 Royal Commission on Health and Public Charities on the high use of over-the-counter medicines on the island: "The obvious conclusion is that a very large portion is used by people who endeavor in this way to make up for what they lack in skilled medical and nursing services."[36] The 1915 remark of one colonial governor of Newfoundland that "every one, by the time he is forty is either a fool or a physician" seemed especially appropriate for the island.[37] Another glimpse of how geography could shape the particulars of medical care is seen in the practice of a doctor in the outport of Twillingate. His celebrated readiness to operate, even for the slightest suspicion of appendicitis, was intended to preempt a "flare up" when a person was out of range of medical help, perhaps fishing. In fact, the phrase "geographic appendix" to describe preventive surgery became fairly well known there. Whether some might see this as what has been called "macho medicine" on the part of male physicians is open to discussion.[38]

Although no doubt exists that, on both sides of the Atlantic in the early 1900s, rural residents with limited access to physicians relied heavily on homemade remedies, commercial remedies were having an increasing impact, even among the poor. In the Highlands and Islands of Scotland, as an example, the 1912 Dewar Commission on health care reported that a "brisk trade in patent medicines [had] developed in recent years and, more particularly in the case of quack medicines of American manufacture." This was said to be due to the fact that the "Americans are more expert advertisers than the British."[39]

The extensive use at the time of commercial over-the-counter medicines has been similarly found for other disadvantaged rural areas, including Appalachia.[40] As in Newfoundland, these medicines clearly led, despite their expense, to some edging out of the harvesting of plants and preparing remedies in the kitchen.[41] No doubt exists that commercialism drove and reshaped self-care for reasons such as limited local supply of herbs, the saving of time in making remedies in the kitchen, and the persuasive promotion of over-the-counter medicines through both advertising and the authority of "famous" companies and of drugstores. Some of these issues are touched upon in Chapter 3, though space does not allow discussion of such ramifications as shifting some health care decision making from the women in the household and the ultimate undermining of the sense of community and self-sufficiency in rural living.

One factor encouraging the use of over-the-counter medicines, at least in larger communities, was their availability not only from druggists but also from doctors' offices, the more so if the latter were in the doctors' own drugstores—as was not uncommon in North America around 1900. Although an office was frequently a separate room in or next to the store, it has been said that most doctors in rural Kansas around 1900 "had drugstores and wore whiskers and examined patients as they were seated besides the counter in view of other customers and loafers."[42]

Rural situations prompt critical appraisals of doctors and their prescribing habits. The opinion that rural health care, because of isolation, was inferior to that in urban areas was commonplace. In the mid-twentieth century it was said that rural general practitioners in Britain suffered by being distanced from "good clinical medicine."[43] This was no different from the United States and Canada, though making generalizations about doctors and their standards of care, particularly in the early decades of the 1900s, is fraught with difficulties. Diverse educational backgrounds were undoubtedly one issue, as evident in Newfoundland with its doctors from England, Scotland, Ireland, the United States, and Canada at a time (circa 1890s to 1920s) when medical education was changing everywhere, albeit unevenly, to incorporate more laboratory medicine and basic science. It is clear that practicing in rural backwaters did not necessarily mean a doctor vegetated and became woefully out of date; in fact, the isolation seemingly increased the conscientiousness of some physicians in reading medical journals.[44] On the other hand, the negative or ambivalent reputations of physicians in the eyes of many patients (Chapter 4) confirm variable quality of care.

Public acceptance and respect of doctors in the first half of the 1900s depended on many factors beyond the authority derived from their special education and scientific medicine's growing public appeal. Particularly relevant to the present account is a patient's confidence in a doctor's prescription and "bottle of medicine," and, perhaps, a doctor's sensitivity to locally popular home remedies, as has been documented for at least one small-town physician in the southern United States.[45] That many doctors were seemingly able to reconcile a "scientific" approach with established traditions—an accommodation that was part of their "art of medicine"—undoubtedly contributed to the heroic images of the "country doc" that had emerged, along with those of the sympathetic general practitioner, around the world.

Doctors in Newfoundland often encountered horrendous traveling conditions on their routine housecalls. Such accounts added to the writings of physicians of the time, such as *The Horse and Buggy Doctor* by A. E. Hertzler.[46] The most celebrated Newfoundland tale was by Wilfred Grenfell, who on Easter Sunday in 1908 was stranded with his dogsled on an ice pan floating out to sea. He saved his own life by killing and skinning three dogs for their warm hides.[47] This, with his own published account, contributed to Grenfell's image of manliness, confirmed him as a hero, and fostered his international reputation as a missionary doctor.[48] There is little doubt that many doctors from outside Newfoundland were drawn there to work in what were viewed as "frontier" conditions in the North, as they might have been drawn a little earlier, in the United States, to the "West." Hazardous journeys were part of the challenge that commonly brought appreciation from patients, though physician frustration often existed when the medical problem was found to be minor, or even more so if the patient had recovered.[49]

The "frontier" conditions perhaps encouraged stereotyping of people. This is particularly evident in Newfoundland where overseas doctors, seemingly tinged with urban arrogance toward rural life, often painted less-than-flattering pictures of rural communities compared with the capital city of St. John's. Condescending reminiscences about the 1930s to 1950s point to a widely perceived cultural divide—similar to the "other side of the tracks" in American towns—with obvious implications for health care.

> On my arrival in St. John's almost all the people I met shook their heads sadly and did their best to dissuade me from proceeding to my isolated assignment on the South-West Coast. When I eventually got there I readily understood why. These were depression days and I found near-starvation everywhere around me. And while sophisticated city-dwellers will find this hard to believe, I can assure them that witches still flourish in the outports. Many a patient has assured me that my labours would be in vain because a witch had caused his illness and taking off the curse was the only cure.[50]

Missing from such comments is any appreciation that even adjacent communities might differ substantially in social and economic conditions, which in Newfoundland invariably depended on the success or failure of the fishery in a particular locality.

Rural/urban social differences also offer a window to examine how conventional health care was provided to relatively impoverished people. Leaving aside the important role of nurses, providing care was a constant challenge for doctors on both sides of the Atlantic. Collecting fees (including for prescribed medicines) was a frequent problem for doctors. One solution in Newfoundland prior to national health insurance was the "book" (or "blanket" or "contract") system. Commonplace, but not unique to the island, it had analogies to the small club systems and medical associations with flat annual fees that existed from the end of the nineteenth century in the Scottish Highlands and Islands.[51] The book system was based on the payment of a set fee per year per family for all necessary medical services, but able-bodied adults who were unable to pay the annual premium contributed "labour or in kind."[52]

The book system raises the question of charity practice for poor patients by doctors, invariably an intriguing mix of altruism, necessity, and a contribution to their social standing.[53] Doctors sometimes marked their prescriptions "charity," at least in North America, and one must wonder if that carried a stigma.[54] The book system did not mean that charity was not practiced, but it did buffer any stigma, particularly through the acceptance of payment other than money.

The Newfoundland cottage hospital scheme—six hospitals opened in 1936 with others to follow—not only took medical care into rural areas but also provided what might be called "silent" government charity. Such hospitals, not unique to Newfoundland (those in Scotland were said to be the principal models), invite comparisons with the 1920s' and 1930s' development of many small town hospitals in the United States, especially those in rural areas, notably the Carolinas.[55] Further, as specialty medical practice developed from the 1930s onward, the small town hospitals became important in attracting specialists to a town. In contrast, cottage hospitals generally remained the territory of local general practitioners. That rural Newfoundlanders were sacrificing time and money in the 1950s to visit physicians in St. John's, even if they could find one locally, reflects lay demands for specialization everywhere. In fact, the island had relatively few specialists before the 1970s, even in St. John's, but Newfoundlanders perceived town doctors to be more up to date with new specialist knowledge than their rural counterparts.[56]

That specialty practice was generally centrally located added to a long-standing issue about maldistribution of health care. In 1976, one observer of the U.S. scene noted that the complaints of the 1920s had not changed in fifty years. "Maldistribution of health care to economically and geographically isolated groups" was said to owe much to physicians' greater concern for individual patients rather than with social/community problems. The "solution for geographically dispersed and culturally diverse populations such as ours will probably never be easy."[57] The same can be said today.

PUBLIC/COMMUNITY HEALTH

Although the interest in public health in this book lies primarily in legislation to safeguard the public from "poisons," "narcotics," and other medicinal substances (see Chapter 4), I comment here on how public health affected attitudes toward diseases and treatment.

The first half of the twentieth century in Britain and North America saw much emphasis on public health reform with increasing government involvement. In Britain, this extended beyond concerns with, for example, infectious diseases and adulteration of food to the effects of the environment on health, a trend that increased the social and political role of medicine.[58] That this was less evident in the United States, at least until the 1930s, cannot be divorced from the republican individualistic spirit. As one historian said of the early decades in the United States, the 1920s saw a "sharp break with the social and political reform spirit of the Progressive movement" of the early years of the century such that "federal provisions for veterans' care, along with those for maternal and child health, stood out as conspicuous exceptions in an overall pattern of official indifference to human needs."[59]

The United States, of course, had particular, intractable regional problems, little different from those in Newfoundland, that were linked with widespread poverty, widely scattered population, lack of industrial development, absence of local government, and relatively few doctors. All this bred many efforts to improve public health, especially to deal with infectious diseases by, for instance, immunization programs. Broadly based reform movements that encouraged confidence in conventional medicine were promoted by a diversity of schoolteachers, reform-minded laypeople and organizations, physicians, public health nurses, and trained midwives as much as by governments.[60] At the Royal National Mission to Deep Sea Fishermen in St. Anthony (known as the International Grenfell Association after 1914), there was the special influence of the social medicine of physician Wilfred Grenfell from his arrival in 1892 until his death in 1940. By then concerted government efforts were made to deal with major health problems in rural areas, though perennial gulfs between concepts and implementation continued.[61]

Everywhere, messages (e.g., learn from the new medical science and avoid germs by controlling flies[62]) questioned the efficacy of many traditional home remedies as well as the promotion of commercial over-the-counter medicines. In consequence, there was often a real dilemma for sufferers from, for instance, tuberculosis, especially acute in Newfoundland, over whether to take over-the-counter remedies when physicians and others, perhaps friends and relatives, constantly proclaimed that they were part of the social evil of quackery (see Chapter 3). This was undoubtedly the case in the well-studied Appalachian region in the United States with its comparable social conditions to Newfoundland.

Once tuberculosis had faded as a major problem by the 1960s, Newfoundland's social conditions led to a totally different public health concern (more often labeled a community health issue) in the second half of the century, namely stress.[63] This concern—a "diagnosis" that gathered momentum with the popularization of Hans Selye's work in the 1950s—and the whole issue of mental health contributed, in the second half of the century, to the emergence of community psychiatry, the burgeoning influence of tranquilizers and anti-depressants, and the growing preoccupation with prevention and lifestyles.[64] In Newfoundland, stress was not just an issue for individuals, but also for communities as a whole; indeed the notion of healthy communities, which was increasingly discussed in health care literature from the 1980s, has been enriched by the Newfoundland experience.[65] A particular issue is the rapidity of change felt by so many people during the last half of the twentieth century, more so in some places than others. In Newfoundland, industrialism, wage labor, and the cash economy came rather late and slowly to the island. This led, through a series of events, to major upheavals among rural communities in the 1950s to 1970s, many of which were subjected to a program of resettlement, whereby entire communities, houses and all, were moved to "centres of development."[66] Such centralization, leaving many "ghost" communities, did improve access to education, health, and various community services, but many lives and communities were radically changed with a further loss of traditional medicines. For some people, it meant "being ashamed of being a Newfoundlander and of being from the outports. Our generation, we lost that pride."[67]

COLONIALISM

The last topic raised here as a regional matter is colonialism. Although this seemingly has less relevance to practices in Britain and the United States, it does prompt questions about attitudes in these countries; this is because, in recent years, historians have become increasingly interested in the nature of power and dependence, even in countries where tropical medicine has always been central to the colonial story.[68] The phrase, "Britain's oldest colony," often used to describe Newfoundland, refers to the period from 1583 until 1949. Unlike countless other British colonies, Newfoundland did not progress to independent nationhood.

This sense of "being colonial," of being dependent, was reinforced in many ways. For instance, as already mentioned, issues arose when members of the U.S. military in Newfoundland in the early 1940s clearly looked for reform when they saw serious public health dangers, especially venereal disease. Newfoundlanders, in fact, often suffered from the negative attitudes of "outsiders" that commonly reflected a lack of cultural understanding. Talking about British nurses in Newfoundland in 1934, one Briton bluntly said: "Newfoundland girls won't do—they have no authority with the people."[69]

The biggest issue for the island was the suspension of its self-governing dominion status in 1934 in favor of an appointed six-member commission that governed on behalf of the British government for fifteen years until the 1949 confederation with Canada. In large measure, Commission Government was precipitated by the undermining of the island's financial solvency by the burdens of World War I and the depression of the 1930s; adding to this were serious health problems among the population, notably the scourge of tuberculosis. Often associated with poor nutrition—an additional widespread problem in the island—tuberculosis was just one factor contributing to the sense that Newfoundland was backward, at least compared to elsewhere in North America.

In a settler colony such as Newfoundland, with a small, relatively homogenous population and comparatively few aboriginal people,

British colonial policies were not overtly evident. With small numbers of doctors, even maintaining the style and attitudes of British medical institutions was hardly possible. Moreover, native or racial issues did not reinforce the philosophy of the eugenics movement, widely discussed in Europe in the early decades of the twentieth century, that wished to ensure white superiority. On the other hand, it was implicit in many ways; Wilfred Grenfell, for instance, extolled the finer Anglo-Saxon characteristics of Newfoundland fishermen, yet made clear how poverty and ill health took their toll. In so doing he spotlighted that the "human race is degenerating and that the changes of decay are most marked among the most civilized people," meaning the British.[70] Ironically, islanders were constantly reminded of the slogan "British is Best," subtly reinforced among Newfoundlanders by, for example, the special value placed on British education, the importance attached to teaching about Britain in Newfoundland schools, the British merchandise conspicuous in Newfoundland stores, the arrival of countless British physicians and nurses, and the missionary/social work of Wilfred Grenfell.[71]

Did the constant reminders of colonialism contribute to attitudes—class attitudes—toward a doctor and his prescriptions? It is impossible to say with any certainty. However, feelings of dependence, perhaps of inferiority, were seemingly in tune with one characteristic often noted by physicians, namely that Newfoundlanders (particularly those living in rural areas) had marked deferential attitudes toward authority, especially toward priests, merchants, and doctors.

Yet being colonial was not all negative. Pride also existed in being part of the British Empire; for instance, photographs of British royalty adorned many homes and "British Empire Product" was proclaimed on bottles of "Munn's Genuine Newfoundland Cod Liver Oil"—the company noted in a patriotic British publication, *The Romance of Empire Drugs* (c. 1932). This noted "the superiority of Newfoundland cod-liver oil, which should encourage wider use of this important product of the oldest colony in the Empire."[72] One druggist recollected in the late 1990s, "Maybe some felt this idea of a colony, of being a little inferior, but that was not applicable to my family. Everyone was as proud as could be of what they were, where they came from, what they had."[73]

Amid what were evidently mixed feelings over colonialism, Newfoundlanders' sea-faring lifestyles did foster an independent spirit.

The island's position as a fish exporter in the North Atlantic had a long history of trade with, for instance, the Caribbean and with the United States, mostly via Boston. With regard to medicines, links elsewhere were strong, at least for imports. In 1905, the British *Pharmaceutical Journal* noted that "trade" between Newfoundland and the United Kingdom had recently increased, although not so much as between the island and the United States (from where "medicinal foods" were imported) and Canada (which provided "proprietary medicines").[74] In contrast, "crude drugs and chemicals" were almost all obtained from the United Kingdom and were considered by Newfoundland health care professionals to be of better quality than elsewhere.

One feature of the Newfoundland scene, the repacking of bulk products under a drugstore label—for example, "Acid Tartaric/A. W. Kennedy, Ph. C./St. John's NF"—was a commonplace practice, as was the preparation of distinct over-the-counter "specialties" by some stores.[75] For instance, just as "British made" was part of the empire mind-set for the British, so did Newfoundland products contribute to a sense of identity on the island. Dr. F. Stafford's drugstore business was just one well known for its own specialties, such as Stafford's Liniment, Prescription "A," and Phoretone Cough Cure, though the Stafford name became more synonymous with a range of essences—almond, butterscotch, ginger, and others.[76] Such local products were commonplace until Newfoundland became a Canadian province, when they largely disappeared because they failed to meet new regulations.

The demise of locally or regionally marketed over-the-counter medicines, which brought with it some loss of a sense of place and identity—as was certainly the case in Newfoundland—became commonplace elsewhere. The emergence of company buyouts and twentieth-century, global pharmaceutical manufacturing and marketing—sometimes viewed as a new medical imperialism or a new colonial power—contributed to this. Whether the loss of regionalism affected general public confidence in medicines is impossible to say; however, it was an aspect of the long-standing dichotomy in which some individuals always favored "local" over "foreign" (exotic) remedies.[77] It is noteworthy that this issue was raised again in the final decades of the 1900s by the growing popularity of Chinese herbs in Western countries.

WRITING THE STORY

In offering comments on the issues and problems faced in writing a complex story, we also add some further detail to the background, particularly in explaining the attention given to pharmacy.

Limitations in Selection and Interpretation

If an exhaustive account of the social history of medicines were possible, it would become tedious if only because of the diversity of practices, theories, issues, and the rise and fall of so many treatments. This account, then, is necessarily selective and excludes, for instance, any discussion of specialized hospital treatment (e.g., for cancer), if only to allow sufficient space for the principal concern, everyday usage.

The process of selecting topics and themes for this book was challenged by the overwhelming amount of scientific and other literature on medicines and medicine taking, as well as by differing interpretations of the nature of change, and what influences it.[78] Although this book constantly acknowledges that the nonmedical and medical factors shaping the use of medicines are commonly inseparable, space severely limits consideration of many direct and less direct or more subtle influences, as important as they are to the total picture. For instance, we omit detailed discussion on the development of medical education (especially on therapy) and on medical research, which can be key elements in a physician's choice of remedies for his or her patients. Hospital medicine, too, is hardly mentioned, though it has been a particular factor in the public validation of medicines, especially in the second half of the century, not only through hospital-based research, but also through patients expecting or demanding, from their general or family physician, the same medicines as prescribed by hospital specialists. Nor do we consider the topic of vaccines and vaccination, which could also illustrate many issues raised in this book.[79]

Such specialty areas of medicine as epidemiology (particularly as it expanded from a preoccupation with infectious diseases into human ecology) have also to be omitted, though they have been an important factor behind the growing numbers of patients treated for hypertension, for example. Further, epidemiology, in conjunction with nutrition and environmental studies, pinpointed "new" conditions (for example, allergies) that also demanded and expanded the use of medications.

Much of the material that I must skate over would add confirmation to one characteristic of the story of medicines, indeed medicine as a whole, that we do emphasize: namely, ever-present uncertainty. Epidemiology, for instance, contributed to confusion and anxiety among both health care practitioners and the public through announcement after announcement of new associations between risk factors and disease states or medications. Other areas of research within medicine that were increasingly prominent after the 1950s—medical sociology, medical psychology, and medical ethics—highlighted uncertainty as they challenged medicine, not so much about treatments but about the situations (e.g., very brief consultations) during which most treatments were prescribed. Omitted, too, except in passing, are such considerations as general societal concerns and worries about technology, or at least the way governments and the industry were seemingly slow to deal with public concerns. One example was the use of diethylstilbestrol for fattening cattle despite known health hazards.[80]

What is left, as I endeavor to illustrate, is still a bewildering range of factors shaping the nature, prescription, acceptance, and validation of medicines by physicians, patients, and the public in general. Amidst this, it needs to be made clear that, without personal testimony from patients or a physician's own insight into his or her prescribing habits, understanding specific decisions about treatment must remain uncertain. Although the broad patterns of factors affecting decision making are made clear in this account, as well as why certain medicines might be chosen over others, this only illustrates a spectrum of factors, a selection of which could explain why a Mr. Brown or Ms. Smith used a particular medication, perhaps an idiosyncratic one, or even failed to use a physician's prescription.

Determining and understanding a particular physician's treatment patterns also leaves much uncertainty, though perhaps less so during the last decades of the twentieth century, when those working under insurance schemes were pressured by professional practice guidelines, insurance companies' policies, and public concerns with accountability to conform to standard treatment guidelines (e.g., in prescribing antibiotics). Physicians who departed from "normal" patterns of prescribing—and this has always happened—were increasingly challenged to defend their practices.[81] Some physicians have always been more conservative than others in their prescribing; indeed, they may be doubtful about many medicines and hence more resistant to the requests or demands of patients than liberal prescribers. Some physicians, too, may be particularly careful to tailor a remedy to the likes and dislikes of the patient rather than solely to his or her particular medical condition, though this was more common before the 1960s.

Last in this catalog of omissions and limitations, it has to be said that comparisons between the two sides of the Atlantic are often short on detail or incomplete and leave many questions to be pursued. This reflects not only space limitations, but also the need for much more basic research, especially into government/industry records, many of which are not yet accessible to historians.[82] At least the globalization of medicine means that information from one country is always relevant to that of another.

Druggists and Drugstores

Compared with physicians, the influence of *druggists* (the term used in most of this book rather than *pharmacists*[83]) in validating medicines is perhaps less obvious and deserves special comment. Pharmacy has a conspicuous and significant place in the present account, beyond offering some insight into what went into, say, a bottle of medicine (dispensed or over the counter) taken away by the patient. Until the last decades of the twentieth century, druggists commonly accepted the physicians' authority as primary in medicines. This reflected a long history of uneasy relationships between physicians and druggists, who were commonly divided by education and social class.[84] It is well remembered, in the first half of the century, that if a patient had a question about the prescription, the druggist would say nothing about its action and instead refer the patient back to the doctor. As in Newfoundland up to the late 1970s, if customers questioned the value of the medicine they were taking, a druggist's response might be: "What did the doctor tell you? I can't go against the doctor."[85]

Despite this acceptance of physician authority, drugstores were the place where individuals could get a sense of the variety of medicines available, and also where they made choices, perhaps with the druggist's advice. Moreover, up to the 1950s or so, druggists not only dispensed physicians' prescriptions but also counter-prescribed, dispensed their own compounded medicines, sold a vast range of over-the-counter medicines (but not from open shelves), and developed community roles for their drugstores. Further, they helped to protect the public from poisons, narcotics, prescription-only medicines, and poor-quality or ineffective preparations. All this led to a respected standing in their communities and their authority in what was seen as "minor" medicine.

A commonplace question, however, within pharmacy—at least in the United States, Britain, and the former British Empire—is whether the authority of druggists was diluted by tensions between professional responsibilities in health care and the overt business activities that were a conspicuous part of drugstores. After all, drugstores from the nineteenth century onward sold toiletries, garden seeds, photographic materials, and much else outside of health care needs, as well as (in North America at least) running a soda fountain. Moreover, the early decades of the twentieth century saw the growth of "cut-price" drugstores on both sides of the Atlantic that added to existing tensions for the profession.[86]

Newfoundland makes a noteworthy comparison with elsewhere in that the tensions may have been less of an issue, at least until the last decades of the twentieth century. Then, interestingly, such tensions were illustrated in the refusal of many pharmacies, despite public pressure, to stop selling tobacco before a grace period of five years. The particular circumstances of Newfoundland sharpen questions about the relationship between the quality of pharmacy practice and education on both sides of the Atlantic. On the island, educational standards of druggists (central to which was an apprenticeship until the late 1960s) were substantially less exacting than those in Britain, the United States, and the rest of Canada until the 1980s. One has to question the sincerity of constant proclamations from druggists— albeit mostly disappearing around the 1950s or so—about the quality of their medicines and the accuracy of dispensing. Typical proclamations (also common throughout the rest of North America and the British Empire) were: "Physicians and Family Recipes filled with accuracy, promptness and neatness," or "Our stock of Medicines is complete, warranted genuine, and of the best quality."[87] However, any question about quality and professional/business tensions has to consider, as will be seen, the relatively small number of druggists and drugstores—as in small towns elsewhere—until the last decades of the 1900s.

By the 1960s dispensing practices that had been changing slowly for some years had shifted to preparations (mostly tablets) manufactured by pharmaceutical companies. Dispensing the "bottle" of medicine, an ointment or powder, for instance, was fading. New professional roles were being forged in consequence of the avalanche of potent medicines after 1950, and, in consequence, pharmacy education changed dramatically. With a new emphasis by the 1970s on the pharmacist as the expert on medicines, as well as for other reasons, Newfoundland, despite its small population, opened in 1985 a school of pharmacy upholding national standards. Nowadays, pharmacy offers far more extensive education about medicines than is received by medical students and junior doctors.

Noticeably, this new role of medicines or "drug" expert, alongside new dispensing practices, coincided with changing shop appearances and with it the atmosphere where people generally obtained their medicines. "Old" though elegant fittings and the distinctive shop-filled odor of medicines gave way on both sides of the Atlantic to utilitarian self-service shelves of over-the-counter medicines. This was accentuated when national chain drugstores, which offered supermarket-style discount services with much promotion of nonhealth items (even junk foods), outnumbered privately owned (independent) drugstores. Such chains, coming later to St. John's than to towns of comparable size in North America, met the same criticisms as elsewhere, namely that they offered a relatively impersonal service. All such changes raise questions about whether the public in general sees nonprescription medicines as being different from general merchandise, and whether they recognize the community druggist as a medicines expert.

We must mention here one particular role of the drugstore, at least up to the 1950s, namely the sale of products that were used for *preparing* medicines in the home or for placing in the home medicine chest or cabinet (for example, packets of herbs, chemicals such as iodine and Mercurochrome, and arrowroot starch for invalids' foods).[88] Further, druggists dispensed "family receipts," for instance, a family's favorite formula for a cough medicine or even a furniture polish.

In many ways, druggists have had manifold roles in the diverse practices of self-care. In Newfoundland, these extended to offering advice and supporting—directly and indirectly—self-sufficiency and other such values associated with Newfoundlanders as resourcefulness, pragmatism, and prudence.[89] Such values contributed to a feeling of distinctiveness, of self-consciousness in Newfoundland. Although this has not been studied to the same extent as has, for example, the distinctiveness of the Southern United States, William Faulkner's comment, "You can't understand it. You would have to be born there," is as apt for Newfoundland—indeed for many other places—as it is for the South.[90] Today, while pharmacists offer advice on self-care, it can perhaps be described as generic with no sense of contributing to a feeling of belonging to a particular place.

Resources

Oral History, Manuscripts, Popular Books

Aside from "traditional" printed sources, the interpretation of trends and attitudes in this account owes much to oral history garnered from formal interviews and informal discussions with doctors, pharmacists, and laypeople (especially elders) over a number of years. Oral history has become an important resource in recent years in examining twentieth-century health care.[91] On the other hand, such history is sometimes considered to be "raw history," which is certainly the case when there is a failure to take into account such limitations as lapses of memory, memories softened through rose-tinted spectacles, and interpretations of the past shaped by biases and hindsight. However, because of the considerable number of informants used for this study over many years, some common patterns in everyday practice emerge that can be supported or interpreted by the printed record or, conversely, can add to or help to navigate the overwhelming amount of literature that has been printed by medical and nonmedical publishers since World War II.

In some respects, manuscripts serve a similar role to oral history in so far as they both add to, and often need to be interpreted by, the published record in order to assess whether the information is generalizable. Unfortunately, patients' medical records, from private rather than institutional practices, even when they exist for the historian—such as the ones used in this book for the late 1950s—are often too meager in detail to reveal a physician's thinking. However, even limited information adds to our knowledge of the spectrum of prescribing practices that is generally difficult to determine, albeit easier with the computerized data of medical insurance records. Physicians' prescriptions are more readily available for study and prescriptions written up to the 1950s are used extensively in the present account. While they offer many invaluable insights into prescribing habits, a major limitation is the difficulty, often impossibility, in correlating them with specific clinical situations.

The spectrum of published sources used in the account is evident from the endnotes, but a word is appropriate on the popular works, increasingly abundant from the 1960s, many written by journalists. Even the most cogent and well researched dwell on the negative aspects of medicine, and it is not surprising that they are commonly chastised for being one-sided. Historians are often uncomfortable with the muckraking—heroes versus villains, or underdogs versus government/big business—tone of such books, which often oversimplify the situation. However, the issue in this book is a cumulative influence of negative comment on the public that has undoubtedly contributed to the growing questioning of medicine and medicines.[92] Moreover, this questioning is seen as especially influential at times, such as helping to turn prescription-only tranquilizers into a social problem.[93]

Advertisements

The growth of consumerism in health care, already evident in the early twentieth century, is well illustrated in advertisements of over-the-counter medicines, a further illustration of the power of the media in shaping lay attitudes not only to medicines but also to the medical profession and health care in general. Liberal quotes, taken from advertisements, especially from the earlier decades of the twentieth century (see Chapter 3) may well amuse today's readers. Certainly most claims are excessive and seemingly had no foundation in clinical experience. In fact, countless contemporaries—not just physicians—also found them outrageously misleading. Historians have commonly followed this view in writing on "quackery," and, in so doing, tend to emphasize the gullibility of the public, sometimes, it seems, with an air of professional or academic snobbery.[94]

Charges of gullibility, even if not altogether inappropriate, commonly marginalize the vulnerability of the sick, ignore the possibility of effectiveness, and dismiss the context in which over-the-counter medicines were promoted. Commonly overlooked is the "pedigree" many medicines acquired because of overlap with physicians' prescriptions and the advertising that referred to such popular theories of disease as autointoxication and acidosis in the body—theories accepted by many physicians until at least the 1940s. Although advertisers often oversimplified and extended such theories so that they were mere caricatures of the originals, by the 1930s an overall change occurred in the character of advertising in Newfoundland reflecting the curbing of the more extravagant promotions in the exporting countries. Unlike exports to large, major markets, there seems to have been no adaptations of labeling and advertising for Newfoundland. Thus Newfoundland could receive the same over-the-counter medicine under either U.S. or Canadian regulations, e.g., Dr. Chase's Nerve Pills from the United States, and Dr. Chase's Nerve Food from Canada.[95]

Also relevant to advertising changes was an emerging emphasis on health, beauty, and wellness—seen in increasing numbers of soap (including germicidal and deodorant soaps), toothpaste, and cosmetic advertisements—such that Newfoundlanders, scanning advertisements originating in Britain, the United States, and Canada, were encouraged to emulate the lifestyle of the respectable middle class, despite difficult economic times.[96] This is reflected particularly in the pressure promotion of vitamins to maintain health by avoiding the threat of subclinical deficiencies.[97] In addition, many laxative advertisements also began to emphasize health rather than the treatment of specific ailments: Andrews Liver Salts, for example, was promoted in 1937 for "daily Good Health!"[98]

Although newspapers reveal a lively sense of commercialism, it is impossible to say how many people were influenced by the advertisements.[99] Illiteracy always has to be considered in all countries, and it was high in Newfoundland; furthermore, many of the literate must have passed over the advertisements, especially those of the early 1900s that were written as tedious and lengthy news items. On the other hand, the repetition of a simple picture of a box of Gin or

Dodd's Pills—the same boxes that were readily seen in general stores or drugstores in every community—reinforced their presence. It should be added that newspaper readership was often extended through secondhand copies; in rural Newfoundland, these moved between communities via constant boat travel and might even have been read while being pasted on inside walls as insulation against the winter cold.[100] Commercial promotion readily found its way into everyday conversation and into the oral tradition, which has always been a central part of rural community life, particularly where illiteracy was high.[101]

Newspapers dominated advertising, but promotion also depended on the extraordinary range of ephemera used by enterprising manufacturers, including annual almanacs, magazines, store catalogs, medicine labels, songbooks, postcards, blotting papers, and home medicine books distributed by medicine manufacturers such as the R. V. Pierce and Chase companies. In 1900, Newfoundlanders could freely obtain, to give one example, Pierce's *People's Common Sense Medical Adviser* by sending "stamps to pay expense of customs and mailing *only.* Send 31 one-cent stamps for paper covers, or 50 stamps for cloth binding."[102]

Some specific comments on almanacs are appropriate here because they were distributed free in the hundreds of thousands in North America and reached the smallest rural communities. Many, such as Grier's, which advertised multiple medicines in the Southern United States, were well known throughout the 1900s, as were Chase's and Dodd's, which became Newfoundland favorites. Although the overt treatment claims of early twentieth-century promotions had generally disappeared by the 1960s and 1970s, the advertising continued to sustain long-standing popular beliefs. Dodd's, for example, still promoted its Kidney Pills for backache and tiredness with claims that they restored energy and dealt with weakness. The company printed testimonials from all corners of Canada. In its 1960 almanac, for example, "21-year old Miss Jean Ford, 75 Alexander Street, St. John's, Newfoundland," stated, "After working [in a food processing company] I used to feel too tired to go out and lacked energy." Naturally, she ended up saying, "I wouldn't be without Dodd's now and I hope they help other women as they have helped me."[103]

Any consideration of promotion must mention specifically the entrepreneurship of agents. Newfoundland illustrates this well with the extraordinarily successful Gerald S. Doyle (1892-1956). Through his wholesale company, Doyle distributed, from 1919 onward, many over-the-counter medicines throughout Newfoundland mostly to general stores. A consummate salesman, Doyle not only advertised innovatively and widely but also personally visited coastal community after community peddling his products by boat.[104] It is certainly not surprising that with his promotion, over-the-counter preparations such as Dodd's Kidney Pills and Dr. Chase's Nerve Food became very much part of Newfoundland traditions and were well remembered by Newfoundland seniors at the end of the twentieth century. If one accepts William Osler's dictum at the beginning of this chapter, much of the desire to take medicines rests on entrepreneurship and commercialism.

Chapter 2

Prelude: Seventeenth to Nineteenth Centuries

FRESH DRUGS, MEDICINES, &C. &C.

The Subscriber has imported from England in the Brig, Charles, a fresh supply of excellent DRUGS, MEDICINES, &c. which, with his former Stock on hand, makes a general supply of DRUGS, PATENT MEDICINES, SPICES, DYE STUFFS, PERFUMERY, and such articles as he has hitherto kept for sale. . . . Practitioners in Town and Out-harbours will be supplied on the most liberal terms, and a credit of six months will be given to those of approved credit, if required.

1830 advertisement to Newfoundlanders[1]

INTRODUCTION

Although the focus of this book is on the twentieth century, the time from the early-seventeenth-century British colonization of North America to the end of the nineteenth century opens up topics that have a bearing on the sense of modernizing treatment that came with the early years of the twentieth century as well as raising recurring themes in the history of medicines. I comment, albeit briefly, on the discovery of new medicines, the social validation and persistence of some medicines despite erratic reputations, uneasy relations between self-care and doctors, the gradual simplification of doctors' prescriptions, the slow shift to chemical rather than plant remedies, and the growing commercialization and growth of the pharmaceutical industry.

AN EARLY SEARCH FOR NEW REMEDIES

Trying to Be Self-Sufficient

Over the years much has been written on whether the New World environment, with its mixing of cultures, produced new ideas and practices in health care and, more generally, throughout society; what is clear is that medical practice in the New World maintained close parallels with those in the Old World.[2] Certainly, as in other British North American colonies (e.g., Jamestown, 1607, and Plymouth, 1620), permanent settlers in Newfoundland—at Cupids (1610) and Ferryland (1621)—relied heavily on imported conventional medicines.[3] In the early years, Newfoundland colonists had little interaction with native people and were unlikely to have acquired any knowledge of medicinal properties of local plants from them; indeed, this route to "discovery" may have been less significant in other North American colonies than sometimes supposed.[4] Nor did slavery contribute to transmission of African knowledge of medicines as happened in the West Indies and the southern United States. Yet the rich written record for the two Newfoundland colonies makes clear that there was much reliance on local resources (mostly herbs and some animal products) that were cultivated, harvested from the wild, or trapped. After all, the colony proprietors expected their investments to become as self-sufficient as possible and to lead to profitability. One potential source of riches was new medicines.

The transatlantic "drug trade" was well developed in the sixteenth century between the West Indies, Central America, and Spain.[5] British trading, too, started even before the first permanent British North American colonies were established. In 1602, for example, one of Walter Raleigh's ships returned to England with a cargo that included sassafras, China root, benjamin, sarsaparilla, cassia lignea, and an unknown strong bark.[6] British planters, entrepreneurs/explorers, and physicians/naturalists actively sought new species or an economically valuable drug, such as sarsaparilla, that had a large European market.[7] Hopes were soon dashed in Newfoundland. On August 20, 1612, Henry Crout wrote that he had seen sarsaparilla, but in insufficient quantities: "I have had sight of some in this country, but it is in veries small not worth the gathering except I may find it in other places."[8]

Even without a potential export, local resources still had to be explored to deal with times of shortages of food and medicines. In part, these times were one and the same, for much emphasis existed on the inseparability of diet and health. William Vaughan (1617), for instance, who had a vested interest in Newfoundland during its early settlement, made this clear in his *Directions for Health, both Naturall and Artificiall.* He recommended: "observe a good diet, [and you] neede no artificiall Physicke, for these after a sort are contraries. The one preserves the bodies frame fresh and free from withered corruption: the other offendeth Nature."[9]

Plants, especially pot herbs that served dual roles as "nutrition" and "medicine," were certainly cultivated from imported seed in the early colonies.[10] Planted in Cupids were "Hysope, Time, Parsely, Clarie, Nepe, french Mallowes, Buglosse, Collombines, Wormewood, &c," and also "of 3. yeares old of my sowing, likewise Rosemary, Fenell, Sweete marierum, Bassell, Purselyn, Lettise."[11] Although such a list is not known for the later Ferryland settlement, Edward Wynne (1622) commented on a "kitchen garden" of beans, peas, raddish, lettuce, kale or cabbage, turnips, and carrots, to which he added, "and all the rest is of like goodness."[12] There is every reason to believe that "the rest" included pot/medicinal herbs, some possibly tried in treating scurvy, a major problem facing the settlers.

Scurvy and the Search for Remedies

The search for remedies for scurvy, not unrepresentative of situations in other colonies, is of special interest in any consideration of how medicinal properties of plants were discovered, as well as the survival of remedies ultimately recognized as of doubtful value. A constant question in the history of medicines is whether a new medicine or regimen emerges from trial and error, a chance observation, or theory. A related matter is whether theory shapes how experience is interpreted; further, in the twentieth century, as becomes clear later, the validity of personal experience was seriously questioned by a scientific approach to determining whether a new product was therapeutically effective.

Constant fears of scurvy undoubtedly drove the search for treatments.[13] Robert Hayman (c. 1628), residing in another Newfoundland settlement at Harbour Grace, wrote:

> Those that liue here, how young, or old soeuer,
> Were neuer vext with Cough, nor Aguish Feauer,
> Nor euer was the Plague, nor small Pox heere;
> The *Aire* is so salubrious, constant, cleere:
> Yet *scurvy Death* stalke heere with theeuish pace,
> Knocks one downe here, two in another place.[14]

Hayman may well have had in mind conditions in the hot southern settlements of Virginia where malaria and yellow fever, in taking a heavy toll on life, hindered settlement. In contrast, concerns in Newfoundland centered on the dangers of cold and cold winds, which were viewed as a cause of scurvy. For instance, eight men died of scurvy in the severe 1612-1613 winter at Cupids, all between January 27 and March 11 (when diet became increasingly restricted in variety and possible quantity), and among the many sick at Ferryland during the winter of 1628-1629, nine or ten deaths were attributed to the disease. In addition, there must have been isolated cases from time to time as reflected in Hayman's line: "[scurvy] knocks one downe here, two in another place." Severity of the condition also varied considerably, some only being "touched" by it: "Brigs and Owen hath bin touched with the Scuruie, but are now well recouered."[15]

It is, of course, impossible to say whether all the cases of "scurvy" were what today would be diagnosed as a vitamin C deficiency. Although responses to dietary treatment were evidently part of the diagnosis, an open mind must be kept on other possible conditions or other dietary and nondietary deficiencies.[16] Nor can it be said whether early diagnoses were made. In fact, these were not easy since initial symptoms are nonspecific—for example, lethargy and dry skin that appear as body stores of vitamin C (which normally hold off overt symptoms for weeks) become low; however, the fear of the disease could well have meant that any symptoms were quickly viewed as incipient scurvy, and preventive advice implemented.[17]

Local Plants

Settlers undoubtedly brought with them much knowledge of contemporary treatments for scurvy. Scurvy grass *(Cochlearia),* for instance, was a well-established remedy in Europe for what was diagnosed as "land" scurvy, a form of scurvy considered distinct from "sea" scurvy. Thus it is no surprise that the plant was mentioned in the first report (1610) of treatment—by a surgeon—in Newfoundland, in which a fisherman (apparently not a permanent settler) was "very well amended."[18] Unfortunately, it is not known whether the administered preparation of scurvy grass was from the surgeon's chest or was gathered locally. The latter assumes the scurvy grass that John Guy— the settlement leader at Cupids—identified at the time was a species of *Cochlearia* (if not the recommended *C. officinalis*), even though it was probably not common around Cupids.[19] Guy certainly made considerable effort to locate the plants, as when on a voyage to Trinity Bay: "we fownde good stoare of scurvie grasse" on an island at the entrance to Mounteagle Bay.[20] On another occasion (February 18, 1613), Henry Crout related that settlers went by boat to Harbour Grace "to search for scurvie grasse for our company [who] are sick."[21] Not surprisingly, in view of the season, he later added (March 2) that the boat returned without finding any.

The scarcity of true scurvy grass obviously encouraged interest in substitutes or alternative remedies, many of which were known in European medicine, notably brooklime *(Veronica beccabunga)* and watercress *(Nasturtium officinale)*. However, these were unavailable locally to Newfoundland settlers.[22] A clear sense of the settlers' diligent search for other remedies comes from John Mason's remarks (1620) about trying such local herbs as "certain great green leaves growing in the woods," "a great root" growing in freshwater ponds and a "pretty root" with a blue stalk.[23]

Trial and Error, and Theory

Particularly noteworthy in connection with the settlers' search for scurvy remedies is the apparent trial-and-error approach—always considered to be a significant aspect of early drug discovery. It was the strategy hinted at by Richard Whitbourne (1620), who said that many settlers finding themselves ill "bruised some herbs," strained the juice into beer or wine, and were restored to their former health.[24] However, a trial-and-error search for new plants is so open-ended that settlers were likely conceptually guided by at least one of three ways. One was analogy to plants known in their homeland, for similar plants (usually other species) were long recognized to have the same properties. One Newfoundland settler indicated he learned John Gerard's (1597) *Herball,* "by heart," although he added this did not help with the "many fair flowers I have seen here, which I cannot name."[25]

A second "guide" to identifying new medicinal plants was reliance on sensory characteristics to determine the so-called qualities of a plant—namely hot, cold, moist, and dry—long part of the theory of humors to be rebalanced in disease states associated with the ancient teachings of the Greek physician and writer, Galen. Sensory characters, then, such as taste and odor, were used to identify whether a plant was "medicinal," a practice still known to some herbalists in the late twentieth century.[26]

In connection with sensory properties, it is appropriate to ask whether the aromatic pot/medicinal herbs cultivated at Cupids were chosen with particular medicinal purposes in mind. After all, the number of herbs that settlers might have brought across the Atlantic was almost unending. Were some thought to be helpful for scurvy on theoretical grounds or, for that matter, other conditions? R. E. Hughes, in his discussion on "The Rise and Fall of the 'Antiscorbutics,'" makes clear that land scurvy—in contrast to the characteristically "hot" sea scurvy—was considered a "cold" disease (in terms of Galenic theory), and thus required "'hot' antiscorbutic herbs such as the various [Cruciferous plants] as a counteracting agent."[27] In fact, the three antiscorbutics considered by Hughes (scurvy grass, watercress, and brooklime) can be characterized as hot and dry, as are eleven of the fifteen herbs in Mason's list of pot/medicinal herbs. Although Gerard and other writers listed medicinal properties for all of Mason's herbs, it is noteworthy that only one, wormwood, seems to have been generally recommended for treating scurvy;[28] no evidence has been found to prove their use in Newfoundland.

A third "guide," somewhat speculative, in the search for remedies relates to the belief at the time in a close relationship between diet and health.[29] Perhaps more than one settler had a hunch that a particular food was good for a particular medical condition, a possible reason for the "trial" (or "experiment," as it was referred to) of turnips in Newfoundland. Although the trial bears no relationship to modern trials of medicines, it was a deliberate effort to see whether a specific plant was useful in treating scurvy. In the early years of settlement in Cupids (April 1613), turnips—grown for food and kept in the ground under snow all winter—were eaten by sufferers of the disease. Despite the positive results, which led the settlers to believe they were effective, and despite being a good source of vitamin C, turnips failed to become a frontline treatment in Newfoundland or elsewhere. As with so many recommended scurvy remedies, turnips received only occasional later mention in the vast scurvy literature—hardly a social validation.[30]

This early story of scurvy in Newfoundland is, in some ways, an instructive footnote to a larger account of a vast number of plants recommended for treating the condition, many of which can now be justified by their vitamin C content. However, few became widely or generally used remedies; even citrus fruits, after they were given prominence following the "clinical" work of British naval surgeon James Lind (1753), who found them to be especially effective, were not widely accepted. Lind reported a "clinical trial" now viewed by historians as a significant development in approaches to drug discovery. He evaluated six "acidic" treatments on patients with scurvy on the basis of his theoretical belief that the condition was associated with alkalinity of the blood. Although lemons and oranges were found to be most effective, the other five treatments were not devoid of activity. In a sense Lind "merely validated the *status quo*," rather than proving the efficacy of lemons and oranges above all other treatments.[31] Clearly, social acceptance and validation depended on a range of factors. What would seem to have been especially significant, but not evident in the story of turnip, was a widely accepted conceptual basis for usage, either as part of popular or conventional medical culture.

Spruce Beer and Its Inconsistent Reputation

Spruce beer was another enigmatic product in the search for new remedies for scurvy. Although the beer, even in places where it was not readily available, acquired a higher profile than turnips as a scurvy treatment, its general acceptance waxed and waned for two centuries as it wavered on the boundary between foods (in this case beverages) and medicines. Generally well known wherever spruce trees grow, no reference to it has been found to its use in the early years of the Newfoundland colonies, though surgeon James Yonge referred to the "tops of spruce . . . steept in beer" on his visit to Newfoundland in 1663.[32] That the beer was seemingly well known at the time to North American colonists is suggested by John Josselyn's comment in his *New-England's Rarities Discovered* (1672) that the tops of green spruce boughs, boiled in beer, "is assuredly one of the best remedies for the scurvy."[33]

At the time, spruce beer was merely one of a number of "antiscorbutic" beers prepared by adding "scorbutic" (then meaning antiscurvy) herbs to beer (and sometimes boiling them) or fermenting fresh plant material. Such beers were also known as "diet drinks," which were medicated wines, ales, meads, and wheys commonly used in chronic illnesses and some as antiscorbutics. John Quincy, in discussing diet drinks (but no mention of spruce beer) in his *Compleat English Dispensatory* (1719), said that he was giving more space to them than to other preparations "because this seems to be most for the Service of common People, who are not willing, or cannot well have recourse to the [apothecary] Shops for every dose of Physick they take."[34]

A strong Newfoundland association with spruce beer becomes clear by the time of the visits to Newfoundland of James Cook from 1763 to 1767, and of Joseph Banks in 1766 when he described it as the "common liquor of the country."[35] This was echoed thirty years or so later by another visitor, Aaron Thomas, who enthusiastically referred to that "grand and important article, not only in Newfoundland, but in the habitable world!—It is Spruce Beer! In this Country it is the principal beverage of the people."[36] Clearly its reputation at the time was as a beverage rather than a specific medicine for scurvy, but, like beer in general, it was clearly viewed as a healthful drink.

An interesting question is whether the observations of Banks and Thomas could have any bearing on James Lind's apparent puzzlement (in his eighteenth-century account of scurvy) about the "healthfulness of Newfoundland, the northern parts of Canada, and of our factories at Hudson's bay." In those parts of the world, Lind added, "the scurvy was formerly more fatal to the first adventurers and planters, than it was ever known at sea."[37] Lind, in fact, had high praise for spruce beer (he made no mention of turnip) as treatment for "inveterate scurvies, or perhaps more properly obstinate eruptions on the skin, many of which bear a great resemblance to those of the true scurvy." For the cure of these, Lind continued,

> the Newfoundland spruce beer, made of the black spruce, either
> fresh or dried, or from its essence, is an excellent medicine. The

beer must be drank daily, and the parts affected with the eruption bathed with it night and morning.[38]

There is no doubt that the spruce beer at the time was fermented as in Banks' Newfoundland recipe, which was to "take a half hogshead and put in nineteen gallons of water and fill it up with the essence [an extract of black spruce boughs and molasses]. Work it with balm or beergrounds and in less than a week it is fit to drink." Banks also indicated that other drinks were made from the beer, one by adding egg and/or sugar, suggestive of a diet drink.[39]

It is unclear to what extent spruce beer maintained its popularity in nineteenth-century Newfoundland or elsewhere. In general, references to it do not suggest a mainline reputation, even though nineteenth-century editions of William Buchan's long-lived *Domestic Medicine* (first published in 1769) continued to mention it as a drink for scurvy patients, though "whey or butter-milk" was favored.[40] Perhaps a sense of ambivalence reflects uncertainties about its usefulness (and, for many people, its rather unpleasant taste). Rare is the enthusiasm of American G. H. Napheys (1875) in his *The Prevention and Cure of Disease:* "Spruce-beer is an admirable remedy in scurvy, and a wholesome, agreeable drink for those exposed to the disease. It was used successfully by Captain Cook . . . to preserve the health of his crew."[41] Napheys might have called on the fact that it was still recommended as a precautionary measure to ward off scurvy as late as the 1850s, when ships were searching the Arctic for Sir John Franklin's lost expedition.[42] Napheys' recipe included ginger and allspice for palatability—a reflection that, from the mid-nineteenth century onward, spruce beer was probably seen more as a general dietetic preparation (in the same context as ginger beer or molasses beer), but useful for warding off scurvy.[43] A 1905 book on "curative foods from the cook; in place of drugs from the chemist" noted that "spruce beer or beer of the Norway [black] spruce fir, or 'Sprouts Beer,' is an agreeable and wholesome beverage, very useful against scurvy, and for chronic rheumatism."[44]

Despite such accolades spilling over into the early twentieth century, interest was seemingly fading. Despite a long history and persistent reputation as a preventative/therapeutic drink, spruce beer faded from use in the last decades of the 1800s in consequence of a spectrum of factors that included the growing popularity of tea as a beverage, spruce beer's association with the lower classes, and physicians' general condemnation of "folk" remedies. But perhaps of greater significance was inconsistent activity. Vitamin C concentrations in foods are now known to be dramatically altered by, for instance, boiling and drying. Specifically, when made by fermentation, spruce beer contains no vitamin C. In one experiment, a fresh infusion of black or white spruce leaves (initially containing 55 mg vitamin C per 100 g leaf) had a concentration of 14 mg/100 ml, but after fermentation the vitamin content had virtually disappeared.[45] Thus, spruce beer was useful only on the basis of vitamin content when prepared, as was sometimes the case, by infusing spruce tops in beer. Of course, any "positive" results helped to perpetuate what was evidently an inconsistent reputation. Nor, perhaps, was there an appreciation that spruce tea made from spruce tops and spruce buds—a recognized tonic and chest medicine in places such as Newfoundland—was significantly different from the beer as a medicinal product.

INTERFACES: CONVENTIONAL MEDICINES, SELF-CARE, AND COMMERCIALISM

In integrating conventional medicine and self-care, the scurvy story straddles two aspects of health care that have long had an uneasy relationship. For example, the once extraordinarily popular *Domestic Medicine* by William Buchan received mixed receptions on its 1769 appearance. By "laying medicine open," many doctors considered Buchan a heretic.[46] This view, despite some lightening of attitudes, persisted during the nineteenth century on the basis that popularizing conventional medicine undermined physicians' authority; further, the view was promoted that home medicine was generally ineffective and could be ignored. Something of this is reflected in, for example, Benjamin Ellis's (1849) *Medical Formulary* when it stated that "dietetic preparations and beverages for the sick" are "trifling" formulae to physicians, but if the latter paid more attention to them they would "place the patient more completely under [a physician's] control."[47] In fact, at the time, physicians as a whole were beginning to pay more attention to such nutritional products due in part to changing treatment regimens and a decline in aggressive therapies. For instance, in the practice of physician James Langstaff (1825-1889) of Ontario, milk (cold or boiled, diluted or straight) was the second most cited "drug" in the 1870s.[48] Yet amid such trends, physicians' attitudes toward self-care generally remained ambivalent, all the more so as the profession mounted vigorous opposition to patent medicines (Chapter 3) as "better" medicines became available and new ways of administering medicines (e.g., hypodermically) emerged that were generally administered or supervised by physicians.

Generalizing about physicians' attitudes is problematic because of the broad spectrum of practitioners throughout North America—apothecaries, surgeons, surgeon-apothecaries, physicians—that existed from the seventeenth to the nineteenth centuries.[49] Despite the different titles (and educational backgrounds), all offered services as *general practitioners,* a term that was established in the first half of the 1800s (by which time an "apothecary" was likely to be practicing solely as a druggist). Local circumstances could determine the type of available practitioners. In Newfoundland up to the early 1800s, they were usually "surgeons" who served fishing crews or the army and navy and relied on conventional medicines from Britain or France.[50] Some, stationed at garrisons on the island, provided care to the civilian population. By around 1800, a few—in consequence of developing a private practice amid a slowly growing population—were staying on the island.

By the early nineteenth century, some such surgeons might have owned a drugstore and pursued the entrepreneurial spirit common to large numbers of North American physicians. A detailed advertisement in the *Newfoundland Mercantile Journal* in 1826—"Selling off by Mr. Dobie, Surgeon"—is not unrepresentative of advertisements found in newspapers elsewhere at the time. Dobie, in apparently selling the contents of a drugstore, advertised "a vast quantity of very superior medicines, just Imported from Mr. D's London House" (a wholesaler), and a wide range of other wares. Noteworthy are his promotional comments that reflect the growing, albeit still small, city of St. John's: "A chest of gum arabic—for the attention of the confectioner and dress-maker;" "some rouge—often used by theatrical practitioners &c;" "Potash, truly economical in the washing of clothes—Mr. D. would be glad to draw the attention of ladies, in the management of houses, to this highly useful article;"

> Mr. D. hopes [with regard to paints, etc.] that the enlightened people of Newfoundland will not be backward in economically improving their Dwellings. . . . Paint preserves the timber, as paper has been found to harbor bugs. The chemical washes are not

only more economical but healthier, and in the United Kingdom are in more general use.

The advertisement continued:

> Argand Standing, hanging and bed-room lamps, (and also the Aromatic Pastile Cups, for sick chambers, and to diffuse a pleasant and grateful flavor in Rooms where there are or have been dinner parties,)—their use is real economy, independent of a very grand object—the preservation of the sight.[51]

Gradually, the number of medical practitioners increased with the expanding population. Some were sons of Newfoundland doctors, though apart from local apprenticeships they were educated elsewhere. Others were nonmilitary practitioners (some recruited as company medical officers) arriving from England, Ireland, Scotland, and the United States. The turnover of practitioners was relatively high and the overall number remained low during the nineteenth century. Only forty-eight were registered in Newfoundland in 1896 (under the first medical act of 1893), of whom fourteen were in St. John's.[52] Given such circumstances, self-care and the services of lay practitioners were a necessity for countless Newfoundland residents, as in innumerable communities elsewhere, that continued into the twentieth century (see Chapter 4).

The Commercialism of Self-Treatment

Amid a gathering momentum of change in nineteenth-century health care, commercialism was significant—an expansion of trends already clear in the eighteenth century. Two types of manufacturing companies became dominant. One manufactured patent medicines only, often promoted with massive advertising campaigns, especially in newspapers. (Very few of these medicines, it should be noted, were patented. The term *proprietary* is more apt, as is the current term, *over the counter,* as used throughout this book.) In contrast, companies such as Burroughs Wellcome in Britain and Parke, Davis in the United States, which emerged into prominence in the late nineteenth century, increasingly advertised many of their products to physicians only ("ethical" pharmaceuticals as they came to be known). Such companies slowly established reputations for a commitment to scientific research and quality control behind new medications. As altruistic as this may sound, it was good business practice in light of the growth of scientific medicine and the authority of physicians over the next few decades.

From the public's viewpoint, over-the-counter medicines were the most readily available. Products of successful (and some less successful) American, British, and Canadian companies—e.g., J.C. Ayer, Beecham, and Lydia Pinkham—reached many places, Newfoundland included. The secret formulae of the majority of such preparations raised concerns, not the least of which were over quality and safety. In fact, in the absence of appropriate legislation (see Chapter 4), the English-speaking world of the nineteenth century was largely dependent for quality and safety of over-the-counter medicines on responsible commercial practices and the ethical mind-set of druggists.[53] The growth of the over-the-counter medicine market, even in small towns, had been evident in St. John's since surgeon Dobie's 1826 sale noted earlier. Although many doctors during the century continued to dispense their own medicines—indeed this was commonplace on both sides of the Atlantic—increasingly a livelihood could be made as a druggist alone.

Druggists, or chemists and druggists, to use British terminology, appeared in Newfoundland for the first time in the 1820s. The first were Thomas McMurdo, the London Medical Establishment, and Alfred Wilson, all of whom came to St. John's.[54] In 1840 a surgeon by the name of O'Dwyer informed the "inhabitants" of St. John's and the outports that he had "disposed of all his interest in the Shops, now carried on by Mr. J. C. Bunting and Mr. H. Findlayter, Apothecaries, Druggists." O'Dwyer indicated that he was to "devote the entire of his time to the Practice of his Profession," at his residence or at his "surgery," "where the children of the Poor will be Vaccinated gratis."[55]

Of these, McMurdo's was to become the best known Newfoundland drugstore until the 1960s. An 1833 McMurdo advertisement, directed to "the Inhabitants of St. John's and the Out-ports of the Island," offered a wide range of merchandise from the old country, including "PATENT and CHEMICAL MEDICINES from the first Houses in London, Edinburgh and Glasgow," along with pickles, spices, dry paints, and jam and jelly pots.[56] Later advertisements, often very detailed as in an example from 1864 (Box 2.1), reflected expanding commercial products and competition.

The story of drugstores from the nineteenth century onward in both North America and Britain is one of an expanding array of merchandise, albeit during the nineteenth century such merchandise fell mostly within the limits of health and beauty, though with many ex-

---

BOX 2.1. 1864 Advertisement from Apothecaries' Hall, St. John's, Newfoundland, Thomas McMurdo and Co., Family and Dispensing Chemists

Have always on hand a large and select Stock of Drugs, Chemicals, English and American Patent Medicines, etc., and every article connected with their line of business, which they can confidently recommend to the public.

Arrowroot, Sago, Robinson's Prepared Groats and Barley, Isinglass, Gelatine, Du Barry's Ravalenta Arabica Food, Flavoring Essences, Candied Lemon, Orange and Citron Peels, Sweet and Bitter Almonds, Barwick's Baking Powder, Coloring for Jellies, Blanc Mange, etc., Spices of all kinds, Lazenby's Pickles and Sauces, India Rubber, Tortoiseshell, Buffalo and White Horn Dressing Combs, Ivory, Small Tooth Combs, Hair, Nail, Tooth and Shaving Brushes, Silver Top and Cut Glass Smelling Bottles. Delcroix and Low's Perfumery, Glycerine, Almond, Windsor, Castle and Sand Soaps, Corn and Bunion Plasters, Gold Beater's Skin, Court Plasters, Hair Dyes, and Pomades, Bears' Grease, Lip Salve, Cold Cream, Eau de Cologne, Rimmel's Toilet Vinegar, Rowland's Macassar Oil, Rowland's Odonto and Kalydor, Trotter's Tooth Powder, Saponceous Tooth Powder, Barnett's Cocaine, Barnett's Kalliston and Tooth Wash, Plate Powder and Silver Soap, Lemon Kali, Henry's Magnesia, Effervescing Citrate of Magnesia, Dinneford and Murray's Fluid Magnesia, Benzino and Benzine Collus, Wax Papura, Float Lights, Enema Instruments in Variety, Disinfecting Fluids, Powder, Boxes, Puffs and Violet Powder, Dye Colors; Soda and Seidlitz Powders, Coward's Seidlitz Powders, do. do. Townsend's and Ayer's Sarsaparilla, Vermifuges, Worm Lozenges, Keating and Locock's Cough Lozenges, Swedish Leeches, Turkey, Honey Comb, and Bath Sponges.

Fresh Seeds from the best houses for Field and garden.

Medicine Chests Supplied and Refitted on the shortest notice.

All the English and American Patent Medicines of Repute.

Source: Hutchinson's Newfoundland Directory for 1864-65, St. John's: McConnan, 1864, p. 154.

ceptions such as photography, books, and grocery items.[57] Druggists were unquestionably at the center of much change in health care practices as, under one roof so to speak, they dealt with family recipes, long-standing and new orthodox medications, over-the-counter medicines with international, regional, and local distribution (often advertised in Newfoundland as "English and American"), botanical and homeopathic medicines, medical apparatus (e.g., inhalers and enema pumps) for use in the home, medicine chests, trusses, toiletries, health/beauty aids (perfumery, fancy soaps, and sponges, etc.), and grocery/dietetic items (e.g., arrowroot, corn, sage, Robinson's Prepared Groats and Barley).

Of these items, the story of the ubiquitous medicine chest is instructive. Advertisements from Newfoundland "chemists and druggists" throughout the nineteenth century commonly noted the sale of sea or family medicine chests—presumably imported, but possibly locally made—"put up," fitted, or refitted at "shortest notice."[58] Such commercial chests had a long history; family chests, used more by the middle and upper classes, became increasingly popular from the mid-1700s onward in Britain and Europe. By providing conventional (as distinct from "folk") medicines for use in the home, they contributed to the incorporation of standard medical treatments into self-care. Some of the guides to the chests also made clear that one reason for owning a chest was to have medicines at hand when a doctor visited.[59] By the early twentieth century, however, the chests contained only prepared medicines or first aid, as if the issue of medicines had been passed over to physicians. Thus McMurdo's 1915 advertisement for "A Medicine Chest for 30 Cents" was for

> minor accidents and emergencies that may crop up in any home any day. . . . This wonderful little box contains a small package each of Absorbent Cotton, Gauze Bandage, Adhesive Plaster, Johnson's Toilet and Baby Powder, Johnson's Digestive Tablets, Menthodonna Corn Tips, Allen's Toothache Plasters, Shaving Cream Soap, Synol Liquid Soap, and a Mustard Leaf.[60]

At the same time, given the special needs of Newfoundland fishers, ships' medicine chests continued to be sold.

Modernity

The changing character of the medicine chest fits with a sense of modernity emerging around 1900. Standards of medical practice varied considerably throughout the nineteenth century, but James Langstaff, the Ontario physician whose detailed records from the 1850s to 1880s have been thoroughly analyzed, was probably not unrepresentative of many.[61] He was wide-ranging in his practice, incorporating, albeit cautiously, new remedies such as salicylate, chloral hydrate, aconite, bromides, and electromagnetism alongside long-standing treatments that included bleeding. Eventually, many of the older treatments became less popular or were pushed aside by new treatments. In many ways, Langstaff combined the enthusiasm often given to new remedies derived earlier in the century (e.g., morphine, quinine, and strychnine) with the cautious approach many practitioners give to novel products.

If his practice reflected a judicious combination of the old with the new, one senses a quickening of change from the 1880s. Even before aspirin was introduced in 1899 by the German company Bayer, other analgesia/fever remedies (e.g., the coal tar derivatives, phenazone [Antipyrine], acetanilid [Antifebrin], and acetophenetidin [phenacetin]) had found ready markets and are seen as milestones in a changing *materia medica* that ultimately, if slowly, led to the virtual sidelining of countless plant remedies by conventional medicine.[62] Moreover, companies such as Burroughs Wellcome, contributors to the beginnings of industrial pharmaceutical research, had a greater impact in Britain and North America with a range of intensively promoted new products.[63] With all this came questions about effective approaches to discovery that challenged the idea of the empirical trial-and-error approach said to characterize early discoveries, though, as said previously, conceptual considerations may well have been at play.

Cod-Liver Oil

In closing this chapter I return to the complex issue of validation with comments on cod-liver oil, including its "modernization" as it moved into the twentieth century. The oil permeated conventional Western medicine and self-care, but, as with spruce beer, a strong local association with Newfoundland adds noteworthy detail to its history. Moreover, unlike spruce beer, it shows how social validation could be sustained over the years by new "scientific" knowledge amid a changing therapeutic scene.

Cod-liver oil entered the materia medica of conventional medicine in the late eighteenth century when some physicians in Manchester, England, reported that the oil, obtained from Newfoundland, relieved "cases of chronic rheumatism, sciatica, and those contractions and rigidities so frequently the consequences of exposure to damp and cold."[64] However, despite continued interest by some physicians, the oil cannot be said to have become a fashionable remedy until the 1840s, by which time it had become something of a panacea, though particularly for "rheumatic, gouty and scrofulous cases," and with a reputation as a strengthener whenever there was a "deficiency of tone." One telling statistic is that, during the 1850s, it was given to nearly one-fifth of the patients admitted to Boston's Massachusetts General Hospital, while at St. George's Hospital in London, costs of the oil became an issue in the decades following a favorable 1849 report of its use for phthisis (tuberculosis).[65]

By mid-century, the oil had also become part of self-care on both sides of the Atlantic, at least for the treatment of invalids. For instance, Emery Souther (1848), "Chemist and Apothecary, Corner of Green Street and Lyman Place, Boston," promoted "real purified oil" obtained from fresh livers with an ethically interesting comment:

> [the] manufacturer has permission to refer all invalids, who may desire it, to various individuals who have used the oil. For obvious reasons, a parade of their names in a pamphlet might be unpleasant to them, but they will be given to any who wish to consult them before using it.[66]

Souther's reference to pure oil raises an issue highlighted by the Newfoundland story. Until well into the twentieth century, countless Newfoundlanders still produced their own supply of "raw oil"—if not rendered from livers in the kitchen, then by rotting livers in a barrel, so that the oil rose to the top of the horrible smelling goo. Although this homemade oil was, for many, an extremely unpleasant product—said to leave a flavor like that of putrid fish and to give a strong taint to perspiration—many Newfoundlanders considered it to be stronger and more healthful (and it was also cheaper) than preparations of "purified" oil, such as Doyle's Newfoundland Oil and

Brick's Tasteless.[67] Such "pure" preparations—the ideal being fresh, "white," or pale yellow oil with no odor of putrefaction—emerged in the nineteenth century. By the 1860s, of three drugstores in St. John's advertising cod-liver oil, J. J. Dearin noted the sale of "Pure Cod Liver Oil for Medicinal Uses, by Wholesale and Retail."[68] At the time, the oil was largely viewed as a dietetic aid, and it is significant that the oil's principal reputation in Newfoundland became as a general tonic, strengthener, and preventative (to build up "resistance" or, from the 1950s, "immunity").[69] The culture of taking the oil (especially for children) up to the 1950s is well remembered: "my mother made us drink cod liver oil; it was a strengthener;"[70] "we always had to have porridge, and after we had our porridge, we had to have cod liver oil;[71] "cod liver oil was our number one medicine. That was for everything: mother used to render it out herself from the cod liver and she'd store away so many bottles for the winter."[72]

By 1900 or so, the public's dilemma of whether cod-liver oil was best viewed as a food or a medicine—typical of many debates today over whether herbs are nutraceuticals or medicines—is reflected in both medical textbooks and public media. G. F. Butler (1900) stated categorically that the "oil is a food and not a medicine,"[73] but a 1902 advertisement in Newfoundland's *Evening Telegram* for Scott's Emulsion of Cod Liver Oil read as follows:

> Tell a man it's a food and he doesn't want to pay for it. Tell him it's a medicine and he says it doesn't look like it. Then tell him it's both a food and a medicine and he thinks you're playing some game on him. Yet these are the facts about Scott's Emulsion of pure cod-liver oil. It is the cream of cod-liver oil, the richest and most digestible of foods. The food for weak stomachs. The food for thin bodies and thin blood.[74]

Science wove in and out of the cod-liver oil story. For example, explanations (invariably disputed) of its "medicinal" activity—iodine and phosphorus content—were in the news in the late 1800s, though many later writers continued to see it as an "alterative," that is, a substance believed to be therapeutically effective in a nonspecific way without a known basis of action.[75] Science is also evident in the competition between manufacturers for the "best oil" (for example, in guarantees of purity). The only Newfoundland contribution, albeit a minor one, to the late nineteenth-century development of the pharmaceutical industry (i.e., outside small-scale production in drugstores) was, in fact, with cod-liver oil. By around 1900, when the world market for the oil seemingly accepted that Norwegian oil was medicinally superior, efforts were made to improve or modernize the Newfoundland product. In 1905 it was said that, "with a more general adoption of scientific methods, Newfoundland manufacturers will be fully able to compete with their Norwegian rivals."[76] In so doing they also had to deal with rumors that Newfoundland oil was adulterated with corn, seal, or whale oil in times of short supplies.[77] Newfoundland rebuttals argued that any adulteration was done in Liverpool or London, and that Newfoundland oil was prepared under stringent standards of quality as a result of new assay techniques.

Vitamins, however, were to become the key issue in terms of the new quality and medicinal value of the oil, made clear in promotion and modernized packaging. In Newfoundland, as in the rest of North America, tonics were not widely replaced by vitamins until the 1960s or later. Nevertheless, vitamins began capturing the popular imagination from the 1920s onward, and soon became very much part of the cod-liver oil story. For example, in 1942: "For Vitamin A and D take Brick's Tasteless."[78] This obviously contrasted with the convenience of taking vitamins alone as Newfoundlanders were being told in 1947: "'8 vitamins in ONE Capsule.' Take Only one Capsule Each Day."[79] It is of particular interest that the issue of whether cod-liver oil was to be considered a food or medicine was also argued with great intensity in the United States in connection with vitamins, as well as whether they could be sold as foods in grocers or only as medicines in drugstores.[80]

Although much of the story of cod-liver oil from the 1920s onward is linked to the recognition of its vitamins A and D content and the emerging knowledge of the physiological role of vitamins, it cannot be assumed that dosages were always appropriate. In commenting on one family's use of the oil for rickets in the 1930s (by which time the specific value of the vitamin D content for the condition was well known), physician Robert Ecke related one story: "'I gives 'em cod-liver oil,' says the mother, 'six spoons a day.' I wondered [thought Ecke] if this would be the only case in the world of cod-liver resistant rickets. 'How long?' ask I. 'Since Thursday,' says the mother."[81]

That cod-liver oil's local and international medicinal/health food reputation was stronger than, say, that of spruce beer reflected a much broader base of explanations through which it was validated by the public. Perhaps, too, effectiveness was an issue. Another milestone in the cod-liver oil story is discovery of the presence of gamma linolenic acid in the last years of the twentieth century, along with clinical trials validating the value of the oil for rheumatoid arthritis.[82] This is a far cry from the pre-1950s, when cod-liver oil was, in part, validated by the widespread belief that weakness was a fundamental medical problem, as discussed in the next chapter.

Chapter 3

Medicines for Weakness:
1900 to c. 1950

"I'm weak doctor, I've had four flus this winter"

Olds OPDism[1]

WEAKNESS AND SOCIAL CONDITIONS

Dividing history into centuries is commonplace and convenient, albeit quite arbitrary. Certainly the optimism of the opening years of the twentieth century—the new face and style of Edwardianism in Britain, the progressive era in the United States, and a relatively golden economic age in Newfoundland—encouraged a sense of modernism, a new era of medical development. Textbooks came with such titles as *The Modern Materia Medica*.[2] Yet most people saw relatively little change in prescribed treatments or those purchased over the counter. Significant carryovers from the 1800s were the generally well-known classes of remedies considered to fortify, strengthen, and/ or revitalize the energy of the body (or parts of it). Such products included foods considered to have medicinal or specific health effects (health foods), general tonics, and treatments promoted for tuberculosis, chlorosis, anemia, asthenia, nerves, women's disorders, the stomach and gastrointestinal tract, and kidney conditions.

This vast range of preparations for such conditions, both over the counter and prescribed by doctors, illustrates particularly well the social validation of medicines. All medicines, in one way or another, were rationalized as dealing with weak conditions. In fact, the very existence of a huge number of medicines to deal with weakness validated, in a reciprocal way, that weakness was a basic medical (and social) problem. Reinforcement of this came from conventional medical teachings (for example, about female weakness), as well as such social trends as eugenics, which argued the white race was in decline, the evangelism of health reformers about moral and social problems in society, and the growing authority of physicians and druggists who prescribed or recommended the medicines. That a circular argument existed was not particularly evident owing to the many distinct categories of treatments.

The medicines for treating weaknesses considered in this chapter were generally available in Britain, the United States, and Canada. Almost all were imported into Newfoundland, where two factors—the high incidence of poor nutrition and tuberculosis—accentuated the weakness concept. Neither factor was unique to Newfoundland, nor was the association often made between poverty and tuberculosis. In fact, social conditions in rural Newfoundland during the first half of the century had analogies to, for example, the Appalachian region, much of the southern United States, and the Highlands and Islands of Scotland, as mentioned previously.

The twentieth-century market economy was especially slow in reaching Newfoundland's hundreds of fishing outports. The formal economy rested on the "truck" system—an inequitable credit system that bound fishermen to privileged merchants. This essentially cashless economy obviously encouraged informal bartering, borrowing, and exchange of goods. One problem, not experienced by Southern Appalachia, for example, was that Newfoundland's short growing season made it almost impossible to live off a "spot of land" through subsistence farming.[3]

Some people always managed to fare better with the informal economy than others, especially in supplying food for the table and escaping "the hungry month of March." This expression, well known in Newfoundland, referred to the time of year when vegetables were no longer available, and pack ice perhaps prevented boats from replenishing supplies in many communities. Except for hunting, the women in the family did much to overcome limited diets based on staples of salt fish or salt meat, white flour, and molasses. A vegetable garden was key, especially as root crops—if stored properly in root cellars—could be eaten throughout the winter. By springtime, as in more favorable climates, "spring greens" arrived. Newfoundlanders commonly relished dandelion leaves, though rarely before May: "I like [dandelion] better than any [and some folks cultivated it.] My God we were as strong as bulls from eating that stuff."[4] Other resources for the table were berries gathered in the late summer, murres (known as "turres" in Newfoundland), moose, caribou, and seals, as well as domesticated cows, goats, or sheep. The nutrition *potential,* then, of the informal economy was considerable but subject to family ingenuity and character, as well as seasonal luck and fortune.[5]

Amid these circumstances and the hard work of fishing and drying and salting codfish, a slim safety margin between adequacy and poverty contributed to Newfoundland's high incidence of such vitamin-deficiency diseases as beriberi, scurvy, and rickets, even after the 1940s. It was a situation that caused the island to be seen as a poor and backward colony. Many believed—all the more so after "accessory food factors" (to be called vitamins) were recognized—that such nonspecific symptoms as malaise and weakness were closely correlated with inadequate nutrition.[6] "Some called it lumbago [but it was] just starving hungry, no nourishment at all."[7] This seemingly lay behind the characterization of Newfoundlanders by various immigrant physicians as "peculiarly unintelligent with regards to medical matters" (1908), "apathetic" (1937), "somewhat slow in mental reactions and lacking in initiative" (1945), and of "low I.Q." (1951).[8] Newfoundland lethargy, apathy, and nervousness were often linked to mild vitamin B_1 (thiamine) deficiency after its isolation in 1926.[9]

Associated with nutrition problems in almost every Newfoundlander's mind was the high incidence of tuberculosis. In fact, while the worldwide impact of the disease in the first half of the twentieth century has been studied in detail, its decimation of the Newfoundland population, especially between 1900 and the 1950s, remains a relatively unknown story. Reference to the situation in Ireland, where so many Newfoundlanders had roots, is appropriate. It has been said that Ireland was "unique among the nations of the British Isles, and one of the few developed countries to see mortality from tuberculosis still rising" around 1900.[10] Yet the situation was the same in Newfoundland, where it peaked a little later.[11] Although by 1900 a bacterial infection was well accepted as the cause of the disease, Newfoundlanders often associated the condition with "starvation": "I have no doubt in my mind that it killed them all; they used the word tuberculosis which was wrong."[12] Others saw it as resulting from "weak lungs." With most small communities only accessible by boat, medical care presented problems. Few could be treated in the "San" (sanatorium), so home care was necessary and widespread, although in 1936 it was described as a "grim joke" because of the problems of poor diet and sanitation, as well as the "habits and the social customs of our people."[13]

Countless Newfoundland families nursed a family member with the disease. Dilemmas arose with over-the-counter remedies, because "messages" of hope in the vigorous advertising contradicted much public chastisement of the remedies. British- and Canadian-trained physician A. E. Rutherford denounced "advertising quacks' patent medicines and other secret remedies" in a 1909 lecture to Newfoundlanders, as did countless other physicians and vigorous lay campaigns on both sides of the Atlantic.[14] In Newfoundland, Aubrey Tizzard remembered the death of his sister from tuberculosis in 1939, after five years of confinement at home, and countless different kinds of over-the-counter medication:

> The last medicine she received arrived a few days before she died. There were several bottles from a distributor in Change Island. Some were to be taken orally and others to be rubbed on the flesh. She took a little and my mother rubbed her with the liniment a few times but it proved of no avail.[15]

PREVENTION AND TREATMENT

Before looking at prevention and treatment choices, the various expressions for and the meanings attached to "weakness" need comment. It was explicit or implied in references to constant fatigue, run-down feelings, general malaise, debility, the need for more energy and nourishment, building up wasted tissues, as well as "weak nerves," "weak lungs," and other organs. Such different diagnoses, often self-diagnoses, were sometimes of little significance in practice, at least so far as such medicines as "tonics" were "general purpose" treatments for all forms of weakness.

Weakness, too, could be described as "asthenia," particularly among physicians. This was a legacy of the classification of diseases by the reactionary eighteenth-century Scottish physician John Brown. Brown divided diseases into two broad categories: asthenic diseases (viewed as a deficiency of natural energy or excitability) and sthenic (in which the body had an excess of excitability). Asthenic conditions, characterized by weakness, were to be treated by stimulants such as a solid diet and medications, of which Brown favored opium, camphor, musk, and ether.[16] By the early twentieth century this Brunonian classification system had become outmoded, but a few medical textbooks and journal articles continued to refer to asthenia until the 1920s. Suggested treatments focused on "nervous excitants" or stimulants such as tincture of nux vomica (containing strychnine) and arsenious chloride.[17] Other texts ignored the concept or used the term to define particular states, for example, asthenic pneumonia.[18]

The pervasiveness of the concept of weakness is also reflected, implicitly if not explicitly, in the health and fitness messages during the early decades of the twentieth century. These came from the disease prevention teachings of the health and hygiene (or health and fitness) reformers. Although essentially the same as those from public health teaching, health reformers emphasized individual responsibility to maintain one's own health.[19] To help attain this, it was said, one needed a simple knowledge of the organs of the body and of the physiological role of the blood in order to appreciate the importance of appropriate diet, exercise, and fresh air.

In his 1909 lecture to a rural audience on "Health and Hygiene"— on "how the laws of health relate to maintaining the health of various organs of the body"—A. E. Rutherford stated that "prolonged concentration of the mind on any one pursuit or occupation, demands an increased supply of blood to the brain at the expense of the other organs which are thereby starved of their regular fuel." This meant that "brain workers" needed regular exercise. He advised:

> If time or weather will not permit of a smart walk after meals some form of gymnastic exercise should be practiced at home— but above all, get all the fresh air as possible into the lungs between the dinner table and the desk.[20]

In fact it was a time, on both sides of the Atlantic, of barrages of messages about keeping fit and building up strength through physical exercise—messages that were often combined with much advice on diet, sleep, mental vigor, and so on. Recommended exercise ranged from sports, home gymnastics, and calisthenic exercises to body building promoted by the likes of Eugene Sandow, Bernarr Macfadden (sometimes described as the "father of fitness"), and Charles Atlas, who became household names.[21]

Rutherford's lecture also paid attention to diet. In fact, a pillar of health reform teaching had long been to ensure appropriate nutrition, often vegetarianism, for the purpose of acquiring good health (and overcoming weakness), or even to control sexual drive.[22] Critics of vegetarianism, who argued that it limited muscular power, based their arguments on the "new" nutrition science that, as it developed from around 1840, correlated the chemistry of food with animal physiology.[23] The new science, which determined the appropriate proportions of fats, carbohydrates, proteins, and minerals (and within a few years vitamins) for both healthy and sick individuals, shaped much popular health education, the commercial promotion of "health foods," as well as widespread interest in diets, including many fad diets.[24]

Although it is impossible to say exactly what the impact of all this was, it was undoubtedly limited in many places, as in Newfoundland because of illiteracy and poor economic means. Nevertheless some exposure occurred (see Box 3.1), probably not much different from elsewhere, especially after experiences with recruitment for military service for World War I, when some 47 percent of Newfoundland volunteers and 57 percent of conscripts were rejected as medically unfit to serve.[25] Similar concerns—some said it was shock—arose over recruitment in Britain and the United States.[26] Aside from a "health through fitness" promotion by schoolteachers and public health nurses, the Church Lads' Brigade (CLB) in Newfoundland had significant influence: "They had a great gymnasium and there was an awful lot of boys went to the gym, and they used to have drill nights two nights a week."[27] Such activity resonated with the mind-set of Christian manhood (or muscular Christianity centering around sport and exercise for moral health) that had a widespread following from the last decades of the nineteenth century up to the 1920s, certainly in Britain and the United States.[28] Just what the impact was of muscular Christianity on Newfoundland is unclear, despite one influential exponent, Wilfred Grenfell, who arrived in Newfoundland and Labrador in 1892 with strong roots in its practice.[29]

Much of the following discussion, on the vast array of medicines that directly or indirectly focus on weakness, can appear as something of a "laundry list." However, it is the smorgasbord of products,

Box 3.1. Health and Fitness

Health and fitness messages reached Newfoundlanders through local news-papers with advertisements for such writings as those by bodybuilder Bernarr Macfadden, and the sale of equipment such as the "Loop Developer," used by "the Territorial Army," for increasing arm strength when worked with five min-utes daily. (G. Knowling, advertisement, *Daily News*, December 2, 1910, p. 6.) Newspaper editors also passed on health messages, such as the following:

ALPHABET OF HEALTH

Abstain from intoxicating liquors
Breathe good air
Consume no more food than the body requires
Drink pure water
Exercise daily
Find congenial occupation
Give the body frequent baths
Have regular habits
Insure good digestion by proper mastication
Justify right living by living right
Keep your head cool and your feet warm
Late hours are a destroyer of beauty
Make definite hours of sleep
Never bolt your food
Over-exercise is as bad as under-exercise
Preserve an even temperament
Question the benefit of too much medicine
Remember, "An ounce of prevention is worth a pound of cure"
Sacrifice money, not health
Temperance in all things
Under no condition allow the teeth to decay
Vanquish superstition
Worry not at all
X-tend the teachings of this alphabet to others
Yield not to discouragement
Zealously labor in the cause of health and gain everlasting reward

Atchison Globe

Source: The Daily News, December 1, 1915, p. 7.

taken together, that reinforced weakness as a basic medical problem. It is noteworthy, too, that many of the preparations survived vigorous criticism from the 1890s onward; in the United States, for example, they faced a crusade that included grassroots support from women to protect the public from dangerous and fraudulent medicines, an effective muckraking campaign by journalists exposing fraud, deceit, unsafe and ineffective remedies, and ambitious bureaucrats with whom legislation was power. A net consequence was the Pure Food and Drugs Act of 1906, which paved the way for the Canadian Proprietary and Patent Medicine Act that became operative in 1909.[30] Such controls, however, only partly met expectations of safeguarding the public. Many people remained skeptical and critical of both the surviving medicines and countless new ones, especially since controls on therapeutic claims remained minimal for some time. On the other hand, countless remedies remained widely used and are fondly remembered by many seniors today. Such circumstances prompt the questions: To what extent were druggists and their customers torn by conflicting messages and information, as with the tuberculosis remedies already mentioned? Did druggists see ethical dilemmas in selling preparations criticized by many of their peers and by the medical profession? Or did they rationalize their sale because such remedies were seemingly widely accepted and validated? Specific responses to these questions would take this book beyond an account of medicines, but the discussion as a whole will suggest that the critics of quack medicines failed to understand the popular beliefs and attitudes that validated them. After looking at the variety of medicines, I suggest that the promotion of so many "panacean" remedies could find much validity at the time, alongside the concept of weakness.

THE MEDICINES

"When I had anaemia, I had cereal every day; I could eat it all day long."

Olds OPDism

From "Health" Foods to Tonics

RALSTON'S HEALTH FOODS
Once Tried Always Used

Brekfast [*sic*]	Food Pancake Flour
Barley Food	Hominy Grist [*sic*]
Health Crisps	Cereal Coffee[31]

This 1907 advertisement, from a Newfoundland grocery, is just one indication of the pervasive advertising of foods and food products as a means to maintain health, to build up strength, and to treat symptoms such as weakness, tiredness, sleeplessness, nervousness, and the run-down feeling.[32] Although not strictly medicines, health foods were seen to be on the borderline of medicines/foods at the time (Chapter 2).[33] Moreover, they featured in physicians' dietetic regimens and did much to reinforce the concept of weakness, particularly by emphasizing the building of strength—hence the discussion here.

Breakfast Cereals and Flours

Breakfast cereals, initially associated with American health reformer John Harvey Kellogg (1852-1943), became health food icons. His first cereal, granola—introduced in the 1870s—was quickly followed by a host of flaked, toasted, and other prepared grains manufactured by Kellogg and his competitors. Their commercial promotion on both sides of the Atlantic was invariably linked to health and appropriate nutrition in keeping with Kellogg's own lifestyle of "hygienic" practices such as vegetarianism, abstinence from alcohol, quelling sexual desires, and much more.[34] Newfoundlanders were bombarded with advertisements. During the early 1900s, they read mostly about Grape-Nuts ("a compound made of Wheat, Barley, Salt and Yeast") not only as a nourishing food but also a treatment for specific health issues. In 1907, the cereal was promoted as a source of vital energy and for "tissue repair." This was justified by the view— well established by the mid-1800s—that phosphorus was an essential component of the brain and nervous system. Because of the phosphorus "stored up in wheat and barley by nature," Grape-Nuts built up "brain and nerve"[35] and strength to deal with problems of "sluggishness, sleepiness, [and] inability to think clearly."[36]

Although by the 1930s such overt treatment claims for cereals and other breakfast foods were very much tempered in consequence of legislation in the United States, Britain, and Canada, notions of weakness in one form or another were sustained by cereal advertising, for example, Scott's Porrage Oats, "Scotland's Favourite Food," offering "Health and Strength."[37] Many Newfoundlanders, too, continued to "add" the island's favored tonic/strengthener, cod-liver oil, to their porridge.

White or brown flour? "There were people who couldn't eat this brown bread; we could, so [Mother] made us eat it. So she would give them our white bread or white flour within reason for their brown flour."[38] In 1909, the medical textbook *Diet in Health and Disease* stated that the chief objection to breakfast foods "is the cost, which is far greater than the same amount of food prepared from the cereal itself."[39] The chief source of calories for Newfoundlanders, many of whom could not afford cereals anyway, was white bread. Intriguingly, some resisted eating brown bread, despite its promotion as a health food and tonic; such resistance offers an illustration not only of the dismissal of authority—frequent in the story of medicines—but also the constant difficulty of health promotion, especially in trying to change lifestyles.

By the early 1900s, to the chagrin of physician J. M. Little, working at Wilfred Grenfell's Mission in St. Anthony, Newfoundland, white rather than brown flour was in general use on the island. As knowledge of vitamins was emerging in 1912, he wrote a significant article, "Beriberi: Caused by Fine White Flour."[40] In noting that many people lived "from hand to mouth being always on the verge of poverty," Little emphasized their limited diet—often "flour, tea and molasses to see them through the winter." He made a strong case that white flour was a principal culprit of beriberi and added that "the 'old stagers' of this country who remember the days when 'brown flour' was the diet, say that this trouble was unknown among them."[41] Eating the "correct" flour (that is, whole wheat rather than white) had, in fact, been part of the teaching of various health reformers in the nineteenth century, from American Sylvester Graham (of Graham Cracker fame) onward.[42] Little is more likely to have been aware of this than of a 1911 brown bread campaign conducted by a British newspaper, *The Daily Mail,* this campaign drew on the pioneer investigations of Frederick Gowland Hopkins, which stated that protein, fat, and carbohydrate were alone insufficient to sustain life.[43]

One consequence of the Newfoundland work of Little was the intensive promotion of brown flour by Wilfred Grenfell and his colleagues.[44] However, by the 1920s success was unclear,[45] just as *The Daily Mail* campaign had failed to alter the long-standing consumption patterns of bread in Britain. Histories of bread emphasize the relative stability of the dominant position of white bread in the hearts of British consumers, to which one can add many Newfoundlanders.[46]

Given the simmering incidence of beriberi throughout Newfoundland, it is not surprising that the brown flour problem came to the fore as a national issue during the Great Depression years of the 1930s. Whether advertisements, from various wholesalers and bakeries, that emphasized the general health benefits of brown flour had any persuasive power is impossible to say. At least they were explicit: Quaker 100 percent whole wheat flour was described as a "Natural Tonic," while Walsh's Brown Bread was advertised in 1937 for

> BODY-BUILDING Would you be strong and virile, able to walk 40 miles on occasion, do a hard day's work without tiring. You can do it, ask some of your husky friends for their secret, 10 to 1 the answer will be BROWN BREAD.[47]

Such promotion almost certainly had little impact on those who "were starving to death on this six cents dole thing."[48] Ultimately, the government substituted brown for white flour supplied to all dole recipients.[49] Many, however, continued their antipathy, perhaps for understandable reasons. Not only was the brown flour often adulterated with grit, but many felt that brown flour reaffirmed a lower social status. A prophetic letter from the office of the prime minister of Newfoundland (November 10, 1933) to physician Charles Parsons stated,

> you remember the trouble that arose when cocoa, a nutritious beverage, was introduced instead of tea. The same prejudice apparently applies in the case of brown or whole wheat flour. It will no doubt be overcome in time but it would be exceedingly difficult to try to force the people to use it before they have become gradually accustomed to its benefits.[50]

Around 1940, an American physician in Twillingate, wrote that "by some strange perversion many [Newfoundlanders] attributed their ills to brown flour, when actually it was a cure for them."[51] Amid the continual dismissal of authority, the view of one lecturer on home economics in the early 1930s might have been relevant, namely that the general public is "inclined to regard nutrition as a complex subject too involved for them to try to understand."[52]

A "resolution" to the brown versus white issue, and a short circuit to academic debate on the precise links between malnutrition, illhealth, and low income, came in June 1944 when, amid the stresses of World War II, white flour on the island was enriched with B vitamins (riboflavin and niacin) and iron.

Foods and Nutritive Drinks for Children and the Sick

Doctor when your sick you're not well [and need building up]

Olds OPDism

The level of promotion of cereals and brown flour as health foods during the early decades of the twentieth century, often paled in comparison with that of "foods" for infants, children, the sick, the elderly, and anyone else needing more strength to get through the day. My remarks in this section do not cover the intense debates over the most appropriate artificial milks—very much embedded in children's health reform movements—though they were all promoted to build *healthy* babies, in some places implicitly to ensure future citizens were fit to defend the Empire. Physicians, too, acquired new expertise and authority.[53]

Milk and malt products. One of the more widely advertised products in Newfoundland newspapers and in such medical journals as the British *Practitioner* was Benger's Food for Infants, Invalids, and the Aged, which was "expressly devised to be used in conjunction with fresh milk."[54] A mixture of wheat flour and pancreatic extract, it competed with twenty-five or so other products by 1910.[55] In its promotion to the general public, Benger claimed to develop "delicate infants into strong robust children," but it was also a restorative, the *safe* food in illness sanctioned by the medical profession: "Even in Fevers and illnesses with inflammatory symptoms such as are present in Enteric Fever, when the giving of correct food is of highest importance, Benger's Food is right."[56]

That many infant foods contained malt as an aid to digestion reflected its reputation as a food/tonic from the last decades of the 1800s onward. Prepared from barley treated to stop sprouting, malt was available in countless products as malt alone, as cod-liver oil and malt (e.g., Maltine, and Diamalt with Cod Liver Oil which masked the taste of the oil), and as malt breakfast foods and innumerable nutrition drinks. Ovaltine—"scientifically prepared from malt, milk and eggs" and providing "every necessary nutritive element"—was a popular "tonic food beverage [to build-up] brain, nerve and body."[57] The name "Ovaltine" did not indicate the presence of malt, unlike "Coco*malt*," produced by the U.S. company R. B. Davis. When mixed with milk, Cocomalt became one of the best-known health drinks in Newfoundland between the 1930s and 1950s.[58] The intensive promotion of Cocomalt to children in the United States—with Buffalo Bill jigsaw puzzles, Buck Rogers adventure books, and promotional comics—seemingly did not reach the island. However, with repetitive advertising in local newspapers and the government's policy of Cocomalt distribution to schools, this was hardly necessary. The cocoa provided "strength and energy," the eggs built "muscle and bone," and malt aided "digestion." It was also "rich in iron, vitamin D, calcium and other food essentials."[59]

The basic advertising message was that malt (made from barley) was a nutrient "in wasting diseases," of which tuberculosis was the best known. Noteworthy features of malt in connection with its use for weak digestion were the diastasic and diastatic values, "scientific measurements" used in promotion to physicians that added a scientific "pedigree." These values were determined by the amount of starch converted into maltose and dextrin by the enzyme diastase; high amounts of the latter were often extolled in advertisements to physicians,[60] as were the most effective extraction methods (e.g., for Kepler's marketed by Burroughs Wellcome)[61]

Meat extracts. Beef extracts were equally if not more popular than milk and malt products, at least among adults, for their strength-building reputation. Beef tea, often made at home, competed with many commercial preparations. In the early 1900s, Newfoundlanders could read U.S. advertisements about Armour's Extract of Beef with "a rich beefy flavor." "Nervous and Tired People" would find that the "mildly stimulating effect of a cup of [Armour's] Beef Tea restores the spirits, strength and energy without disagreeable after effects."[62] On the other hand, the British product Bovril—a meat juice extracted so as to retain the "fibrin, gelatin and coagulable albumin"—with its remarkable "body-building powers," was much more intensively promoted in the island.[63] Newfoundlanders could certainly identify with 1902 advertising that stated: "In Damp and Chilly Weather a cup of hot Bovril erects a fortification in the system that bids defiance to the inclemencies and keeps out the diseases that follow in their wake."[64] Later advertisements (1930s) were in similar vein, albeit less specific: "Keep fit on Bovril. Bovril stands supreme as the great supporter of the people's health. BOVRIL Gives Fitness."[65]

Physician prescribing. To what extent did doctors encourage the health foods just discussed? Did their authority foster the belief that weakness was a pervasive problem? By 1900, physicians were probably taking more and more interest than in previous decades in dietetic preparations for the sick. In this they were not only pushed by manufacturers, but also by the growth of "scientific nutrition" that, by the early 1900s, brought with it specialist textbooks for physicians, chapters in general textbooks of therapeutics, and information in the handy compendia—e.g., Martindale's (1906) *The Extra Pharmacopoeia*—consulted by physicians and druggists. Newfoundland doctors, too, in constantly facing the serious issues of poor nutrition and tuberculosis, must have been especially receptive to the bombardment of health food and cod-liver oil advertisements in medical journals they received. For example, around 1910 readers of *The Practitioner* were assailed by Bovril (and the unseasoned Invalid Bovril), Möller's Hydroxyl Free Cod Liver Oil (for "all wasting diseases, rickets, tuberculosis, the most reliable restorative"), various malt extracts, Wincarnis ("a delicious and nourishing wine tonic . . . said to be a scientific preparation of choice wine, extract of meat and extract of malt"), Diamalt with Cod Liver Oil, Miol ("the most scientific nutritive food for general use"), and Angier's Emulsion (petroleum with hypophosphite).[66]

For public consumption, the authority of doctors was often invoked in advertising. In 1912, for instance, Newfoundlanders were told that Virol was recommended and prescribed by doctors all over the United Kingdom, and that it was "used in 500 Hospitals for Consumption, Anaemia and Rickets,"[67] and that "when your physician tells you to take SCOTT'S EMULSION you may rest assured that his decision is the result of confidence, built upon experience."[68] No evidence exists that Newfoundland physicians wrote many prescriptions for health foods except for children (malt and cod-liver oil and Virol containing bone marrow with malt, egg, and lime), but little doubt can exist that they and druggists often encouraged the use of such products, readily available in drug and general stores, to supplement prescriptions.[69]

Tonics

"80 year old asked, 'How do you feel now?' Pause. 'Well, my dear man, I believe I could kill a man right here if he made me mad enough.'"

Olds OPDism

Of the countless medicines promoted for general weakness or, more specifically, for "weak nerves" or "weak hearts," tonics were central players among medicines prepared in the home, purchased over-the-counter, and prescribed by physicians. An eclectic group of preparations, tonics—according to an 1896 medical textbook—maintained and promoted body tone "through improving appetite, digestion, assimilation, secretion, circulation, composition of the blood, invigorating the muscular system, and promotion of the nutrition of nerve-centres and fibres."[70] Many, with bitter or astringent tastes, already had a long history of use in a variety of conditions with weakness as a feature. For instance, eighteenth-century stimulants to treat asthenic conditions or to purify the blood—concepts that continued to underpin many twentieth-century uses. The long history of tonics, sustained as much by the oral tradition as printed text, contributed to social validation.

While it would be both impossible and tedious to discuss the countless tonics here, two groups, spring tonics and bitters, illustrate the rationale and use of many. Spring tonics, well known on both sides of the Atlantic, persisted longer in rural Newfoundland than in most other places. Their special place in the island's culture perhaps owed something to the privations of winter weather, the often inclement springtime, and dietary deficiencies. It was, after all, reported in 1921 that the "first seasonal signs of the effect of restricted diet appeared at the end of March and beginning of April. . . . A sudden increase in nervous instability was evident at this season."[71] Perhaps this is what one Newfoundlander meant when saying, "I used to have fits especially when my blood turned from winter condition to summer."[72] The actions of spring tonics were generally viewed as blood purifiers, but some also saw the need to clean out the gastrointestinal system in the springtime with castor oil, for example;[73] senna, a milder laxative often viewed as another blood purifier, was equally popular.[74]

Commercial tonics competed with, and in many homes pushed aside, such home-prepared items as sulfur and molasses and teas made from "cherry," "dogwood," "juniper," and "pine."[75] Cod-liver oil was also used as a home tonic and a commercial tonic:

> Now that to all appearances we are to have an early spring [1925], and it is the time when one does not feel quite alright a bottle of any of the following will pick you up very quickly. Wampole's Extract of C.L.O. [a restorative, fortifier]—$1.20; Compound Sarsaparilla [blood purifier]—$1.00; Quinine Iron Tonic [a bitter tonic]—50c; Compound Hypophosphites [a tonic]—50c and $1.00.[76]

Although tonics sold as bitters were commonly viewed as spring tonics/blood purifiers, their high alcohol content contributed to their popularity during prohibition times (from 1917 to 1923 in Newfoundland). Newfoundlanders had imported choices besides locally produced Stafford Mandrake Bitters.[77] As with Wilson's Herbine Bitters, the laxative properties of such tonics were extolled in advertisements or on the container labels for a variety of ailments (e.g., dyspepsia, sick headache, and constipation) by "removing impurities which tend to disrupt the natural functioning of the bowels."[78] Another competitor, Dr. West's OK Bitters ("Compound of the extracts of roots, herbs and barks combined with the purest old Bourbon Whiskey"), focused more on invigorating the digestive organs.[79]

Fortifiers for Specific Diseases: Building Resistance

Tuberculosis

> "My cousin, he was supposed to have TB, they were testing him, I suppose his lungs must be weak or something."[80]

Tonics were used for both general ill health and for specific medical conditions in which lack of energy and weakness were cardinal symptoms. Above all, the scourge of tuberculosis during the first half of the twentieth century encouraged their use whatever other treatments were tried. Moreover, tonics and other medications—restorers of strength and vitality—fitted very much into the widely touted concept of building resistance. Marmite, for instance, was promoted in the 1930s for "increasing the resistance to infections of all kinds."[81]

The concept of resistance came into prominence with the establishment of the germ theory of disease in the last decades of the 1800s, and the consequent rapid development of innumerable vaccines. It was fostered in some degree by the emergence of a "germ panic" between 1900 and 1940,[82] though advertising tended to focus more on killing "dangerous," or potentially dangerous, germs lurking everywhere in the home, on flies, and so on. Disinfectants became part of everyday life, as when looking after tuberculosis patients: "I used a lot of lye water . . . you don't want to catch any germs, so everything you touch you wash it in lye water, washing dishes, everything like that, put a little drop of lye into everything."[83] But aside from killing germs, the need to build up resistance to overcome weakness—perhaps a weak chest—was a common enough theme. It could be accomplished by strengtheners (e.g., iron tonics); and Father Morriscy's No. 10, "better known as a lung tonic," proclaimed in 1910 to "really tone up and strengthen the lungs," as well as,

> the whole system giving the vitality needed to fight off lung diseases. Even in cases of Consumption it has proved very helpful. It arrests the decline and builds up the system at the same time that it helps clear the passages of mucus.[84]

Other preparations, such as Dr. Pierce's Golden Medical Discovery, sounded more specific by considering "How the Body Kills Germs." It was a "germ-killing substance" in the blood (presently unknown) that was dependent on putting the body and blood in a healthy state.[85]

One other product, promoted to overcome weakness and to build up resistance, stands out as one of the most intensively advertised preparations in Newfoundland during the first half of the twentieth century. This was Ferrozone, an iron preparation of ferrous vanadate in sugarcoated pills.[86] As a 1905 advertisement—captioned, "How to get consumption"—stated,

ninety per cent of the "lungers" contract consumption by allowing power of resistance to fall so low that a favorable condition
for the development of the bacilli is provided. . . .Where there is
weakness and debility, there you find tuberculosis. For developing strength and building up the weak, nothing equals Ferrozone.
(See also Box 3.2.)[87]

BOX 3.2. Ferrozone

A variety of medicines for tuberculosis were advertised, especially up to
around 1910. Ferrozone, one of the most widely promoted iron preparations in
Newfoundland, touched on weakness in various ways in this 1907 advertisement.

SUNKEN CHEEKS, BLANCHED LIPS
USUALLY INDICATE CONSUMPTION

Those hollow cheeks, that feeble walk, sunken chest and woebegone, va-
cant expression, to most people are evidences of the work of consumption.
Even the small hacking cough, night sweats and wasting of the body, so popularly accepted as indications of the same dread scourge, are in many instances entirely misleading. Nine-tenths of these so-called "consumptives" are
only cases of underfeeding.

Especially in children and young girls there is a sad lack of appetite, no vitality, cheeks are pallid. Many adults are just as bad, because they, too, starve the
body.

Before you and your children get beyond the reach of medicine commence
treatment with Ferrozone, the best appetizer and most nutritive tonic known.
Ferrozone creates an appetite keen as a razor; it simply makes you eat, and
besides it strengthens digestion so much that all food is assimilated and at
once converted into nourishment for the blood, brain, nerves and muscles. The
general health is thus built up in a marvelous way by Ferrozone, which overcomes weakness and debility in both young and old.

The systematic use of Ferrozone, together with fresh air and exercise, will in
a short time restore any person in poor health.

Whether weak through worry, over-work or disease, whether your case is recent or chronic, Ferrozone will permanently cure. In every case it is successful
because it contains more actual nourishment than you can get in any other way.

No matter what the age or sex, as a nerve builder and general body
invigorator, Ferrozone is the best medicine. It pushes back the feeling of old
age and puts the elasticity and vim of youth into systems that ordinary remedies fail to rebuild. This is not mere theory, but a claim reinforced by overwhelming evidence.

Source: The Evening Telegram, December 17, 1907, p. 2

It was also advertised with such tag lines as "Makes the weak strong, the sick well," "Weakness foe of the aged," "Ferrozone for bracing health," and "A wonderful tonic and strengthener."

In the face of all this, the prevailing view of physicians was that prevention and treatment of tuberculosis was accomplished less by medicines than by rest, fresh air, and nutrition—the core of sanatorium treatment. As Newfoundland physician A. E. Rutherford explained to a rural community in 1909:

> Consumption is *not* cured by advertising quacks' patent medicines or other secret remedies but solely and exclusively by the judicious use of fresh air—sunshine—water—abundant and good food, e.g., milk, eggs, meat, vegetables and fruit, and the help of certain medicines, used sparingly, when the aforementioned measures and diet are not in themselves sufficiently powerful to combat the disease.[88]

Aside from the impracticality of Rutherford's diet suggestions, the deep-rooted belief in tonics and the intense promotion of many of them were strong inducements to dismiss such advice. Rutherford's dismissal of over-the-counter medicines would have included general chest medicines that did not necessarily make claim to kill germs. Ayer's Cherry Pectoral (from the successful J. C. Ayer and Company in the United States) was just one cough medicine touted for consumption. As many other advertisements stated, coughs and colds could lead to consumption and had to be prevented or dealt with promptly. "It's the neglected cold that is the parent of consumption."[89]

Rutherford would not have included cod-liver oil in his castigation of remedies, for, as mentioned in Chapter 2, among both physicians and laypeople it had a particular reputation—aside from its general action as a "strengthener"—in the treatment of tuberculosis. He might, however, have felt that the commercial preparations were unnecessarily expensive. Some of the latter, such as the well-advertised Park's Perfect Emulsion, containing "Cod Liver Oil, with Hypophosphites of Lime and Soda and Guaiacol," mentioned consumption in their promotion: "You may have consumption very badly, but your chances for recovery are good if you use a remedy that will nourish your body, reconstruct your wasted tissues, and destroy the principle of the disease."[90] Another advertisement read, "Losing flesh is not a good sign, but it is a timely warning" to take the "excellent nutrient."[91] Scott's Emulsion of Cod Liver Oil was just as explicit: "Consumption is less deadly than it used to be [hardly the case in Newfoundland in 1907]. Certain relief and usually complete recovery will result from the following treatment: Hope, rest, fresh air, and—Scott's Emulsion."[92]

One general chest medicine merits comment for a particular cultural link with the island. Sprucine, which consisted of "spruce gum, wild cherry, hoarhound and tar," was said to be invaluable when taken "with cod liver oil in the first stages of consumption."[93] Frequently advertised in the early 1900s, this resonated with the kitchen medicine tradition in Newfoundland not only because of the cod-liver oil but also because the spruce, abundant on the island, had a reputation as a tonic and chest medicine. "Get spruce boughs, clean boughs, and wash them and steep them out and then drain off the water. . . . Take a drink, it would give you a good appetite."[94]

Chlorosis and Anemia

> Patient wants a blood test because "it must be low." "Why must it be low?" "Because when I sticks a needle in myself I don't bleed nearly as much as [I] used to."
>
> Olds OPDism

Two conditions, chlorosis and anemia, with marked symptoms of lethargy and tiredness, have a key place in the weakness story. Chlorosis, because it faded and disappeared as a diagnosis after the 1920s, has fascinated and vexed historians for some time.[95] It is, in fact, an especially intriguing example of how approaches to diagnosis and treatment are affected by general social and scientific trends, which, in this case, included women's emancipation, laboratory medicine, and iron metabolism research.[96]

William Osler described chlorosis in 1892 as "an essential anaemia met with chiefly in young girls, characterized by a marked relative diminution of the haemoglobin."[97] Making the diagnosis dependent on a laboratory determination of hemoglobin concentrations (as was happening at the time), rather than from a patient's history and physical appearance, encouraged the view—accepted by more and more physicians around 1900—that administering iron was all that was needed for treatment. Successful results then became part of the diagnosis; one consequence was that chlorosis and anemia (hitherto an adult diagnosis) were increasingly seen as one and the same condition.

In contrast, some practitioners held onto the view that chlorosis was due to the failure of young women to adjust to the increasing pace and character of modern society; in consequence, treatment had to embrace what was often called moral management: rest, exercise, attention to diet, and treatment of symptoms.[98] Aside from iron, the latter might include, as one 1904 medical textbook advised, "laxatives, preferably mild salines, rank next in importance to iron," bitters to stimulate appetite and treat "superacidity of the gastric juice."[99] Notions that chlorosis could be due to some form of chronic autointoxication (see later discussion in this chapter in the section Digestives/Laxatives) could also influence some physicians' prescribing habits.[100]

Just how Newfoundlanders and the public elsewhere were "educated" into combining chlorosis and anemia into one condition rather than two cannot be explored here, except for noting that advertising might have played a part. Amid the early 1900s' promotion of innumerable iron preparations in the 1900s, occasional references to chlorosis *and* anemia can be found, for instance, Serravillo's Tonic (quinine and iron wine) "cures Anaemia, Chlorosis, Debility."[101] The popular Ferrozone, already noted in connection with tuberculosis, also referred to both conditions (Box 3.3).[102] In contrast, advertisements such as for Dr. Williams' Pink Pills (reported to contain ferrous sulphate, potassium carbonate, magnesia, powdered licorice, and sugar)[103] did not mention chlorosis, but "Wasting Anaemia. A Trouble that Afflicts Thousands of Young Girl's."[104] Ultimately, by 1910 or so, chlorosis generally disappeared from advertisements in the Newfoundland newspapers.[105]

Given all this, the distinction between chlorosis and anemia probably had little significance for most Newfoundlanders. All that mattered was medicines for the blood. As one Newfoundland senior remembered: "You used to get blood pills . . . to build up your blood. You'd be always feeling tired, then once you'd take them, you'd be O.K."[106] Such comments echo the language of advertisements, e.g., Ferrozone in the 1930s, promoting a "blood maker" to deal with

> ## BOX 3.3. Ferrozone, Chlorosis, and Anemia
>
> ### A WONDERFUL TONIC AND STRENGTHENER
>
> Said a druggist today: "No doubt about it, the tonic that gives best results is the biggest seller, and that is Ferrozone. It enriches and purifies the blood, restores strength and energy to the feeble, and is a scientific reconstructor that was always popular. In Chlorosis, Anemia, Tiredness, Langour, Brain Fag, Indigestion and Dyspepsia its action is prompt and satisfactory cures always follow. Yes, I recommend Ferrozone to my customers because I believe it is the best tonic and strengthening medicine that money can buy." Large boxes cost 50c. Thos. McMurdo & Co., St. John's Agents.
>
> *Source: The Evening Telegram*, December 24, 1902, p. 3.

weakness, nervousness, and the run-down feeling, and Dr. Bovel's Iron Tonic Pills "Make a rich red blood."[107]

Physician prescribing. Did physicians reinforce the popular use of tonics and fortifiers? The answer is "yes." Throughout the first half of the twentieth century, tonics were a common "bottle of medicine." They were unquestionably a key part of the armamentarium of physicians, though the frequency and pattern of prescribing could vary from doctor to doctor and from place to place.[108]

The most commonly prescribed tonics in Newfoundland, at least until the 1940s, were iron preparations. Although many prescriptions in Newfoundland were written for women (both "Mrs." and "Miss"), it is unlikely they were all for anemia, for the "tonic" action of iron was considered to be due not only to improving the blood but, around 1900, to the persistent idea that it had a general action on the body.[109] Physicians, amid dozens and dozens of recommended prescription formulae and of commercial preparations of iron, had their own favorites; some, perhaps, were preferred for specific conditions, such as the popular Blaud's Pill (mostly iron carbonate) as the first choice for chlorosis.[110] Many physicians seemingly favored iron/phosphorus compounds, not uncommonly prescribed with arsenic and strychnine. Patients, too, had their favorites, finding some preparations more agreeable (perhaps less indigestion or constipation) than others.

One of the most common prescriptions in Newfoundland up to the 1930s or so was Easton's Syrup ("Syrup of Iron Phosphate with Quinine and Strychnine"), with a solid reputation as a tonic (a "nervine tonic"), especially for nervousness and general weakness.[111] The original formula was, as the name indicates, a syrup, but by the early 1920s a marked shift to the prescribing of Easton's Syrup tablets was under way, a reflection of a gradual trend away from liquid medicines to tablets, which were more convenient to take and offered more accurate dosages than "spoonfuls." Noteworthy is the prescribing of Easton Syrup Tabloids, the particular brand name for tablets marketed by British company Burroughs Wellcome. One consequence of the shift—sometimes seen as a negative one by physicians—was that the "tailoring" of iron preparations to the needs or preferences of individual patients became limited to the dosage provided by a tablet (or multiples thereof). Furthermore, the liquid Easton's Syrup could be readily adapted by adding other phosphorus or iron preparations such as iron phosphate compound (containing the phosphates of iron, calcium, sodium and potassium) or phospho-lecithin, the latter recommended specifically for exhausted nerves.[112] Some physicians also prescribed cod-liver oil or malted cod-liver oil to be taken with Easton's—a double tonic as it were.

The just mentioned Iron Phosphate Compound, often prescribed alone by Newfoundland physicians, albeit "disguised" for the patient by the pharmaceutical Latin of the prescriptions, was, in fact, available over the counter as the well-known Parrish's Chemical Food. An example of common ground between many conventional and over-the-counter medicines, it became especially popular for children until the 1950s. Countless versions of the Chemical Food (modifications of Parrish's original formula) were marketed by companies as well as by individual pharmacies. At least three local Newfoundland brands were marketed, the labeling of which raises interesting questions about the quality of professional services.[113]

Nerves

"Me nerves is teetolly gone, doctor." "I have arthritis. I have it in my head and every nerve in my body."

Olds OPDism

The appearance of the expression "Oh! me Nerves!" on a 1990s Newfoundland souvenir mug testifies that although the term *nerves* has been commonplace elsewhere on both sides of the Atlantic, it has enjoyed a particularly widespread use by Newfoundlanders. Since the early 1900s, the term has covered behavior that seemed outside the individual's normal pattern, or a reference to vague symptoms and feelings that overlapped with a general diagnosis of weakness; for example, listlessness, the run-down feeling, the blues, restlessness, and irritability that might be occasioned by a variety of events such as a poor day's fishing, menopause, or a bereavement. It covered much more than a physician's diagnosis of nerves as "anxiety" or "depression," as commonly made in the second half of the 1900s (see Chapter 5); at the same time, although often worrisome to the sufferer, it generally carried little stigma, certainly not that of mental problems.

Newfoundland seniors rarely remember the preparation of specific "nerve" remedies in the home—one exception being to eat "raw eggs, or brandy and eggs."[114] A variety of tonics were tried up to 1950 or so, but the over-the-counter Dr. Chase's Nerve Food (or Nerve Pills if imported from the United States) was preferred. This product cornered a substantial market among many competitors marketing nervines or preparations for "weak" nerves, the latter coming to the fore in the last decades of the nineteenth century with the increasingly popular diagnosis of neurasthenia. Weak nerves was commonly defined as a "condition of weakness or exhaustion of the nervous system giving rise to various forms of mental and bodily inefficiency."[115] Interestingly, American physician George Beard, a significant figure behind the rising popularity of the diagnosis, saw it as a weakening or weakened condition akin to anemia.[116] William Osler and others also talked of an impoverishment of a nervous force. Such impoverishment could stem from excessive demands on the brain, digestion, and reproduction commonly attributed to the fast pace of "modern" life. On the basis of a pattern of symptoms, neurasthenia was diagnosed as general or limited to particular organs (hence "cardiac" and "gastric" neurasthenia). Interpreting vague and shifting symptoms could be difficult and commonly shaped by different theoretical concepts held by the practitioner.[117]

Although a diagnosis of neurasthenia has been commonly associated with women patients—some commentators have viewed it as a medical diagnosis imposed on women in consequence of male physician dominance—Osler was one who said that it occurred "chiefly in men"[118] (see also Box 3.4). However, that was in 1892, and, as he and

---

BOX 3.4. Gender, Neurasthenia, and Nervous Conditions

There is a sense that in the late 1800s and early 1900s, women were targeted as sufferers from neurasthenia and nervous weakness because of their reproductive physiology. However, manufacturers of over-the-counter medicines were always intent on marketing their products as widely as possible. Testimonials in, for instance, the many editions of R. V. Pierce's *The People's Common Sense Adviser* featured men as prominently as women.

Nor were men ignored in newspaper advertisements. For instance, a large 1917 advertisement with the banner headline, "The Man Who Has Not Slept Is Irritable and Nervous," played on the theme that "more and more people are crowding into the cities, living huddled together in poorly-ventilated houses and taking insufficient exercise. The blood becomes thin and vitiated, and with a little extra strain the nerves collapse."

Source: The Evening Telegram, December 15, 1917, p. 10.

---

other physicians struggled with a spectrum of symptoms that did not always allow differential diagnosis between hysteria and hypochondria, women and neurasthenia began to receive more attention.[119] American physician Silas Weir Mitchell's writings and celebrated rest cure contributed much to this.[120] In fact, by the early twentieth century medical treatment was widely downplayed, fitting in with the therapeutic conservatism not uncommon at the time. Physicians were told that "drugs are of little value [for neurasthenia] except in meeting underlying conditions (e.g., anaemia) and treating specific symptoms," but even this medical treatment had its skeptics.[121]

Despite the acclaim given to treatments such as Mitchell's rest cure and psychotherapeutic approaches in general, only the affluent could afford them.[122] Little place existed for them in Newfoundland, though attention to diet and general health maxims, including sleep and rest, might have been tried by any physician, perhaps more so at the Grenfell Mission influenced by Grenfell's own brand of muscular Christianity.[123] Yet even this faded by the 1920s or so, as the diagnosis of neurasthenia became less fashionable with the growing belief that it merely covered a physician's ignorance.[124] The condition was increasingly seen not as a disease entity but as a symptom complex. Language such as a "nervous person" became more common; that still left questions of weakness with respect to a person with "very little energy in reserve" and "exactly the opposite of strong and vigorous."[125]

Phosphorus compounds. Skepticism about phosphorus-based medications among textbook writers and others did not dampen their popularity as over-the-counter medicines and physicians' prescriptions.[126] By the final decades of the 1800s, many were established as tonics especially for "certain diseases of the nervous system that are dependent on exhaustion rather than upon organic changes,"[127] and for a few other conditions, such as tuberculosis and anemia, advocated from time to time.[128]

It is noteworthy that a range of breakfast cereals and over-the-counter medicines containing phosphorus compounds kept their "importance" in the minds of the public and physicians. Mention has already been made of (1) Grape-Nuts (the "phosphate of potash" makes "brains and keeps them in repair"),[129] (2) two iron-phosphorus preparations, Easton's Syrup and Parrish's Chemical Food, and (3) Park's Perfect Emulsion of Cod Liver Oil, which contained hypophospites of lime and soda; the latter ingredients were promoted for "a stimulating action upon nervous systems, and to increase digestion and nutrition." Not surprisingly amidst all this Newfoundland seniors remember taking "phosphites" as a "blood tonic."[130] References to phosphorus seemingly brought a veneer of "scientific" validation. Constant references were made to phosphorus being a constituent of brain and nervous tissue, while, in the previtamin era, it had been suggested that the loss of phosphorus during the preparation of polished rice caused beriberi in the Far East. By extension, phosphorus was implicated in other conditions: "We have similar diseases in the United States, but we call them inanition, anaemia, neurasthenia, nervous prostration, paralysis, death."[131]

Physicians were constantly reminded of phosphorus preparations by a bombardment of advertisements in medical journals, such as "Maltine with Hypophosphites," "Fellows' Syrup of Hypophosphites," "Glyphocal (Squire's Glycerophosphate Syrup)."[132] Given the social conditions, physicians in Newfoundland may well have been more liberal prescribers of phosphorus compounds than in other places.[133] Their tonic prescriptions commonly included Elixir Glycerophosphates Compound and Phospho-Lecithin.[134] The latter (a commercial brand of lecithin—an organic phosphorus compound—widely endorsed by 1900 for building up the nervous system) was promoted as being more effective than inorganic phosphorus compounds. Lecithin was also available in various over-the-counter preparations or nervines. One was Assaya-Neurall, which was promoted over many years. In 1922, it was still described as "The *New* Remedy for Nervous Exhaustion which contains Lecithin (concentrated from eggs), the form of phosphates required for nerve repair." It was promoted for treating neuralgia, nightsweats, sleeplessness, indigestion, and hysteria.[135]

No account of over-the-counter preparations—at least with respect to Newfoundland—can omit further comment on Dr. Chase's Nerve Food: "When your nerves would get bad, you'd take a couple of boxes of them and you're all right again."[136] Whether it contained lecithin or another phosphorus compound is uncertain, but it is noteworthy that Newfoundland knew it mostly as a "food" that was recognized for building oneself up.[137] A concept that nerves required special nutrition emerged around 1900, bolstered by the discovery that a factor in food was necessary to prevent the symptom of polyneuritis in beriberi.[138] In fact, the Chase formula was changed around the 1930s to include the antiberiberi vitamin B_1. Much of Chase's advertising focused on the theme of rebuilding the wasted nerve cells that resulted from improper nutrition.[139] "The doctor says . . . the nervous system [is] run-down for want of proper nutrition" (see also Box 3.5).[140] Similarly for anemia: "I thought it was only for the nerves, whereas what I need is something to enrich the blood." "Well" [came a reply] "that is exactly what Dr. Chase's Nerve Food does."[141]

From the early 1920s onward Chase became even more aggressive in its advertising—perhaps due to Gerald S. Doyle, who had become a company agent in Newfoundland. Promotion, directed mostly to women, linked a range of conditions to nerves or weakness; for example, eye strain broke down the nervous system, and postpartum recovery was a state of weakness. Advertisement messages included: "My heart would palpitate, I had weak spells"; "My Hands Trembled and I Could Not Sleep"; "There Were Many Things Which I Could Not Eat."

Aside from weakness, one advertisement in 1932 added an interesting spin to the "food theme" by focusing on "From Angles to Curves" as a sign of health:

There is no encouragement for the "skinny" ones, for the more feminine form is making a definite come back. A rounder bustline, boneless back, fuller upper arms and broader shoulders. If you are to regain weight, worry and irritability must be avoided and more rest, sleep and relaxation sought.[142]

The changing fashion in "feminine beauty"—in line with generally rising body weights in the United States and Britain—had, in fact, been used in earlier advertising, such as the 1922 promotion in Newfoundland of Ironized Yeast recommended to women as a way to become as "Plump as you Please . . . to have a body deliciously alluring in its attractive curves."[143] Nutritional issues, too, were behind the promotion of the beverage Instant Postum. Although not promoted as a specific remedy for nerves, it was part of the long history of attacks on the dangers of caffeine in coffee and tea. Instant Postum saw coffee as a "definite poison producing headache, heart palpitation, paralysis, nervousness, or some other fixed disease."[144] Resulting nervousness was said to take its toll in various ways, such as being "too nervous to drive a car." "If you would quit tea and coffee and use Postum your nerves would steady up. [And] there's no drug in it—that's where it's got tea and coffee beat by a mile."[145]

BOX 3.5. Advertisement for Dr. Chase's Nerve Food—For Nervousness and Female Weakness

SHE WAS PALE, WEAK, AND VERY NERVOUS

Mrs. Benj. Hatfield, 77 Hillyard St., St. John, N.B., writes: "For three years I was a sufferer from extreme nervousness and female weakness. I was pale and weak, had no appetite and would sometimes faint two or three times a day. I underwent a very painful operation and for seven weeks was under the doctor's care but he seemed unable to help me.

Despairing of recovery, I took the advice of a friend who told me that Dr. Chase's Nerve Food would build me up and make me strong and well again. I continued this treatment using in all sixteen boxes, and believe that I am as strong and well as ever in my life. As a result I cannot say too much for Dr. Chase's Nerve Food. The testimonials I see for it are not half strong enough.". . . On every box will be found portrait and signature of Dr. A. W. Chase.

DR. CHASE'S NERVE FOOD
M. Connors, St. John's, Newfoundland, General Agent

Source: The Evening Telegram, December 15, 1902, p. 2.

Medicines for Women and Men

"I got my feet wet picking berries in the burnt woods and my periods stopped." "When was your last period?" I don't rightly
know but I think it was about bakeapple picking time."

Olds OPDism

If advertising copy for tonics and treatments for nerves often implied greater weakness and nervousness among women than in men,
it was sharply reinforced by the widespread advertising of female
remedies for "women's weaknesses." Dr. Hooker's Female Cordial,
for example, was a treatment for "Weakening Disorders of the Female Generative Organs in ailments not requiring surgical treatment."[146] Up to the 1920s, women could well have felt overwhelmed
by intensively promoted products such as U.S.-manufactured Dr.
Pierce's Favorite Prescription and Lydia E. Pinkham's Vegetable
Compound. Both reached Newfoundland, as did Orange Lily ("a sure
relief for women's disorders"[147]), Dr. De Van's Female Pills, and Dr.
Hamilton's Pills. The latter, sometimes promoted for "women with
weakness," was a drastic purgative of "mandrake and butternut" suggestive of the many "remedies" for abortion.[148]

Dr. Pierce's Favorite Prescription—one of a range of medicines
marketed by the R.V. Pierce Company of Buffalo, New York—imparted
"strength to the whole system and to the organs distinctly feminine
[the uterus especially]." In 1907 "overworked, worn-out, run-down,
debilitated teachers, milliners, dressmakers, seamstresses, shop-girls,
house-keepers, nursing mothers, and feeble-women generally" were
singled out as needing it—language that also reflects the general attitude toward the sufferers of neurasthenia.[149] *The People's Common
Sense Medical Adviser,* the home medicine book that was part of
Pierce's promotion machine for many years, elaborated on "female
weakness" as "nervous prostration, or exhaustion"—in effect neurasthenia—considered to be caused by congestion of the uterus and ova-
ries due to overindulgence, overwork, the strain of too many household
cares, or multiple childbirth.[150] In the 1930s the advertising copy for
Dr. Pierce's Favorite Prescription focused more on menopause difficulties that were functional and not organic in origin.

Lydia Pinkham's Vegetable Compound advertisements in the early 1900s spelled out more explicitly the multiple aspects of women's weaknesses: "Weakness of the Stomach," "Spinal Weakness," "Nervous exhaustion"; extreme "lassitude," "don't-care," "nervousness," "melancholy or the 'blues"; "backache," "painful periods," and "displacements of the female organs."[151] Later promotion (c. 1940s to 1950s) focused on "painful menstruation and menopause," but still included references to "nervous irritability" and "restoring strength and energy."[152]

Medicines for men also commonly focused on weakness: "Weak, Tired and Nervous Men," a thinly disguised reference to impotence. Particularly well known was Damiana, sometimes promoted as a nerve invigorator.[153] Newfoundlanders could also write to England in 1912 for a "valuable pamphlet" on Phosphonal, the "Electric Restorer for Men" that restored "every nerve in the body to its proper tension. Premature decay and all sexual weakness averted at once."[154]

Digestives/Laxatives

"I had pains in my stomach last night as big as my fist."

Olds OPDism

"I know men that took bread soda [baking soda] in their lunch and take a spoonful after every meal, and it worked then, it might damage the stomach, but it did relieve it."[155]

The account so far outlines the promotion of an almost countless number of medicines that drew upon and reinforced (individually and in total numbers) weakness as a basic problem. Before commenting on this further, I look briefly at two other groups of medicines, digestives/laxatives and kidney. Although they did not focus on weakness as such, conceptually they were highly relevant, for weakness was one consequence of an untreated digestive disorder.

By 1896 indigestion, or dyspepsia, was recognized as an "American Disease." "In the distribution of diseases among nations," an Ohio physician wrote, "the English get gout, the French syphilis, and the Americans dyspepsia."[156] A diagnosis of dyspepsia, or nervous dyspepsia, varied from physician to physician, but invariably included such symptoms as a sense of fullness, flatulence, coating of the tongue, and perhaps biliousness and headache. In fact, the United States had no lock on dyspepsia. Stomach trouble was ubiquitous, and Newfoundland had its own disorder called "Newfoundland stomach." A syndrome that extended beyond dyspepsia and indigestion to include constipation, irritability, lassitude, and itching and burning sensations, Newfoundland stomach was considered in 1941 to be due partly to "subclinical" thiamine deficiency.[157] Other diagnostic labels for stomach troubles included cramps, flu, and stomach flu. Remedies were ubiquitous and those that were found or prepared in the kitchen remained popular for a long time. Although the most common home remedy in Newfoundland was probably baking soda ("bread soda we called it"), also popular were "settlers" (or carminatives) such as ginger, nutmeg and peppermint essences, and teas made from squashberry or juniper. Stomach flu, generally involving diarrhea and vomiting, was treated in various ways, perhaps drinking lots of cow's milk.[158] However, over-the-counter remedies were also much in evidence.

Typical advertising offered treatment for a "shopping list" of ailments or symptoms, from general malaise to headache arising from a basic gastrointestinal problem that was rationalized by one or more of four overlapping theories to explain why gastrointestinal conditions could lead to various forms of weakness.

Toxin Theories

The most general of the four theories was improper absorption of nutrients due to a "weak" stomach, indigestion (especially when chronic), or biliousness (perhaps due to a "sluggish" or "torpid" liver). Anything less than proper nutrition (impossible if one had a "weak" stomach; see Box 3.6) undermined health, as health reformers and advertisers commonly pointed out.

A second and overriding theory overlapping with the first was that the basic problem was really a buildup of waste matter, generally due to constipation. In turn, this meant that toxins were absorbed into the bloodstream. In 1892 William Osler authoritatively stated that "all kinds of evils have been attributed to poisoning by the resorption of noxious matters from the retained faeces—copraemia—but, it is not likely that this takes place to any extent."[159] However, the heyday of what was to become generally known as autointoxication (some-

82   *A Social History of Medicines in the Twentieth Century*

BOX 3.6. Advertisement for Dr. Pierce's Golden Medical Discovery

Much sickness starts with weak stomach, and consequent poor, impoverished blood. Nervous and pale-people lack good, rich, red blood. Their stomachs need invigorating for, after all, a man can be no stronger than his stomach.

A remedy that makes the stomach strong and the liver active, makes rich red blood and overcomes and drives out disease-producing bacteria and cures a whole multitude of diseases.

Get rid of your Stomach Weakness and Liver Laziness by taking a course of Dr. Pierce's Golden Medical Discovery—the great Stomach Restorative, Liver Invigorator and Blood Cleanser.

You can't afford to accept any medicine of *unknown composition* as a substitute for "Golden Medical Discovery," which is a medicine of KNOWN COMPOSITION, having a complete list of ingredients in plain English on its bottle-wrapper, same being attested as correct under oath

Dr. Pierce's Pleasant Pellets regulate and invigorate Stomach, Liver and Bowels.

Source: The Daily News, July 7, 1910, p. 2.

---

times autotoxemia), came in the first three decades of the 1900s, supported by the argument that the putrefactive toxins arose from intestinal bacteria. The newly won popularity of the theory came about, in large part, through the influence of London surgeon Sir Arbuthnot Lane, backed by the simplicity of the theory and by the new science of bacteriology. Although the theory's impact was almost certainly greatest among the public, many physicians embraced the concept in their everyday practice, certainly until the 1940s and 1950s. Respected U.S. physician Walter Alvarez, who became a popular author of a syndicated newspaper column that reached Newfoundland newspapers, wrote in his 1943 book *Nervousness, Indigestion, and Pain:*

I see many persons with sensations of fatigue, perhaps a temperature of 99.5° F., and perhaps aching muscles or joints, who expect me to find some "poison in their system." Perhaps a physician has told them that this is their trouble, but I cannot find any sign of such poison or any source for it, and in most cases it looks to me as if the cause of the syndrome was a neurosis or possibly a fibrositis.[160]

Alvarez also had little time for "middle-aged women who haunt the offices of physicians complaining bitterly of intestinal auto-intoxication" and who "think their brain is being destroyed by toxins arising in the bowel."[161] And others, he said, would get well if they were not so fearful that they would suffer injury from intestinal auto-intoxication. By 1943, however, Alvarez, after many years of decrying autointoxication, was justifiably able to say that "fortunately, this idea seems to be dying out, and I do not now have to spend as much time combating it as I had to do thirty years ago."[162]

How many Newfoundland physicians accepted the concept of autointoxication is unknown, though one enthusiastically supported a third popular theory, namely focal infection or focal sepsis.[163] In holding that local chronic infections released toxins into the blood circulation, this theory overlapped with autointoxication, as a 1936 surgical textbook made clear when stating that the intestinal tract "may be regarded as a focus of infection."[164] Other focal sites came into prominence—for example, carious teeth, infected tonsils, si-nuses, and middle ear infection, as well as "chronic infection" of the appendix, gallbladder, or cervix—and were more likely to be viewed as a cause of arthritis, mental disorders, and other ailments.[165]

A fourth popular theory can be described as acidosis or the presence of excess acid circulating in the body (not merely hyperacidity in the stomach). This was popularly viewed as being brought on by inappropriate diet (often "acid-producing" foods), which is not to be confused with what physicians recognized as a symptom of conditions such as starvation and diabetic ketosis. Although it is said that notions of excess acid were promoted by food faddists, advertising copy drew on scientific and physician interest at the time in acid-base equilibrium.[166] The theory became pervasive as it rationalized much ill health, malaise and tiredness, and even the use of beauty aids.[167] At least one prominent Newfoundland physician, Cluny Macpherson, had a firm belief in the theory until the 1950s, though most others followed Walter Alvarez:

> Quite a few patients come with the idea that they have "too much acid in their system," and demand that something be done

to correct the situation. I tell them that this is largely a layman's idea with little basis in scientific fact.[168]

One specific acid, uric acid, attracted particular attention, as mentioned in the Kidney Medicines section later in this chapter. First, medicines to strengthen digestion and the roles of laxatives and antacids are discussed.

Strengthening Digestion; Enzyme Preparations

"Strengthening digestion" (with the implication that weakness was a problem) was a common phrase used to promote over-the-counter stomach medicines. Many were "tonics" promoted for "weak stomachs" (see Box 3.6). Generally bitter preparations, they were often used to stimulate the appetite during illness or convalescence. A local product, Stafford's Prescription "A"—proclaimed in 1912 to "strengthen the digestive organs and enable them to assimilate food"—was apparently successful,[169] but an American preparation, Tanlac, was more widely promoted as "the best and safest tonic and system purifier." It stimulated "the digestive system to its proper functioning, so the blood is able to take up fresh building material and is so vitalized as to be able to more thoroughly eliminate the waste products which make you feel all tired out."[170]

Neither Prescription "A" nor Tanlac belonged to another class of preparations based on enzymes ("ferments") that became very popular as aids to "strengthen" the digestive process. From the 1870s onward, such enzyme preparations (e.g., those containing pepsin, pancreatin, and papain) were widely promoted to physicians and the public. They were taken orally or used to prepare such items as peptonized milk and peptonized beef tea.[171] Although Pape's Diapepsin, containing pepsin, for "a weak disordered stomach" was perhaps the best known preparation on the island,[172] Dr. Valin's Digestive Elixir also caught the eye of Newfoundlanders. Promoted by banner-style advertisements in 1905 from druggist "G. J. Brocklehurst, Ph.G., of Carbonear." As "Sole Agent for Dr. Valin's Tonic and Digestive Elixirs," Brocklehurst departed from most advertising in Newfoundland by printing a local testimonial. A Mrs. John Thomas of Carbonear announced, "I am completely cured. For years I suffered acutely from indigestion. I found no relief in the so-called cures that I was constantly taking for this trouble. One bottle of Dr. Valin's Digestive Elixir completely cured me."[173]

Laxatives

"This is my constipation headache doctor, not me normal headache." "Well, me bowels is stuck sir. T'other day I had to force 'em somethin' wonderful."

Olds OPDism

Laxatives were promoted for a wide range of conditions beyond constipation (see Box 3.7), including for women who did not have clear skin and bright eyes. A beauty column noted: "When food is only imperfectly digested, it gives rise to fermentation, clogs the bowels, and renders the blood impure. This results in dull eyes, muddy skin, blotches, pimples and other disfiguring marks."[174] Headaches, including "bilious headache," were a more widespread problem. A 1920s' promotion for Dr. Chase's Kidney-Liver Pills stated that bilious spells came from "eating too much" or "foods which do not agree and by taking too little exercise," causing the liver to become "torpid and sluggish and the bowels constipated. Then comes the bilious spell."[175]

Many would have readily seen a link with autointoxication as they read about torpid and sluggish livers or about the absorption of poisons from the intestinal tract in laxative advertisements. "Decay is not digestion" was a slogan of Cascarets, a chocolate flavored preparation that was sold to correct the problem of weak "bowel-muscles."[176] Dangerous, "sluggish" bowels were referred to in many advertisements. Syrup of Figs, for example, alerted elderly men and women in 1912 to deal with torpid livers and weak, sluggish bowels that "allow decaying waste and poisons" to enter into the blood.[177] One popular laxative commonly prescribed by physicians, calomel (mercurous chloride), needs mention because it represents an interesting example of a medicine's slow demise. Calomel had long had validation with physicians and the public. Although it came under attack in the nineteenth century by alternative practitioners as dangerous in the doses used,[178] many physicians were still prescribing it in the 1930s not only as a laxative but also as teething powders for children, a prepara-

BOX 3.7. Laxatives

Particularly up to the 1950s, laxatives were promoted for much more than constipation. Two illustrative examples:

I. IN WAGES OR PROFIT

Health, sooner or later, shows its value. No man can expect to go very far or very fast toward success—no woman either—who suffers from the headaches, the sour stomach and poor digestion, the unpleasant breath and the good-for-nothing feelings which result from constipation and biliousness. But just learn for yourself what a difference will be made by a few doses of

BEECHAM'S PILLS

Tested through three generations—favorably known the world over this perfect vegetable and always efficient family remedy is universally accepted as the best preventive or corrective of disorders of the organs of digestion. Beecham's Pills regulate the bowels, stir the liver to natural activity—enable you to get all the nourishment and blood-making qualities from your food. As sure as you try them you will know that—in your looks and in your increased vigor—Beecham's Pills

Pay Big Dividends

The directions with every box are very valuable—especially to women. Sold everywhere. In Boxes 25c.

II. NO SATISFACTION IN EATING

Food does you no good. You can't digest—consequently you're afraid to eat; tongue is coated, mouth tastes bad, stomach is bloated. Pretty soon you'll be overcome by weakness and nervous prostration.

Best prescription for your condition is Dr. Hamilton's Pills of Mandrake and Butternut. For dyspepsia and indigestion it is doubtful if a better remedy will ever be devised. These pills bring new strength and vitality to the stomach and digestive organs; they build up the general health and instill such vim and resisting power into the system that sickness is impossible; try Dr. Hamilton's Pill. T. McMurdo & Co., agents for Nfld.

Although Dr. Hamilton's Pills were not promoted as a laxative, mandrake and butternut (noted in the advertisement) were almost certainly known to many members of the public as particularly "strong." As noted under Medicines for Women and Men, it could well have been tried as an abortifacient.

Source: *The Evening Telegram*, December 11, 1912, p. 9; and *The Daily News*, December 30, 1905, p. 6.

tion ultimately recognized as dangerous to the general health of children.[179]

Antacids

No discussion on stomach preparations can omit reference to antacids, the various alkalis used to treat ulcers, heartburn, and dyspepsia. Although references to weakness were rare in their promotion, claims were made in 1932 to restore "normal functioning" and to overcome such problems as sleeplessness and nervousness.[180] At the time, however, confusion existed between antacids for the stomach acidity and the need to treat "excess acid in the system"—the fourth toxin theory mentioned as a cause of countless ailments. However, some preparations referred to both, as did 1930s' advertisements for Alka-Seltzer for "headache-sour stomach" or to "knock out that stomach acidity" to treat "ACID mornings—caused by excess accumulation of acid in your system."[181]

Physicians' Prescriptions

The overlap in constituents in the categories of over-the-counter and prescription medicines mentioned so far was particularly evident with digestives/laxatives. Perhaps this and widespread self-medication with sodium bicarbonate accounts for the relatively few prescriptions for these medicines from some Newfoundland physicians between 1910 and the 1930s, except for tonics to stimulate the appetite and digestive enzyme preparations that were also available over the counter. On the other hand, other physicians were relatively heavy prescribers, including the prescribing of bismuth compounds, even though noted to be relatively expensive compared with other antacids.[182]

Kidney Medicines

"Mother brought child to 'find out if she was a real bedwetter or was her kidney's weak.'"

"Some mornings I can piss over the fence and sometimes I can't get it clear of my boots."

Olds OPDisms

Promotion of over-the-counter kidney medicines (including those for bladder problems) generally capitalized on the toxin/acid theories already outlined. Advertisements such as for Haarlem Oil in 1937, with such captions as "Flush Kidneys of Poisons and Stop Getting Up Nights," suggested the diagnosis of autointoxication.[183] Other advertisements invoked focal infection, as with Dr. Chase's Kidney-Liver Pills for "pruning the appendix," which implied that a "grumbling appendix" might be a site for such infection. At other times, the pills were said to be an alternative to being "rushed" to the hospital for removal of the appendix so as to overcome "the cause and effect of wrong habits of eating and living."[184]

By the 1930s, the theory of too much acid in the system was replacing toxin theories as the dominant theme in kidney advertisements, though the "consequences" of problem kidneys did not change. Time and time again, newspaper readers were told about "kidney acidity" and that "Acid in Your Blood Kills Health and Vigour. Kidneys usually to Blame."[185] Cystex advertisements, for example, proclaimed that everyone who was "old at 40" had to "beware" of kidney acidity:[186]

> Thousands of men and women past 40, and many far younger, needlessly endanger their lives by neglecting to treat serious symptoms of kidney trouble. If you suffer from Getting Up Nights, Leg Pains, Neuralgia, Lumbago, Nervousness, Rheumatism, Puffy Eyelids, Dizziness, Backache, or Burning Bladder Weakness, your troubles may be due entirely to poisoning by Kidney Acidity. Clear out the acids and soothe and heal raw irritated membranes with Cystex and feel 10 years younger.[187]

Given the overlap—confusing to many—among various theories, it is no surprise that kidney advertisements—such as those for antacids—covered more than one theory. Haarlem Oil Capsules, for example, were said to flush "kidneys of harmful acids and poisons."[188]

Uric Acid

"Is there any arthritis in my water doctor?

Olds OPDism

The promotion of kidney medicines frequently focused on ridding the body of one particular acid—uric acid. Widespread acceptance that excess uric acid was a fundamental problem owed much to British physician/health reformer Alexander Haig (1853-1924). From both a suspicion that his personal history of migraine headaches was due to uric acid and his studies of acid-base properties, Haig developed sophisticated theories incriminating uric acid as the cause of many conditions.[189]

Mounting opposition from within the medical profession over Haig's "scientific" interpretations failed to stem popular enthusiasm for what was yet another simple, unitary theory of disease. Although Haig's advocacy of a uric-acid-free diet failed to achieve popularity, North Americans were bombarded as much as the British with advertisements for over-the-counter remedies to treat uric acid problems; indeed many medicines co-opted the theory. For example, advertisements for the iron preparation Ferrozone stated that when "introduced" into the circulation, it would "dissolve the uric acid."[190] Kidney medicines, however, were the mainstay of treating uric acid through removal. Although weakness and nervousness were referred to on occasion, the uric acid was mostly linked to rheumatism. Thus, in 1900 Newfoundlanders read that Dodd's Kidney Pills—to become one of the best-known medicines on the island ("people would go to town on them")—cured neuralgia ("rheumatism of the face" due to uric acid left in the blood by disordered kidneys[191]) or lumbago and rheumatism.[192] Dodd's advertisements linking uric acid and rheumatism were relentless, and continued long after the acid's heyday in the 1930s. For example, the *Twillingate Sun* informed readers in 1942 of the following:

How to Combat Rheumatic Pains

Rheumatic pains are often caused by uric acid in the blood. The blood impurity should be extracted by the kidneys. If kidneys fail, and excess uric acid remains, it irritates the muscles and joints causing excruciating pains. Treat rheumatic pains by keeping your kidneys in good condition. Take regularly Dodd's Kidney Pills—for half a century the favorite kidney remedy.[193]

Physician Prescribing

Although perhaps less obvious to the public than with many other categories of medicines, physician prescribing of kidney medicines—often as mixtures—validated many homemade or over-the-counter preparations. Many constituents were the same (leaving aside dosages), even though physicians' reasons for prescribing were usually very much different from public beliefs. For example, potassium nitrate (niter) was used as a diuretic in Dodd's Kidney Pills; methylene blue, an "antiseptic," was used in De Witt's Kidney and Bladder Pills;[194] and hexamethyleneamine (hexamine), an antiseptic and diuretic, was used in Cystex pills. That hexamine had become a generally popular physician remedy for infections by the 1930s perhaps explains the following "simple and fundamental" objection to Cystex:

> There is no legitimate place for self-treatment of pathologic conditions of the kidneys or bladder. It is sheer madness for persons who have the symptom complex described in the Cystex advertisements to attempt to treat themselves and waste what may well be vitally valuable time before seeking competent treatment based on a rational diagnosis.[195]

By this time (1936), as had been happening for some years, prescription medicines reflected increasingly sophisticated diagnostic classifications of kidney diseases with different prescriptions for problems ranging from acute nephritis to uric acid diathesis.[196] While "weakness" still preoccupied the public mind, physicians often debated over whether to treat for germs as well as for general inflammation for which potassium citrate, diuretin (theobromine solium salicylate), and other diuretics might be prescribed.

PHARMACOLOGICAL EFFECTS, "CASCADES," AND SOCIAL VALIDATION

The constant negative attitudes toward pre-1950 treatments have already been stressed (Chapter 1). When challenged, critics at least recognize the usefulness of various medicines for pain relief (from aspirin to morphine), iron preparations (for anemia), thyroid replacement therapy, insulin for diabetes, effective laxatives, digitalis for certain heart conditions, various sedatives/hypnotics and more—in fact a significant range of medicines. That still left much skepticism of, if not disbelief in, many prescriptions as well as countless home and over-the-counter remedies. Female remedies, tonics, nerve remedies, etc., have all been roundly condemned.

Without suggesting that such attitudes were not justified in many cases, patient acceptance and validation has to be generally recognized, if only from the testimonies to widespread popularity so evident in Newfoundland. So far the possibility of positive benefits arising from specific pharmacological effects has not been addressed directly. Certainly there is no reason to dismiss it out of hand. For example, the two key "female medicines" already considered, Lydia Pinkham's Vegetable Compound and Pierce's Favorite Prescription, contained herbs (e.g., black cohosh) that have received some scientific validation in recent years as relieving certain menstrual and menopausal difficulties. Moreover, the 18 percent alcohol content in Lydia Pinkham's preparation could have offered some level of comfort.[197] As suggested with spruce beer (Chapter 2), occasional positive testimonials—even if mixed with negative opinions—could sustain some level of reputation and perhaps validation.

Cascades of Symptoms

I have made abundantly clear that support for weakness as a fundamental problem owed much to myriad over-the-counter medicines and the reinforcement of the notion from physicians. However, one other significant factor relates to the many medicines. One of the biggest issues for contemporary and today's critics of, for example, Lydia Pinkham's Vegetable Compound, as with so many other preparations, is the "shopping list" of medical problems or symptoms that could be treated by the medicines, such that they were virtual cure-alls. Yet this ignores that the lists made sense to many laypersons, especially in the context of autointoxication. The symptoms fell into patterns—commonly cascades with one symptom following another—as especially evident in the advertising of digestives, laxatives, and kidney medicines. For example, a sluggish intestine or liver and/or constipation could lead first to poor absorption of nutrients or absorption of poisons, then to poor blood, to weak nerves, to bad breath, almost always to headaches, and indeed to other symptoms that were often associated with feelings of malaise. Some cascades were short (e.g., "sour stomach, vile gases, headache" to be treated by Syrup of Figs), but there was always an implication of other problems.[198] Thus kidney medicines were recommended for many symptoms, including restoring the digestive system; Dr. Chase's Kidney-Liver Pills, for instance, "claimed to sweep the poisons from the digestive system and enable the organs of digestion to resume their natural functions."[199]

The cascade analogy, seen by many as fear mongering (which it was), fit with many popular texts of the time on health and hygiene that presented the body in mechanical terms. For example, Wilfred Grenfell's ([1924] 1946) *Yourself and Your Body* followed the theme of "our bodies—combining every kind of machine into one." He wrote:

> It's the only real automatic machinery in the world. Moreover, the units make their own rules; choose some to govern the rest, while they train others to do all the repairing, feeding, draining, tending the pumps, and manufacturing of everything needed from a drain-pipe to a seeing-machine.[200]

Along with Grenfell's thumbnail sketches to illustrate his points, it was easy for readers to understand how one symptom led to another. In fact, they might have read, aside from advertisements, other popular medical writings of the period that spelled out this cause-and-effect "cascade." For instance, one author discusses the autointoxication cascade:

> The absorption of poisons and toxins generated from feces retained in the intestine is the direct cause of many irritable conditions, headaches, neuralgias, some forms of neuritis, and a large and aggravating number of nervous conditions, including insomnia and unrefreshing sleep, nervous dyspepsia, melancholia, heart irregularities of functional origin, and scores of other conditions, which, like the deeds of the witches in Macbeth, are almost without a name, but are none the less material.[201]

The cascades and mechanical concepts also fell in line with seeing the body as an integrated whole at a time when physicians appreciated the psychological component of illnesses, such as neurasthenia and nervous dyspepsia, as they did the role of placebo treatments. In some respects, the cascade of symptom complex reflects a persistent thread in the search for treatment, "a perennial yearning for individuality and holism in therapy."[202] Paradoxically, it was also a time when the medical world was looking for new scientific remedies that were disease specific, or at least was shifting to "rational" formulae. Although this did not fully develop until the second half of the century (see Chapters 5 and 6), it still meant that the distance between medical and lay thinking was growing, an issue that increasingly plagued much of the modern story of medicines.

Chapter 4

Authority and Gatekeeping: 1900 to c. 1950

"I don't compare very favorably with the local doc. He can examine them through their clothes and tell them from the door
what's wrong with them. He gives them much larger bottles of
medicine."[1]

Robert Ecke,
American doctor working in Newfoundland, 1938

Physicians drove much of the criticism noted so far of over-the-
counter remedies. They acquired new knowledge and authority from
significant developments in medical science and education evident to
the public in hospitals, new diagnostic capabilities through laboratory
tests and complex diagnostic technology (e.g., X rays), and new treatments from surgery to insulin.[2] As movies and radio came into their
own, the public was assailed with images of physicians who were totally dedicated to patients—images bolstered by censorship of negative portrayals.[3] New gatekeeping powers, in the form of legislated
control of access to medicines, also lay behind the buildup of public
recognition of medical authority.

The authority of practitioners and, to a lesser extent, druggists and
the trust that went with it were critical factors in the choices and use
of many medicines by Mr. Brown and Ms. Smith. In exploring this,
the role of authority and trust in validation, I look first at some general issues that have particular significance in the validation or dis-
credit of a medicine. Next I consider further extension of practitioner
authority through new gatekeeping roles and prescription medicines,
and finally the role of druggists and drugstores in shaping attitudes to

medicines—after all, the pharmacy was more a point of contact with medicines than was the doctor's office.

AUTHORITY AND PATIENTS' FAITH

Placebos

Any consideration of practitioner authority and whether a patient has faith in such authority must also contemplate the role of placebo action in any treatment. The placebo—long an issue in the story of medicines—is always a likely explanation of unanticipated and erratic outcomes of treatment. Indeed, the reputations of "premodern" medicines have been commonly dismissed as merely placebo. Despite some questioning, it is now generally accepted that, to a greater or lesser extent, placebo action plays a part in all therapies, conventional or otherwise.[4] Discussions on placebos often raise another explanation for the success of the "old, ineffective" medicines, namely that "cure" or improvement was brought about by natural healing processes; indeed, placebo action is sometimes viewed as merely precipitating or harnessing the body's healing powers.

The physiologically inert placebo, used as imitation therapy, has a striking historical pedigree, with the benefits of "sugar pills" becoming part of medical lore, especially in conditions where it was felt that a patient's imagination or mind was involved as a cause of the illness.[5] By the early twentieth century, the phenomenon was well known to and exploited by physicians. William Osler, who made clear the importance of a patient having faith in his or her physician, wrote that in treating neurasthenia, "a placebo is sometimes necessary for its psychic effect."[6] Osler was not the only physician to comment at the time. In 1903 American Richard Cabot indicated its widespread practice when saying that he was "brought up, as I suppose every physician is, to use placebo, bread pills, water subcutaneously [i.e., hypodermic injection], and other devices." He went on to say that how frequently it is used depends on individual practitioners, "but I doubt if there is a physician in this room who has not used them and used them pretty often. . . . I used to give them by the bushels."[7]

In 1905, two years after Cabot's comment, St. John's *The Daily News* carried an item on "Faith Healing":

The influence of faith in medicine is both overestimated and underestimated, according to the type of mind considering it. Physicians are well aware that it can have little effect upon organic disease, like cancer or tuberculosis, but in many nervous and largely imaginary disorders it may have great potency. A Dublin druggist notes that the poorer classes of that city appraise medicines by their looks. They attach little importance to colourless mixtures, however good, but are made happy by a bottle of some herbal extract. And great is the effect if a muddy sediment is to be shaken up before taking in tablespoonful doses every four hours in water.[8]

Although physicians were still prescribing inert placebos in the 1950s, the practice was becoming obsolete due to the growing number of active new medicines. Moreover, placebos became limited to serving as "controls" in clinical trials, such that other uses became generally unacceptable; indeed, they became viewed as unethical, though some moderation of this view emerged in the 1990s.

The Therapeutic Use of Authority

The constant use of the placebo in clinical trials from the 1950s onward encouraged detailed studies that, by identifying countless factors relevant to the placebo phenomenon, revealed its complexity. These factors ranged from practitioner authority to a patient's faith or trust in a practitioner's prescription or recommendation, perhaps fostered by practitioner empathy and other positive characteristics of a relationship. It is noteworthy that druggists, on looking back to the pre-1950s, often feel that doctors' handwritten prescriptions fostered a placebo response as a result of their mystique, and that a tonic prescribed by a doctor was more effective than the same one (e.g., Parrish's Chemical Food) bought over the counter.

In the heyday of prescribing inert placebos, physician authority was consciously used to build a patient's confidence and faith. No less an authority than William Osler stated categorically in 1907 that a "physician must first gain the confidence of his patient."[9] Many specific strategies, aside from cultivating a firm or "authoritative" and knowledgeable bedside manner, were recommended to build confidence—sometimes viewed as "mental therapeutics." American physician A. E. Hertzler commented pertinently in his 1938 book

The Horse and Buggy Doctor: "Regardless of what the old doctor was able to accomplish in a therapeutic way, the sense of security inspired by the doctor's arrival affected the patients favorably. The degree of this influence depended on faith."[10] Measures to enhance this and thereby relieve suffering, "even though we could not curtail the disease," included making patients comfortable, relieving stress, and easing symptoms to promote healing and recovery. Patients' confidence could be high. In 1940, one woman noted that "from the time I was a little girl I always beheld the doctor with a halo."[11]

A significant aspect of confidence building was that the patient recognized a physician's specialized knowledge of therapy. This followed a significant transformation of medicine in the nineteenth century in which a physician's professional identity became identified more closely with specialized knowledge about medicines.[12] This authority could be theoretical or practical, based on empiricism and experience. It is noteworthy that English medicine, in particular with its marked empirical bent, entered the 1900s with great reverence for the formulae of prescriptions used by celebrated, successful physicians, many linked to famed London hospitals.[13] What changed, however, was that the new "science-based" knowledge slowly extended the authority of the prescription to all physicians.

By the 1960s, to jump ahead briefly, the role of physician authority in relation to therapy was being questioned; indeed, an American professor of psychiatry found himself defending the "therapeutic use of authority" in the context of a society in "turmoil."[14] Although this was not a "last stand," the 1970s onward witnessed growing criticism of "paternalistic" doctors, meaning that a doctor expected total authority in decision making without any input from patients. A new emphasis was being placed on a patient's own responsibility in health matters, an echo of the message of health reformers of the early decades of the twentieth century. The physician, too, was increasingly expected to respect the autonomy of patients, which allowed patients to be actively involved in decisions about their own treatment. In fact, the paternalism of the past was often discussed, especially by medical ethicists, as part of "bad," unenlightened times, in contrast to the new, enlightened, "patient-centered" care of the final decades of the 1900s (see Chapter 6).[15]

However, before accepting the widespread condemnation of paternalism in the past, its contribution to validating treatment at the time needs appreciating. After all, "good medicine" in the first half of the twentieth century was commonly considered to involve patient confidence and faith. One historian has noted that paternalism has to be seen as part of the then-commonplace house call, which helped to ensure at least "a human relationship" even if patients asked few questions: "Home visits were different from office visits [up to around the 1950s]; doctors were smaller, patients were bigger, and their families could participate in consultation as they rarely did otherwise." It was noted that the only technology was what the practitioner could carry.[16] Two other commentators have made the challenging interpretation that the post-1970s' emphasis on patient-centered care was not such a major departure from the old "biomedical" model as is generally supposed: doctors in "doctor-centered" relationships were not necessarily any less compassionate, humane, or effective than the new "patient-centered" ones; they "simply located illness in a framework that was less concerned with the process of obtaining narration from the patient." Both approaches, the writers argue, share the same basic premise that there was "an objective reality called 'the patient,' that should be examined objectively in order to devise and apply rational methods of treatment."[17] If dialogue was not such a consideration in the pre-1950s—at least for many physicians—the general practitioner invariably acquired a good understanding of a patient's social concerns and circumstances (class, literacy, income, etc.) from house calls and knowledge of occupation.

Ambivalence Toward Authority

The diversity of practitioners makes it difficult to generalize about the overall role of their authority in therapy. Certainly not everyone accepted the authority of doctors, had unwavering confidence or trust in them, or even recognized the hardships of house calls or the convenience of offices in doctors' homes (as compared to today).[18] Ambivalence about, if not skepticism toward, doctors and their treatments undoubtedly existed. Although historians, in looking at the image of physicians in the United States during the first half of the twentieth century, often see it as a "golden age," opinions vary on the impact of an undercurrent of public concerns. Some would say that for "half a century" physicians were "relatively free from public censure,"[19] but others can read the magazines of the day, and perhaps the uncertainties about medicine expressed in Sinclair Lewis's (1925) celebrated novel *Arrowsmith* (and the subsequent movie of 1931) or A. J. Cronin's (1937) *The Citadel* (movie 1938) as reflecting a significant level of disquiet toward physicians and their medicines (see Figure 4.1).[20] The Newfoundland scene certainly suggests this.

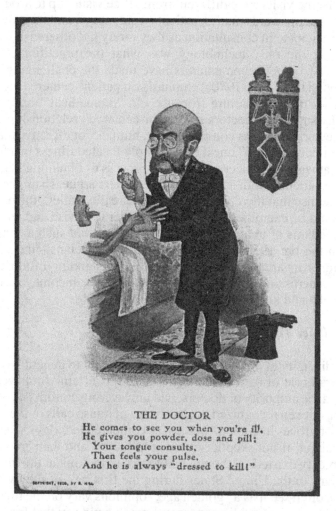

THE DOCTOR
He comes to see you when you're ill,
He gives you powder, dose and pill;
Your tongue consults,
Then feels your pulse,
And he is always "dressed to kill!"

FIGURE 4.1. Physician authority was complex. Social class and sartorial elegance were considerations, as reflected in this comic postcard, copyright 1905. (*Source:* Author's collection.)

The marked deference of rural Newfoundlanders to the authority of the priest, the merchant, and the doctor was noted in Chapter 1. However, a significant difference existed in the nature of the authority. That of the priest and the merchant came from the power—spiritual, economic, and social—they held over Newfoundlanders. With physicians, despite their education and special knowledge, there is a real sense that they had to earn their authority. Many did; some did not.[21] In fact, public attitudes to physicians were not always easy to discern, at least by the physicians themselves. The widespread reluctance of Newfoundlanders—sometimes linked to poor education and illiteracy—to ask questions, certainly up to the 1960s, was viewed by physicians as deference, if not passiveness, and perhaps a mark of their own authority and superiority. However, it did not necessarily mean patients followed a physician's advice.[22] Many people were ambivalent about doctors' medicines and held attitudes expressed in the following story, which even if embroidered is instructive:

> A colleague of mine was visiting on his winter rounds in a delightful village some forty miles south of St. Anthony Hospital. The "swiles" (seals) had "stuck in" and all hands were out on the ice eager to capture their share of these valuable animals. But snow-blindness had attacked the men, and had rendered them utterly unable to profit by their good fortune. The doctor's clinic was long and busy that night. The following morning he was, however, amazed to see many of his erstwhile patients wending their way seawards, each with one eye only treated on his prescription. The other (for safety's sake) was being doctored after the long-accepted methods of the talent of the village—tansy poultices and sugar being the favourites. The consensus of opinion obviously was that the risk was too great to venture both eyes at once on the doubtful altar of modern medicine.[23]

Many Newfoundlanders viewed doctors as a "last resort" for the "simple reason" that many people did not have the money to pay—even the customary dollar or dollar-and-a-half fee up to the 1950s. (Exceptions on the island occurred where a doctor was running a "book system" in which annual payment might be five or ten dollars or more per family).[24] Another reason for doctors being the last resort was simply, as one Newfoundlander said of an aunt, "lack of faith in them, and her mother was the same. She lived to be ninety-three! They would say the same thing, 'Keep going and work it off.' "[25]

Quality of Care

Patients' attitudes toward physicians owed much to the quality, or the perceived quality, of care they received. One historian's view is that U.S. general practitioners "epitomized both the best and the worst about medicine for generations of Americans."[26] In Britain, a 1950 report on the state of general practice was a "condemnation" of it, especially in terms of widespread poor-quality care. Amid criticisms of inadequate premises and of physical examinations of patients, the author frequently witnessed the "bottle of medicine" mentality; " 'bottles' were asked for by almost everyone seen, and were supplied on request."[27] The British report found problems in both urban and rural situations, whereas Newfoundlanders remember the difficulties being mostly among rural practitioners. One representative view, even if somewhat sharper than most, stated the following:

> We had doctors. For most of my growing up there was a resident doctor, but if I may say this, they didn't amount to much. You couldn't get a skilled doctor in a small place like that. You couldn't support them I suppose. So we had doctors that weren't quite finished. Maybe I'm just guessing at that, or doctors that had not made good somewhere else. As far as I remember them they didn't amount to much. I remember three doctors we had. One of them used to drink. The others didn't seem to know too much and nobody seemed to have any confidence in them, so gradually they left and we got along without them.[28]

On occasions, visitors to Newfoundland confirmed the existence of problem doctors: "There is only one physician practicing in Placentia [in 1940], an elderly man, who, according to apparently reliable reports, is neither qualified in clinical medicine nor in public health work."[29]

Patients' lack of faith commonly focused on medicines. Some, with perhaps inappropriate expectations, felt little confidence when doctors offered no treatment other than regular home medicine. One senior remembered being sick as a youngster with what was called "the flu or a bad cold or something"; on being taken to the doctor she could see "that he didn't know any more" than anyone else. His only advice was to "keep me warm and give lots of liquids, but anyone would know that anyhow."[30] Similar situations have been recalled for "muscular rheumatism": "all she was told was, 'Go home and rub it as much as you can with Minard's Liniment' [a favorite over-the-counter preparation]—that's all the trouble he would take with it."[31] At the same time, other people might see such doctor recommendations for home treatments, which included backplasters, poultices, and various nursing regimens, as validation of their usefulness. "We were doing what the doctor would advise you to do: keep you warm, give lots of liquids, don't give you foods that were indigestible, make sure whatever they give you was easy to digest."[32]

Safety concerns with medicines were not particularly high on the agenda, though they were creeping in with new products, even before the tragedy of more than one hundred deaths from a sulfonamide medicine in 1937 (see discussion on sulfonamides, Chapter 5) led to satirical "warning" in a St. John's newspaper (Box 4.1). Moreover, there had always been some worry over opium and the mercury preparation calomel, the latter previously noted as being prescribed by some physicians until the 1950s for its strong laxative action. Advertisements that proclaimed the absence of these substances only helped to reinforce concerns in some people's minds: Carter's Little Liver Pills were "purely vegetable,"[33] while Fletcher's Castoria for children was a "pleasant, harmless substitute for castor oil, paregoric, teething drops and soothing syrups."[34] Attention was also given to alcohol with appeals to those of a temperance mind-set. For example, Pierce's Favorite Prescription—"a true temperance medicine"[35] (see Figure 4.2)—was promoted with such reassurances as "No alcohol and no habit-forming drugs are found in it"[36] or "It contains no alcohol, neither opium, cocaine or other form of narcotic."[37]

Physicians, many of whom dispensed their own prescriptions, varied in their conscientiousness over providing information on safety. Not many had special labels, as did a North Carolina physician (albeit dispensed in his own drugstore in the 1930s). The label for calomel and soda tablets, for example, stated:

No cathartic or laxative of any kind should be taken when abdominal pain, nausea, vomiting or persistent tenderness in the abdominal region are present, as these may be due to appendicitis. Consult a physician. Laxatives and cathartics may be habit forming if used frequently. Replace cover and keep tightly closed.[38]

Lay Practitioners

Any consideration of confidence and faith in physicians raises questions about attitudes toward lay practitioners. Physicians, often supported by historians, have generally accentuated a gulf between "elite" and "popular" practitioners, but many rural patients saw a more fuzzy boundary. Lay practitioners in North America and Britain were often significant for community self-sufficiency.[39] Bonesetters, charmers, and granny midwives in Newfoundland, for example, all had important roles in offering first aid, especially for broken bones ("to splice up bones and put splints on them"[40]), burns, and bleeding, as well as treating ubiquitous warts and advising on and treating sun-

---

Box 4.1. Ambivalence Toward Doctor's Medicines

The following, undoubtedly inspired by the sulfanilamide tragedy, appeared in a St. John's newspaper in 1937 under the title "Dangerous Business."

"Recently we read some sheezes touching a new kind of dope that would cure up dread disease, prove a beacon light of hope. The epitome of science, it was helpful, it was pure, on it we could place reliance as a sure and certain cure. Then the people with rheumatics, tired of lotion, pill and drug, pawned the chattels in their attics so that they could buy a jug. To the drug store they went speeding for this dope so rich and rare; shortly after we were reading of folks, dying everywhere. Someone's figures were mistaken, [a] scientist had muffed the ball, and the countryside was shaken by the tales of bier and pall. And the sad apothecaries who had sold the fatal dope, in a gloom that never varies now in dire repentance grope. And the folks who manufactured this fine cure and forced its sale, find their reputations fractured and they dream of terms in jail. When we are in poor condition it is helpful, it is wise, to consult the learned physician with the keen all-seeing eyes. He will test our circulation, feel our pulses, view our tongues, and size up our respiration with his ear against our lungs. And a grand reflection thrills us while we're gasping in the chair, that our lawyers, if he kills us, will pursue him to his lair."

Source: The Evening Telegram, December 3, 1937, p. 13.

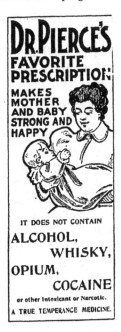

FIGURE 4.2. Advertisement for a "temperance" medicine. (*Source: The Daily News,* July 16, 1900.)

dry matters.[41] Some undertook magical cures in the tradition of cunning-folk.[42] In any case, "you couldn't get access to a doctor, you had to wait weeks, months, to see a doctor, because there weren't that many, they were scarce. And you didn't have the money, another thing, even a dollar or two."[43] It is clear that the reputations of lay practitioners could compare favorably with conventional doctors and even surpassed some.

> Now my brother cut off his finger at the chopping block. There was a little bit of flesh left. There was no doctor to go to, we sent for Uncle Michael Rourke, he came and put Frank's finger on. He never lost his finger, I don't know if he stitched it or what he did, but he never lost his finger and it was hanging. He's eighty-two now.

And people went to Hannah, another lay practitioner, for warts: "Amazing, you know. Doctors have sent them to Hannah."[44]

Although British colonial health care policy in general deliberately marginalized traditional medicine practitioners, the island's limited number of physicians meant that, for many years, this was an impossibility; even when efforts were taken around 1920 to control lay practitioners, only midwives were targeted.[45] Granny midwives—women without any formal training—played an especially major role in rural Newfoundland communities. Although vocationally trained midwives, with government funding for salaries, became increasingly evident in cottage hospitals and remote nursing stations after the Midwifery Act of 1920, granny midwives continued for many years in time-consuming and onerous roles.[46] It was not unusual for them to live with families for days before and after childbirth as they provided general nursing, medical advice, and treatments. As part of a community they were adept at home care and constantly passed on advice about medicines when they did not do the "doctoring" themselves. One former midwife wrote knowledgeably about communities:

> Any family member who was ill stayed in bed, was kept warm, given cough mixture and had their back and chest rubbed with liniment or sometimes kerosene or molasses. If a fever persisted, the doctor was sent for. He had stronger medicine for a cough, and if pneumonia set in, he ordered linseed meal poultices, applied heat to the chest and back for eight days. Then the sickness was supposed to turn for the better or the worse.[47]

Such regimens further helped some people to validate home medicine (e.g., the use of poultices). This common ground between professional and home medicine is also reflected in many of the following treatments recorded in a nursing station (with a trained nurse in attendance) on one day in 1945.[48]

Diagnosis	Treatment
Paralysis rt hand and arm	Massage, exercises
Constipation (whoop cough)	Mineral Oil liquid paraffin
Eczema	Lassar's Paste
Impetigo, whooping cough, rickets	Sulphathiazole Ung, Cod L. Oil
Pneumonia, whooping cough	Cod Liver Oil—laxative (M.O.) [mineral oil]
Rheumatism	Aspirin Tablets. White Liniment

Mastitis	(Opened March 17th) Hot boracic fomentations; elevated breast; advice, i.e., feeding
Debility	Vitamin A B and D
Whooping Cough	Cod Liver Oil
Headache	Aspirins
Burn (Hand)	Sulphathiazole Ung
Sore Throat	Mouth Wash

Only Sulphathiazole Ung. ointment was outside the usual boundaries of popular medical advice and self-care. Liquid paraffin was well known, though not the most popular laxative because of its tendency to seep onto underwear.

Lay practitioners, beyond those generally viewed as "traditional," included clergy, who, for centuries, combined pastoral and health care. In the eighteenth century, Newfoundland had John Clinch (a physician before being ordained), the first practitioner of any kind to introduce Jenner's vaccination to North America (probably before July 1800).[49] A later clergyman, Ernest Rusted, who straddled the nineteenth and twentieth centuries, is well remembered for being called upon by the sick. He had medicines in the house to give away and helped one doctor during surgery by administering anesthetics in local homes. On one occasion he was thanked by a local doctor for his interventions saved the doctor from driving "seven miles to see minor cases who could not afford to pay."[50] The role of the clergy serves as a reminder that, for many people, religion (or spirituality) and sickness were intimately bound in various ways, in particular the issue of faith:

> I remember, we had a neighbour and she was bleeding after childbirth. [In the ambulance] the woman said to me, "Mrs. Corcoran, I'm bleeding to death." The perspiration was just coming out and the blood running on the floor, but I had a green scapular and the medal of St. Anne in my bag. I never asked the lady her religion or anything, but . . . I said, "Now my love, I don't know what religion you are, but here's the green scapular, and you put your faith in that, you'll be alright, don't you worry, the green scapular stops the blood." I said, "You believe in that and you'll be alright." . . . The bleeding stopped.[51]

The last group of "practitioners" to be mentioned here includes entrepreneurs, ranging from the "doctors" in medicine shows to itinerant medicine or health lecturers. Although they hardly contributed to community self-sufficiency, some helped to sustain a popular (now called "alternative") medicine distinct from conventional practice. Compared with other regions of North America, isolated Newfoundland saw relatively few entrepreneurs, but it did see some. For example, E. J. Pratt, a homegrown Methodist preacher and celebrated poet, peddled his universal Lung Healer (containing "spruce tops, wild cherry bark, the rind of fir trees and sarsaparilla") in small coastal communities during the early 1900s.[52] Relatively few of the "newer" nonconventional practitioners, such as chiropractors, tried their hand at practicing in Newfoundland. However, one entrepreneur who was established in St. John's in 1922 complained that a local newspaper would not publish an article he wrote for "fear of offending the Medical fraternity."[53] Aldridge Leathrington Wallis of Gower Street, St. John's, a "Qualified Masseur and Doctor's Assistant," told readers of *The Evening Telegram* in 1912 that he had been treating "local and chronic diseases" for the past three years, and that he had purchased a "new improved Electric Vibrator," which he dutifully extolled.[54]

Depending on locality, the choice of practitioners available to citizens on both sides of the Atlantic could have been wide-ranging, perhaps not much different from the number of alternative practitioners at the end of the twentieth century. In the scale of history, their relative demise in the middle of the century—when the authority of physicians was unassailable in many people's minds—was an aberration.

AUTHORITY AND PRESCRIPTION MEDICINES

Reference has already been made to the mystique of the physician's prescription. One consequence of the emphasis of applying science to medicine was a crusade on the part of many physicians to greater simplify and standardize remedies. Alongside a slow shift toward less complex prescriptions was a creeping change toward the use of more products manufactured by the pharmaceutical industry, many of which were available only through doctors. In commenting on this I see not only growing dependence of patients on physicians, which tended to consolidate their authority, but also a sense of the different approach to medication from that characterizing the second half of the twentieth century.

Patterns of Prescribing

As the 1900s opened, signs of a relatively cautious approach to therapy were in the air. William Osler remarked that "imperative drugging—the ordering of medicine in any and every malady—is no longer regarded as the chief function of the doctor."[55] Although prescribing habits during the first half of the twentieth century have not been well studied, it is evident that much individualism existed, ranging from extreme conservatism to what might be described as prescription frenzy, with most practitioners somewhere in between. However, marking the period are clear efforts to bring more standardization into prescribing. The Newfoundland records, typical of those in Britain and the United States, illuminate not only specific medications in common use (many already noted in Chapter 3) but also a significant decline in multi-ingredient prescriptions and the growth in prescribing manufactured products.[56]

In 1914, Dr. William Campbell commonly prescribed a complex cough/cold/chest remedy typical of many prescriptions at the time; this was a ten-ounce bottle containing up to six active constituents, often compounded in a syrup base along with extract of cochineal to color the medicine red and sometimes spirit of chloroform as a preservative and sweetener. His prescriptions were written in abbreviated pharmaceutical Latin, the use of which was under attack by the 1920s or at least being questioned. A 1925 study indicated that 14 percent of prescriptions were being written in English, a trend that continued.[57] The continued use of Latin, however, was defended on a number of counts. One was that it helped

> to conceal the kind of medicine being taken and perhaps the nature of the disease being treated, from the patient himself, if this be desirable, and also from inquisitive persons who may have a more or less legitimate interest in the patient.[58]

Transcribed in Table 4.1 is a Campbell prescription (c. 1922), with the difficult-to-read handwriting of the same prescription (probably illegible to patients) shown in Figure 4.3 in abbreviated pharmaceutical Latin, and the "strange" (to a layperson) symbols that created for some an almost alchemical "mystique" to the prescription—a mystique often remembered in druggists' recollections of the 1950s and earlier.[59] In fact, the mystique could be enhanced by how the druggist went about "filling" the prescription or compounding the medicine (see section Quality of Dispensed Medicines later in this chapter). The key ingredients of this prescription were the two opium preparations as cough suppressants— compound tincture of camphor (paregoric) and chlorodyne (a well-known morphine-cannabis preparation)—and the tincture of squill as an expectorant.[60] The strychnine hydrochloride was included as a tonic, perhaps to stimulate the appetite. Other physicians might add tincture of hyoscyamus (perhaps as an added sedative or antispasmodic to help with breathing) and Easton's Syrup (for tonic/iron properties). Small variations in ingredients from one Campbell prescription to another suggest that he tailored prescriptions to individual patients' needs.[61]

Although an insufficient number of Campbell prescriptions from later years have been found to allow for any definitive comment about changes, he might well have simplified them over the next few years.

TABLE 4.1. Transcription of Campbell Prescription, c. 1922

Mrs. Bennett

R

Tr. Camph Co	℥ vii ss	Compound Tincture of Camphor	7½ fluid drachms
Chlorodine	℥ viii	Chlorodyne	8 fluid drachms
Tr. Scillae	℥ iii ss	Tincture of Squill	3½ fluid drachms
Pot. Acetas	℥ iii	Potassium Acetate	3 drachms
Liq. Strych Hyd	℥ ii	Solution of Strychnine Hydrochloride	2 fluid drachms
Sp. Clform	℥ ii	Spirit of Chloroform	2 fluid drachms
Syr. Simplex	℥ iii	Syrup	3 fluid ounces
Liq Cocci	m x	Solution of Cochineal	10 minims
Aq.	℥ vi	Water	6 fluid ounces
Sig.	℥ ii ev. 4h		Label it two teaspoonfuls every 4 hours

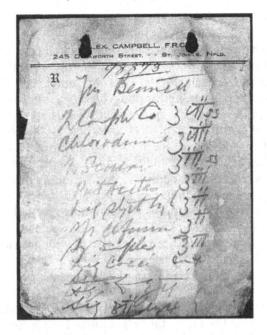

FIGURE 4.3. Dr. Campbell's Prescription c. 1922 (*Source:* Faculty of Medicine archives, Memorial University of Newfoundland.)

On the other hand, druggists' recollections of the 1940s and 1950s, even into the 1960s, mention more complex prescriptions than Campbell's, albeit declining in numbers. ("Now we had them as high as 14 or 15 ingredients in a single prescription.")[62]

The growing trend to prescribing manufactured products is seen more clearly in the practices of another St. John's physician, Cluny Macpherson. Between 1912 and the early 1920s, Macpherson, who was to become one of the doyens of Newfoundland medicine—partly through his fame as the inventor of the gas mask during World War I—commonly prescribed the brands of a number of manufacturers in Britain, Canada, and the United States, for example, H.K.W. and Co. (H.K. Wampole), Parke, Davis, Wyeth, and Burroughs Wellcome. Although such preparations as Creoterpin, Phospho-Lecithin, Hemogan, effervescing sodium phosphate, and paraform were all tagged H.K.W. and Co., Macpherson perhaps prescribed mostly Burroughs Wellcome products, since he often specified "tabloids" when prescribing tablets. You may recall that Burroughs Wellcome coined the term *tabloids* to identify medicine in tablet form.

Macpherson's prescribing was also characterized by relatively few mixtures and certainly no complex ones—rarely more than four constituents even in the earliest (1913) of his found prescriptions. The most detailed, a favored one for coughs/colds, contained potassium citrate, wine of ipecacuanha, spirits of ethyl nitrite, and syrup of tolu and wild cherry (the latter always specified as the Wyeth brand). Quantities of ingredients in the prescription varied for children and adults. Another Macpherson multi-ingredient prescription is worthy of comment because it can be linked to his lifelong interest in acidosis (see Chapter 3). Although labeled for acidosis, its ingredients—acetozone (benzoyl-acetyl-peroxide, an antiseptic), oil of gaultheria (wintergreen, also antiseptic), saccharin (as a sweetener), and water—suggest it was more an intestinal antiseptic to treat gastric and intestinal fermentations caused by bacteria.[63]

The trend of simplification and standardization of formulae, although accentuated in the first half of the twentieth century, was already evident in the last decades of the 1800s in the context of rational therapeutics, at least in so far as this looked at a better understanding of the action of individual substances. Influential American physician D. W. Cathell (1883) wrote:

> In prescribing medicines for the sick it is better to confine yourself to a limited number of remedies with whose uses and powers you are fully acquainted, than to employ a larger number of ill-understood ones. . . . Avoid polypharmacy. It is much better to order some single remedy or a combination of which you know the physiological effect, than to give an indefinite medley on the ancient blunderbuss principle.[64]

This and related messages came to be reiterated time and again, as in the standard U.S. textbooks; for example, the American Medical Association's (1926) *Useful Drugs: A List of Drugs Selected to Supply the Demand for a Less Extensive Materia Medica with a Brief Discussion of Their Actions, Uses, and Dosage* minced no words in noting, "It has long been recognized that the great number of drugs and preparations of drugs presented to the attention of physicians is an evil." It went on to say that "efforts were made by the Council on Medical Education of the American Medical Association and the

Confederation of State Examining and Licensing Boards to restrict instruction and examination in materia medica to the more important drugs."[65] Occasional copies of *New and Nonofficial Remedies,* published under the auspices of the Council on Pharmacy and Chemistry of the American Medical Association, also reached Newfoundland. Appearing annually for fifty years or so after 1905, each volume maintained a list of the most important remedies and was a significant publication in shaping prescribing in the United States and beyond.[66]

Although the trend to simplify prescriptions was inexorable, Mr. Brown and Ms. Smith could still find a vast range of different prescriptions from different physicians, perhaps even their favorite medicine, maybe from a "famous" physician or hospital.[67] That simplification was somewhat erratic is reflected in Morris Bealle's (1949) vehement attack on the pharmaceutical industry and medical establishment in his popular work, *The Drug Story.* He bemoaned that young physicians who met drugs they know nothing about, and do not realize that they have been discarded by their teachers are "tempted to fall into the slugh of unreasoning empiricism."[68]

Ethical Pharmaceuticals, the Bottle of Medicine,
and Placebo Responses

A particular if not immediately obvious contribution from the pharmaceutical industry to standardization was the development of "ethical pharmaceuticals," that is, products advertised to the medical profession alone, not to the general public. They emerged in the last decades of the nineteenth century from companies—e.g., Bayer, E. R. Squibb, Parke Davis, Burroughs Wellcome—as competition to the questionable commercialism and promotion of "quack," secret-ingredient preparations.[69] In fact, the new ethicals hardly led to restraint of advertising—intense pressures from mailings, sales representatives, and free doctors' samples were commonplace by 1900; what changed was the target audience. A noteworthy example is Bayer and its promotion of aspirin first to physicians and ultimately to the general public.[70] Ethicals turned out to be excellent business strategy due to public recognition of scientific medicine and research (much of it centering on quality control) undertaken in many companies.[71] Acceptance of ethicals came readily from physicians (as noted in brand-name prescribing) and their institutions; the American

Medical Association, for example, established nonadvertising of a product to the public as a criterion for inclusion in its widely used annual, *New and Nonofficial Remedies.* Ultimately, ethical pharmaceuticals were a major factor behind the disappearance of "the bottle of medicine."

It is often suggested that the mystique of the bottle of medicine— the end result of a prescription, perhaps written specifically for one patient (i.e., not a stock medicine)—coupled with the authority of the physician, owed much to placebo action. Certainly, there is every reason to think this was a factor behind any reputation, but physiological actions that contributed to symptom relief cannot be dismissed. The extent to which the mystique of medicines persisted in the new ethical preparations products is not easy to say. With them came long scientific names of the new medicines and ultimately new classifications of medicines, commonly linked with new diagnostic categories, far removed from the world of tonics and sedatives.[72] In fact, the mystique of prescriptions changed from the unknown to one of impenetrable science. That is not to say that symbolism, always to be considered in the eye of the beholder and hence a variable issue, vanished. For a Mr. Brown or Ms. Smith, terms such as *magic bullets, comforters,* and *purifiers* might carry special meanings and expectations that contributed to placebo responses. Perhaps this included seeing medicines as tangible substances that helped to demystify a disease since it could be visualized as being attacked by the medicine.[73]

AUTHORITY, GATEKEEPING, AND RESPONSIBILITIES

Legally enforced standards and controls in any profession often have an ambivalent quality in the public mind: whether in the long run the assurance of more predictable and effective professional services will outweigh the risk of fostering special privileges and restrictive practices that may not be in the public interest?

Sonnedecker, *Kremers and Urdang's History of Pharmacy*

In *Opium and the People,* Berridge and Edwards make clear that professional medical dominance runs throughout the nineteenth- and twentieth-century British story of the control of medicines—not only of opium and other narcotics but also of medicines designated as poisons.[74] That is not to say that behind every piece of legislation there is not a complex interplay of other factors such as professional and business self-interests, lobbying (perhaps crusading) by self-interested parties (including consumers), government bureaucracy, genuine concerns for public health, and the need for compromises. In this section, some comparisons between British, U.S., and Newfoundland legislation help to sharpen an understanding of the diverse factors that shaped the regulation of medicines, increased the authority of physicians and druggists through gatekeeping, and limited the public's ability to choose their own medicines. In fact, Mr. Brown and Ms. Smith increasingly found that legislative controls made them more and more dependent on physicians and druggists, though the heyday of this was to come in the second half of the twentieth century.

The following discussion also provides background to questions on whether the increasing protection of the public was excessive. For example, could the controls have been overly influenced by the medical and pharmaceutical professions (always looking for professional authority), which were able to capitalize on societal concerns over, say, narcotic abuse? In exploring relevant issues, four topics are raised: poison and pharmacy legislation, narcotic controls, the emergence of prescription-only medicines, and changes in over-the-counter preparations.[75]

Poison and Pharmacy Legislation

I first look back to the nineteenth century when legislation, emerging on both sides of the Atlantic, contributed to pharmacy's efforts to acquire professional authority. Britain, considered first, offers a relative straightforward story, at least compared with the multiple jurisdictions in the various American states. Our subsequent comments on developments in the United States and Newfoundland then sharpen the picture of how the gatekeeping of medicines underpinned changes in the professional standing of pharmacy, as well as Mr. Brown's and Ms. Smith's ready access to medicines.

Britain

During the first half of the nineteenth century, increasing public concerns in Britain over accidental, suicidal, and criminal poisoning by arsenic and strychnine fueled legislation to "protect" the public. Control of arsenic—widely used in the arts and agriculture (e.g., sheep dressings)—came first with the Arsenic Act of 1851.[76] Despite the many vested interests in the status quo, the new legislation seemingly received little strong opposition.[77]

Amid efforts to extend such controls to other substances, British chemists and druggists made determined efforts to promote their professional standing and authority, something they had failed to accomplish under the 1851 arsenic legislation. For the next few years, in an era of free-trade philosophy that viewed any granting of monopoly power with deep suspicion, the efforts to achieve their goals met with limited success.[78] It was only with the 1868 Act to Regulate the Sale of Poisons and Amend the Pharmacy Act of 1852 that chemists and druggists felt significant developments had been made. Although the short title of the act was the Pharmacy Act, it was, according to one historian, "in all essentials a poisons Act [in which the government] set up a register of chemists and druggists as people qualified to retail, dispense and compound poisons."[79] Not all historians see it quite this way, for they view it less as the government's use of a convenient group of shopkeepers to institute controls and more as a recognition of pharmacy's own efforts to improve its professional standing by giving it responsibility over poisonous or potentially poisonous substances.[80]

Certainly the Pharmacy Act was something of a compromise between two different viewpoints about how to protect the public. One viewpoint was that this was best brought about by stringent controls on sales of poisons (opium was a particular issue), and the other was that full and clear labeling, along with a record of purchases, was all that was needed. One historian described the act as "more a patchwork quilt of amendments than a seamless web of legislative thought."[81] Whatever interpretation is placed on the Pharmacy Act, it established control of a limited number of poisons (see Table 4.2, left column). Although it did curtail the freedom of the individual with regard to poisons, in reflecting the views of John Stuart Mill (1859) in his classic essay, "On Liberty," it was generally felt to be acceptable in order to protect others.[82]

The controlled poisons were listed in a two-part schedule. Those in Part 1 could be sold only if the purchaser was known to the seller or to an intermediary known to both. A detailed entry had to be made in a poisons register. The bottle or other container had to be labeled "poison," along with the name of the substance and name and address of the seller. The labeling requirements applied only to substances in Part 2 of the schedule.[83] No requirements applied to physicians' prescriptions.

A number of concerns arose in the implementation of the Pharmacy Act, especially over the failure to add, despite much public pressure, many other worrisome "poisons" to the schedules—only chloral hydrate (1877) and nux vomica (1882) were added prior to 1900.[84] Why so few were added, given what seemed to be substantial public health concerns that surrounded the 1851 and 1868 acts, is not entirely clear. Although the authority to designate new substances was given to the Council of the Pharmaceutical Society, decisions had to be approved by the Privy Council, and it was this body that delayed the scheduling of, for example, carbolic acid for many years after it was first recommended by the Pharmaceutical Society's council in 1882. Only in 1900, due to the use of the acid in many suicides and pressures from many quarters, did the Privy Council add certain preparations of it to the second part of the poisons schedule.[85] The Privy Council's apparent obstinacy, despite a time of growing preoccupation with living germs (bacteria) and the need to combat them, perhaps rested on such intertwined reasons as a mind-set of free trade (the council had no real interest in the professional aspirations of pharmacy), pressure from the principal manufacturer of the acid (F. C. Calvert and Co.), and prospects of new comprehensive poison legislation. Other reasons, not yet investigated, must account for the Privy Council's rejection of hellebore, vermin killers containing phosphorus, digitalin, nitrobenzol, lobelia, Indian hemp, and nitroglycerine prior to 1900.

Following the Pharmacy Act of 1868, no new poison legislation came until the Poisons and Pharmacy Act of 1908. In consequence of pressure from the medical profession and a new theory of addiction as a disease, the 1908 act tightened controls on opium, albeit through the medical profession.[86] Subsequently, an inexorable trend up to the

TABLE 4.2. Comparison of Poisons Controlled in Britain, the United States (Colorado), and Newfoundland (1868-1886)

Britain, 1868	Colorado, 1872	Newfoundland, 1886
Part 1 (Entry in poisons register and designated labeling)	(Entry in poisons register and designated labeling)	(Entry in "receipt book" and designated labeling)
Arsenic and its preparations	Arsenic and its preparations	Arsenic and its preparations
Prussic acid	Prussic acid	Prussic acid
Cyanides of potassium and all metallic cyanides	Cyanides of potassium and all metallic cyanides	All metallic cyanides
Strychnine and all poisonous vegetable alkaloids and their salts	Strychnine and all poisonous vegetable alkaloids and their salts	All poisonous vegetable alkaloids as strychnine
Aconite and its preparations	Aconite	All atropine &c., and their salts
Emetic tartar		Aconite and its preparations
Corrosive sublimate	Designated labeling only	Tartar emetic
Cantharides		Corrosive sublimate
Savin and its oil	Belladonna	Cantharides and its preparations
Ergot of rye and its preparations	Conium	Savin and its oil
	Cantharides	Ergot of rye and its preparations
Part 2 (Designated labeling only)	Corrosive sublimate	Essential oil of almonds, unless deprived of its prussic acid
	Croton oil	
	Carbolic acid	
Oxalic acid	Chloroform	Opium and its alkaloids, and their salts
Chloroform	Chloral hydrate	
Belladonna and its preparations	Digitalis	Hydrate of chloral and its preparations
Essential oil of almonds, unless deprived of its prussic acid	Ergot	Chloroform
	Henbane	Belladonna and its preparations
	Mineral acids and their pharmaceutical preparations	Phosphorus
Opium and all preparations of opium or of poppies	Nux vomica	
	Opium and all preparations of opium, except paregoric and preparations containing less than two grains to the ounce	
	Oxalic acid	
	Savin oil	
	Sulphate of zinc	

Note: Despite differences, general similarities of the three jurisdictions are striking, even confusion over defining alkaloids. Although all substances listed are poisonous, unlike arsenic, strychnine, and cyanide not all had aroused concerns of use for homicide. Savin and ergot were already known as abortifacients, illegal to use at the time. Cantharides, a vesicant, had the popular reputation as an aphrodisiac.

1950s becomes clear of more and more piecemeal restrictions on the sale of medicines—a trend viewed as part of the general movement of social health and welfare reform during the early decades of the twentieth century on both sides of the Atlantic.[87] Notable milestones up to 1950 were the Poisons and Pharmacy Act of 1908, the 1916 regulation under the Defence of the Realm Act (DORA 40B) (mandating cocaine as the first prescription-only medicine), the Dangerous Drugs Act of 1920 (provision of narcotic drugs by pharmacists acting on a doctor's written prescription), the Therapeutic Substances Act 1925 (regulating the manufacture, standardization, and supply of antitoxins and sera, vaccines, posterior pituitary preparations, and organic arsenicals), and the Pharmacy and Poisons Act of 1933.

Although historians have not yet explored in detail the debates, disagreements, and controversies behind the legislation, one significant development in the Pharmacy and Poisons Act of 1933 was the loosening of the close association between poisons and recognition of pharmacy as a profession. Custodianship of poisons remained with chemists and druggists, but the act was clearly designed to improve "the status of a responsible and important class of public servants, i.e., druggists."[88] The act strengthened the organization, authority, and supervision of the Pharmaceutical Society of Great Britain by making membership of the society compulsory. Important, too, was the appointment of a poisons board, independent from the society, thus avoiding any future conflicts of interest, real or suspected. Given such developments it is noteworthy that it was only with the Medicines Act of 1968 and the Poisons Act of 1972 (dealing only with nonmedicinal poisons) that poison and pharmacy practice legislation were, in a sense, finally separated in Britain, albeit with powers and duties conferred and/or imposed on the profession by these and other acts.

Similarities and Differences of the United States and Newfoundland

It is unnecessary to detail the U.S. and Newfoundland legislation at the same length, only to notice similarities with or differences from the British scene. It has been said that, compared with Britain, early

U.S. legislation was centered less on a preoccupation with poisons than with concerns over the "adulteration of food, drink and drugs."[89] Seemingly, this meant the same focus was not on finding guardians for a limited social problem. Historians suggest that state legislatures in the United States readily responded to the efforts of druggists to improve their professional standing through legislation. As one authoritative study suggests, state pharmaceutical laws were shaped largely by educational, professional, and economic considerations.[90] "Model" laws (1869 and 1900) that were circulated to state governments were not without influence; these made clear the differences between a druggist and "a mere merchant" and the value of pharmacy existing as a distinct profession for the public good.[91] In addition, state legislation, albeit with variations from one to another, commonly did have close analogies with poison control in Britain, for example, druggists had to have knowledge of the purchaser, to use a poison register, and to ensure poisons had distinctive labeling (see Table 4.2).[92]

As elsewhere, the supply of medicines to rural residents in the United States remained problematic—in fact, physicians generally did their own dispensing—and statutes made necessary allowances.[93] Rural needs and local lifestyles (the "use of poisons in killing fur-bearing and other animals") were also reflected in the first and relatively late (1886) poison legislation in Newfoundland.[94] There, druggists were not given the sole role of gatekeepers largely because less than a handful of druggists practiced outside St. John's. Thus it was enacted that *any* certified person could sell a poison so long as the sale was recorded in a receipt book and the item labeled as a "poison." The only reference to druggists in the legislation was to indicate that the regulations did not apply to "any article when forming part of the ingredients of any medicine dispensed" by them. Certification as a seller recognized physicians as citizens of special standing in so far as certificates had to be signed by the president and secretary of the Medical Society of St. John's and countersigned by the colonial secretary.[95]

When the next piece of Newfoundland legislation—the Pharmacy Practice Act of 1911—was established, a clear change had occurred, which might be described as catch-up. Although the act established druggists as custodians of poisons, it was also concerned with the quality of pharmacy practice as a whole.[96] A revealing comment was that Newfoundland druggists were not allowed to practice in the United States.[97] The preamble for the new act stated that it is desirable "to provide for the improvement of pharmaceutical practice in this Colony" and "to regulate the sale of drugs." The act was a slimmed-down version of the objectives of the Newfoundland Pharmaceutical Society (founded in 1910), which echoed pharmacy's concerns everywhere over "professionalism," especially the need to ensure the quality of products and of compounding and dispensing medicines.[98] It was self-evident to Newfoundland legislators and others that, unlike elsewhere, the public had no real way of assessing the professional state of pharmacy on the island.[99]

There was apparently no substantial opposition to the new Pharmacy Act, which remained essentially unchanged until 1954.[100] Minimal concerns over granting a monopoly, of creating a "closed occupation," came with the impractical and quickly discarded suggestion that druggists be obliged to keep a drugstore "open continuously both in St. John's East and West, all day and all night long on every day of the year."[101]

A significant responsibility given to the new board of pharmacy (established under the 1911 act to make bylaws for the practice of pharmacy) was to add "any poisonous drug" or "drugs" to the existing schedule, subject to final approval by the governor in council. That the original schedule remained unchanged (narcotics were controlled under a different act) until the Pharmaceutical Association Act of 1954 might suggest an analogy with the situation already described in Britain during the last two decades of the 1800s. In this case, however, Newfoundland's slowness was linked to the lack of public pressure and to the small size of a professional group with nothing or little to gain from a few additional gatekeeping roles.

Legislation does not guarantee quality of care and it is appropriate to ask here whether Mr. Brown and Ms. Smith, as Newfoundlanders, were well served by their druggists, especially in view of much lower educational standards than in Britain and the United States. Although little evidence is available to assess the quality of dispensing (see Quality of Dispensed Medicines in this chapter), variations in practice were possibly less than in many other places. One reason, still prevailing in the 1950s and 1960s, was that with every druggist knowing one another—all in a relatively small community—peer pressure from the core of leaders contributed to standards. As was remembered:

> We figured we were good; we were damn good. The name on the store said it all. It wasn't Peter O'Mara's Drugs. It was Peter O'Mara, *the* Druggist. I said, "father that's kind of wrong." I said, "you're not *the* druggist." He said, "yes, I am." He said, "a hell a lot of others are not."[102]

Narcotics: Gatekeeping and Control of Medicines

The inexorable path to control of medicines in the first half of the century included narcotics, notably opium (and morphine and heroin), cocaine, and cannabis. The discussion here on additional gatekeeping roles for physicians and druggists also considers whether the general concerns over narcotics helped to create a climate of controls, extending beyond 1950, that spread to medicines in general and psychoactive medicines in particular. After all, terms such as *dependence, habituation, addiction, habit-forming, drug misuse, substance/drug abuse,* and *withdrawal syndromes* have slippery definitions, especially when applied to nonnarcotics—sedatives/hypnotics, tranquilizers, antidepressants, etc.[103]

One difficulty in summarizing the story of narcotic control is the diversity of approaches that have been taken in different countries. For example, during the first half of the twentieth century Britain generally viewed addiction as a medical problem, a disease that could be dealt with through physicians treating addicts; in contrast, the United States and Canada developed policies that criminalized addiction.[104] Clearly this could have consequences for a Mr. Brown or a Ms. Smith depending on whether they lived in Britain, the United States, or Newfoundland/Canada. For example, they could not be prescribed heroin after 1924 in the United States, and in Canada between 1954 and 1985, whereas British physicians resisted such bans.[105]

The control of narcotics, at least opium, commenced long before 1900; however, here we need only mention that the initial nineteenth-century controls on both sides of the Atlantic were generally part of the poisons/pharmaceutical legislation already considered.[106] In practice, although this restricted completely open sales, the early controls made relatively little difference to the overall availability of opiate preparations as medicines, prescribed or over the counter. This changed in consequence of various trends on both sides of the Atlantic. The twentieth century saw a shift in control of narcotics to designating them as illicit substances separate from poisons/pharmaceutical substances. Behind this lay late nineteenth-century concerns over morphine addiction from hypodermic injections (introduced in the 1870s), increasing fears of opium as its recreational use grew around 1900, and hostility to minority groups. Blacks, Chinese, and other ethnic immigrants were singled out with stereotypical mind-sets, for example, that the Chinese spread the opium habit.[107] Such groups, considered a threat to society, were labeled "dangerous classes," as were their activities.[108] Moreover, the significance of the word *dangerous* had extended, by the 1930s, beyond narcotics to a range of other medicines, particularly hypnotics/sedatives.

International concerns over opium trade precipitated the Hague International Opium Convention (1911-1912), which committed signatory countries to restrict the trade and consumption of opium and cocaine and their derivatives to "medical and legitimate uses" and to regulate preparations of certain strengths. The U.S. Harrison Narcotic Act (1914) and Britain's Dangerous Drugs Act (1920) were two consequences.[109] Both acts made it illegal to possess opium- or cocaine-based preparations without a prescription (which could not be repeated, only rewritten) from a physician, dentist, or veterinary surgeon. However, as indicated, distinctly different enforcement policies arose in Britain and North America. In the United States, the Supreme Court ruled that the treatment or maintenance of addicts with opiates (which, it was argued, would help avoid black-market activity) fell outside the bounds of professional practice (and hence of the act), a view about the practice not accepted by British physicians.

The failure of the American medical profession to challenge this loss of professional/clinical autonomy seemingly went alongside a growing wariness over prescribing opiates as, by the 1930s, physicians were exhorted to accept responsibility for preventing addiction.[110] That is not to say the U.S. medical and pharmaceutical professions did not continue to recognize their stake in narcotics control. Physicians' and druggists' views, however, have always been disparate. Although some, druggists in particular, were swayed by the views of pharmaceutical manufacturers that legislation would be hurtful to business, leaders felt that "in addition to aiding public welfare" strict narcotic laws could be a distinct advantage for [professional] development if great care was exercised in their framing."[111] It is unclear whether the "advantage" was seen as acquiring more professional authority through a wider gatekeeping role or helping leaders to purge the professions of unprofessional behavior (e.g., overprescribing opiates) among practitioners.[112]

In Newfoundland, the separation of narcotic and poisons control did not happen as in the other two countries. A sparse population, much of it in small, isolated communities, meant that addiction or recreational use of narcotics, if it existed, did not become a public issue, thus avoiding tension between public health policies and maintenance of public order. When the first narcotics legislation came in the 1931 Health and Public Welfare Act—a consolidation and reform act—it was as a "Narcotics and Poisons" section. This seemingly acknowledged a mind-set that lumped together substances potentially dangerous to health, although initially only the sedative chloral hydrate joined narcotics to be prescribed by physicians, dentists, and veterinarians who had to be of good standing in the profession, not intemperate or addicted to any drugs. Opiate medicines still exempted were paregoric, laudanum, and proprietary preparations under certain strengths, and preparations of opium "sold [over the counter] in good faith for diarrhoea and cholera" so long as they were accompanied by specific directions.[113] Revision of the list did not occur until 1945. Then, belatedly compared with elsewhere, barbiturates, sulfonamides, and ergot, along with new controls on paregoric and laudanum, were added.[114]

Proponents of alcohol prohibition in the United States (which existed from 1920 to 1933), who also lobbied for the control of narcotics, had a significant impact in prohibiting opiate use for the maintenance of addicts.[115] In contrast, alcohol prohibition in Newfoundland (1917-1925)—enacted in consequence of a strong temperance movement—does not seem to have fostered a particular mind-set of narcotics/medicines control.[116] It did, however, as in the United States, add to physicians' gatekeeping roles. "Duly qualified medical practitioners, practicing in the Colony," could prescribe and dispense intoxicating liquors for medicinal purposes, though they were bound by strict controls on maximum amounts per prescription.[117] For example, no more than "8 ozs. per patient" within St. John's and twelve ounces outside; limits were also placed on the total quantity a physician could prescribe in a month. Alcohol "kicks," however, were still available through various tonics ranging from beef, iron, and wine to bitters, all noted in Chapter 3.[118] There is no doubt that prohibition placed ethical dilemmas on the shoulders of temperance-minded physicians and druggists, perhaps affecting a patient's choice of practitioner or drugstore. Some practitioners compromised. When Conrad Fitz-Gerald—a revered and respected physician on the South Coast of Newfoundland—was asked whether he would vote for the "Open Bar" or "Total Prohibition," he replied, "when it becomes necessary for me to vote for one of two evils, I can only vote for the lesser."[119] Interestingly, druggists objected to the government about their new roles in dispensing alcohol, even though it gave them new responsibilities.[120]

Although Newfoundland did not, at the time, jump to employ narcotic controls, its physicians did face growing concerns about certain sedatives and hypnotic medications—a problem faced by physicians outside Newfoundland as well. A somewhat blurred boundary between these drugs and narcotics was emerging by the 1930s, just as the language of abuse of medicines in general became more common.[121] Although it is evident that narcotics fostered a general climate for their control, did this extend to medicines viewed as poisons?

Issues arose over the safety of barbiturates some time after their introduction (for example, Veronal [barbitone] in 1903 and Luminal [phenobarbitone] in 1912). Worries about overdoses in the 1920s and a proliferation of many different barbiturates on the market contributed to strong differences of opinion about safety risks that erupted in the 1930s.[122] A 1934 British study "On the Alleged Dangers of the Barbiturates" concluded that in the absence of complicating factors, no deaths had occurred from therapeutic doses of barbiturates; this, however, failed to convince many that barbiturates were generally safe.[123] Already calls for controls had been made, as in debates leading to Britain's Pharmacy and Poison Act of 1933, when it was noted that barbiturate control was "frequently recommended by coroners;" and in 1934, an editorial in the *British Medical Journal* noted the intense debate at the time in which it was difficult to "distinguish between evidence and advocacy."[124] In 1935, under the enabling legislation of the 1933 act, a poisons board developed a new schedule of prescription-only medicines for substances which "experience has shown are liable to be self prescribed with fatal results." Included were two sedatives/hypnotics based on barbituric acid and sulphonal, along with amidopyrine (an analgesic known to cause agranulocytosis and which could be especially problematic when taken with barbiturates), and compounds of nitrophenol and of phenylcinchoninic acid (used to increase uric acid output).[125] Despite what was apparently a central concern over suicides and overdoses, the shadow of habituation/addiction probably entered into the control of barbiturates, particularly through the influence of physician Sir William Willcox. In frequently demanding controls on barbiturates, he stressed that the "risk of habit formation or addiction is well known."[126]

In the United States, rising concerns over barbiturates in the 1930s—recognizing the British shift in 1933 to prescription-only use and the activities of Willcox—lay behind twenty-seven states enacting laws regulating the sale of barbiturates by 1940; in all but one state they were to be available by prescription only.[127] Newfoundland, as noted earlier, waited until 1945 before introducing controls. Although many reasons exist for the lateness, it is noteworthy that there was still no unanimity about risks. A 1947 editorial in *The Lancet*, the authoritative British medical journal, played down any real problems: "Fortunately, there is little risk of addiction, although habituation and undue dependence can occur."[128] What had developed, however, was a climate of control.

A readiness to control in the absence of an existing social problem is well seen with cannabis in Canada. Controls were introduced in 1923 (compared with 1937 in the United States). Although it has been said that there was no general concern over misuse at the time, and that the only persons familiar with it were in the birdseed and plant industries, fearmongering became a factor.[129] Concerns over its actual availability in the country came about in the 1930s through the self-appointed, vocal "reformer," Janey Canuck who persuaded the legislature to act.[130]

In closing this discussion on narcotics and gatekeeping I jump ahead and look briefly at the 1960s, which saw another peak in the climate of control. Alarm was prompted by the growing recreational use and habituation to "uppers" and "downers"—commonly the stimulant amphetamine which, like the barbiturates ("downers"), had attracted increasing scrutiny since the 1930s—as well as by the widening use of heroin, cannabis, and LSD.[131] In Britain alone, the number of heroin addicts grew over a ten-year period from about fifty in 1957 to 1,299 in 1967.[132] As in earlier years, circumstances precipitated new drug policies on both sides of the Atlantic. One noteworthy consequence was British physicians' loss of much of their clinical freedom, in so far as they could no longer prescribe narcotics for addicts without a special license. Tightening controls was hardly a surprise, for it followed a severe shock to 1960s' Britain and its medical profession. A small number of London physicians—"junkies' doctors"—were exposed as prescribers of massive quantities of narcotics, much of which found its way to the illicit drugs market.[133] Paradoxically, while Britain was shifting away from a policy that saw addiction as a medical disease problem (it was a time when relatively few addicts existed), Canada and the United States (the latter only until the 1980s) moved more toward a medical model of addiction, a shift that is beyond the scope of the present account.[134]

Prescription-Only Medicines: The Early Years

Few people can doubt that one of the most far-reaching features of twentieth-century health care is the heyday of prescription-only medicines in the second half of the century (see Chapter 5). Even so, the removal of many items from prescription-only status from the 1970s onward raises an obvious question: To what extent were the gatekeeping controls really necessary in the interests of public safety? Did they perhaps result more from a climate of controls intended to preempt problems, but which also served the interests of the medical and pharmaceutical professions and perhaps even more the pharmaceutical industry? Would an equally effective policy at least for many products have been to educate the public on how best to use them safely? As will be seen, there are no hard and fast answers to such questions; perhaps the key question is why weren't the issues debated, at least in a public manner, before policy decisions were made?

Increasingly central to the story of medicines and public safety was the growing power of the pharmaceutical industry. Indeed it seems to have been key to the establishment of prescription-only medications in the United States (albeit amid concerns over narcotics and barbiturates, as well as sulfonamides); this came indirectly since it was far from an obvious consequence of the 1938 Food, Drug, and

Cosmetic Act.[135] It seems clear that the pharmaceutical industry promoted the idea of prescription-only medicines (to be marketed with the label "for professional use only") in order to bypass complex warning labels about safety that the FDA, in accordance with the act, was to put in place. This approach was accepted by the FDA as a way to control increasing numbers of dangerous, or potentially dangerous, medicines.

By 1941, the FDA identified more than twenty drugs or drug groups that were too dangerous to sell other than on a physician's prescription.[136] A determination of "dangerous" was based on the consensus of "qualified experts" and "careful consideration," for which the agency appealed to physicians for their experiences, observations, and opinions.[137] This clearly opened the door for the medical profession to control more and more medicines.

Problems arose under the new legislation, particularly druggists selling prescription medicines over the counter (see Chapter 5 for ethical issues in supplying medicines). Ultimately, U.S. Congress was persuaded to legally clarify interpretations of prescription-only medicines. This was enacted in the 1951 Durham-Humphrey Amendment to the 1938 Food, Drug, and Cosmetic Act. This defined a *prescription medicine* as any habit-forming substance, any substance so toxic or harmful that it required the supervision of a practitioner for its administration, or any new substance approved under the safety provision of the 1938 act that had to be used under supervision.[138] Mr. Brown and Ms. Smith might later reflect that, by happenstance, this was in place to catch the avalanche of new medicines arriving in the 1950s and later.

Over-the-Counter Medicines

Although the legislated gatekeeping roles for physicians and druggists impacted on public access to medications, patients saw the more obvious erosion of choices with the disappearance of countless numbers of over-the-counter medicines during the first half of the twentieth century. Yet amid a climate of accepting controls, this seemingly aroused little public concern.

Leading the way in this trend was the intense public pressure that helped to precipitate the 1906 Pure Food and Drugs Act in the United States, and the 1908 Proprietary or Patent Medicines Act in Canada, both of which affected Newfoundland imports since no distinction was made between the home and island markets. Even so, an intriguing number of medicines escaped anticipated controls. For example, the 1906 U.S. Pure Food and Drug Act—federal legislation to control adulteration and safety on an interstate basis—was undermined by a court challenge that found the sanctions on false and misleading labeling did not apply to therapeutic claims. Despite a 1912 amendment to the act, enforcement problems remained. Voluntary changes were precipitated, such as companies making marked reductions of narcotic and alcohol content in many medicines; however, scores of other medicines with high narcotic or alcohol content took the place of those that disappeared.[139] Moreover, the role of the FDA in public education in the 1930s was perhaps not without significance.[140] It is noteworthy that in Britain, in the absence of specific legislation to control over-the-counter medicines, various factors—for example, public and medical concerns with existing products, the influence of the National Health Insurance Act (facilitating access to physicians by the less affluent), the Dangerous Drugs Act (reducing the amount of morphine available in nonprescription medicines), and controls of labeling—contributed to some reform.[141]

The 1908 Canadian act also had a significant impact on Newfoundland. It mandated that the composition of all secret formula medicines for internal use had to be registered annually with the minister of inland revenue.[142] As with the 1906 U.S. act, not all ingredients had to be listed on the label; in fact, the list of thirty-one exceptions (basically those on the poison schedules, Table 4.2) was substantially more than those that had to be listed under the U.S. act ("alcohol, morphine, opium, cocaine, heroin, alpha or beta eucaine, chloroform, cannabis indica, chloral hydrate, or acetanilide").[143] Furthermore, preparations containing cocaine or a high alcohol content could not be registered. The Canadian act led to the disappearance of thousands of preparations. It was strengthened in 1919 by extending coverage to external preparations, expanding the list of prohibited substances, mandating the proportion of scheduled ingredients to be printed on labels, and banning false, misleading, or exaggerated claims on labels or claims to cure a disease.[144] Further controls were added to the latter provision in 1934 by making it an offense to offer for sale or to advertise any remedy as a *treatment* for an intriguingly wide range of conditions, including alcoholism, appendicitis, cancer, diabetes, epilepsy, goiter, heart disease, infantile paralysis, influenza, kidney, gallstones and bladder stones, obesity, tuberculosis, and venereal diseases. As a contemporary observer made clear, a fundamental issue was that the care of such conditions should be under medical supervision only; for example, to use thyroid for certain kinds of goiter "will do more harm than good."[145]

AUTHORITY: THE DRUGGISTS' ROLE

An Ambivalent Picture

I have already discussed the growth of professional authority through poisons legislation; here, in looking at authority and gate-keeping, I focus on the point of contact between the patient (or customer) and his or her medicine, both prescription and over the counter. The specific question is, to what extent did druggists contribute to lay acceptance and validation of medicines? Although druggists' roles in the medicines story have already been emphasized—for example, the commercialization of self-care, offering advice on the choices and the dangers of medicines, checking on the safety of physicians' prescriptions—the opportunities to affect attitudes to medicines needs particular comment. After all, druggists were readily accessible to anyone walking into a drugstore, which, during the first half of the twentieth century at least, was often open long hours, perhaps from 8 a.m. until 11 p.m., as well as offering a night service.

Attitudes toward druggists, obviously relevant to accepting and acting on any advice given, were variable, often neutral. Public images portrayed through the radio and print media offered a somewhat ambivalent picture. Radio druggists in the United States from 1935 to 1960 (with a notable exception of two) reflected a "dull personality, somewhat second class to the physician."[146] A study on the public image of American pharmacists concluded that public opinion of druggists began to decline around 1900, "reaching its nadir in the 1930s. It took an uptick in the following decade, soared in the 1950s, dipped again in the late 1960s, and then began the steady improvement reflected in today's [1990s] Gallup polls."[147] U.S. media comments on pharmacy, at least until the 1940s, were not particularly positive when highlighting growing commercialism in nonpharmacy lines, the questionable supply of alcohol-containing medicines during prohibition, the variations in prescription prices from one drugstore to the next, and druggists' accuracy in compounding physicians' prescriptions.

Although no comparable study exists on the public image of British or Newfoundland chemists and druggists, their second-class status to physicians was clear. One significant difference in Britain was that, as a result of National Health Insurance introduced in 1911, British pharmacy acquired a well-defined professional (distinct from commercial) role in dispensing National Insurance prescriptions. For the first time a substantial number of prescriptions reached pharmacies rather than being dispensed in doctors' offices. Many pharmacies, too, housed "secondary" health occupations, notably chemist-dentist and chemist-optician.[148]

An overriding issue for pharmacy in all English-speaking countries was the impact on the public of its conflict of interest between professionalism and business, a conflict that could encourage views that medicines were no different from grocery or hardware items, despite messages from the growing legislation that they were to be treated differently. Ethical issues were often spotlighted in the pharmaceutical press. The sale of questionable over-the-counter medicines, for example, was often felt to have overridden professional concerns, especially when profit margins contributed to the economic survival of a drugstore. Many a druggist defended this by saying if he did not stock them, the public would just purchase them elsewhere, even from general stores. As early as 1842, Jacob Bell, the acknowledged founder of the Pharmaceutical Society of Great Britain, publicly raised concerns that druggists, who promoted the sale of secret remedies to any great extent, were ethically no better than "patent medicine vendors," often viewed as quacks.[149] The dilemma changed little over the next hundred years or so through the heyday of newspaper advertising of medicines up to the 1930s, when regulations were still relatively lax or not being enforced. Without question, druggists sold many over-the-counter medicines with little knowledge of their ingredients or of their actions beyond the often hyperbolic claims of manufacturers. Yet the very sale of such remedies in drugstores must have added validation to the claims discussed in Chapter 3. Furthermore, the very distinctive atmosphere of drugstores—different from any other store, as becomes clear in the discussion that follows—added an aura that tended to blur distinctions between commercialism and professionalism, at least up to the 1950s. The relatively small profession in Newfoundland illustrates this well, as it also typifies situations elsewhere.

Commercialism Expands

In the first half of the 1900s Newfoundland drugstores combined three elements: the ethos of the more professional, somewhat austere, British chemist and druggist shops that could be found in the fashionable parts of London and major cities; the commercialism and price-cutting that was emerging with chains of pharmacies on both sides of the Atlantic; and the small-town drugstore, serving as a community center.[150] Although competition between the relatively small number of drugstores could be intense, even in Newfoundland's small capital city of St. John's, with its two main streets—Water and Duckworth—running parallel to the harbor, senior pharmacists in Newfoundland remember the 1960s and earlier as relatively genteel times, certainly not cutthroat; indeed, as happened elsewhere, there was much cooperation, at least in loaning prescription ingredients to a fellow druggist who might have run out.[151]

Professional colleagueship in genteel times did not mean the absence of intensely competitive advertising, as intense in Newfoundland as in urban centers in Britain and the United States. What is clear from the Newfoundland advertising is that drugstores were hubs of much seasonal life in the local community. Aside from "straight advertising" of over-the-counter medicines—sometimes merely by appending the drugstore's name as "agent" to an overseas advertisement—a noteworthy feature for many years in St. John's was the regular "McMurdo's Store News." These were informative, chatty newspaper "notices"—a paragraph or so on the "latest arrivals" to the McMurdo drugstore, its "latest shipment" or "arrivals for the Christmas season," as well as information on trends, as when, in 1922, aspirin tablets were said to be "coming more and more in popular use [for] colds, slight cases of rheumatism, neuralgia, face-ache and headache." McMurdo's, like all drugstores, also paid particular attention to dental care and, particularly at Christmas, perfumery and toiletries, but not to the exclusion of, for example, the availability of "new two pound box of Park and Tilford's chocolates" (1912), Oxo cubes (1912), hair tonics (e.g., Quinine, 1917), ice cream (for "close, hot weather," July 1917), hot-water bottles (December 1917), and "breast pumps" (1922).[152]

The advertised medicines—from the United States, Britain, and Canada—were the same as or analogous to those already discussed in Chapter 3; for example, enzyme preparations and "Soda Mint and Pepsin Tablets [that] answer well for such stomach troubles as heartburn, water brash, sourness, distress after eating" (1912). As to be expected, advertising reflected seasonal concerns, such as fly paper in the summer to deal with "carriers of germs" and cold remedies in winter. Drugstores, too, carried their own successful in-house preparations, an indication that a good name could validate a medicine. In 1922 McMurdo's drugstore was selling McMurdo's Compound Syrup of Figs ("a gentle laxative medicine, specially adapted to ladies' and children's use"), McMurdo's Cres Cough Cure ("You cannot afford in summer, any more than in winter, to allow a cold or cough to gain a footing") and McMurdo's Compound Licorice Powder ("a gentle laxative"). As with most advertising, the "Store News" served to reinforce widely accepted concepts within and without the medical profession, such as the value of hypophosphites as a "nutritive" and "first rate nerve food" (see Box 4.2).

Gerald S. Doyle (1892-1956)

Although Newfoundland's highly successful entrepreneur, Gerald S. Doyle, was briefly noted in Chapter 1, further comments are appropriate, for he joins such internationally known entrepreneurs as Holloway, Ayer, and Beecham as candidates for a medicine's hall of fame. Although his fame was local, he illustrates a different path to socially validating medicines. Doyle's special forte was invoking community and patriotic feelings among Newfoundlanders; this translated into many years of successful sales trips aboard his boat, *Miss Newfoundland,* to countless outports—festive occasions with free samples of Life Savers and maybe drinks of rum. A legacy of "stories" about Doyle reveals added elements of showmanship. "One time in Fogo he threw a handful of Tru-Lax packets to a crowd on the wharf and the next day most of them had to stay home 'with the runs'—strong advertising indeed."[153]

Experiences as a youth in St. John's drugstores—he did not qualify as a druggist—stood Doyle in good stead. His career in selling a con-

---

BOX 4.2. Advertising

Drugstore advertising of medicines around 1900 was often long lists of available items, but this disappeared and all advertising became quite specific as in the following from "McMurdo's Store News":

> There are many people who, when the end of the year comes, need a good tonic. For this purpose we confidently recommend a bottle of Nutritive Hypophosphites; the experience our customers have had with it proves its value. Nutritive Hypophosphites is not only a general tonic but a medicine of great value in clearing up a chronic cough and preventing bronchial troubles, as well as being a first rate nerve food. Two sizes (about 50 and 100 average doses respectively), 50¢ and $1.

Source: The Evening Telegram, December 27, 1922, p. 4.

---

siderable range of over-the-counter medicines, health products, and a few sundries began around 1919 when he became a Newfoundland wholesale agent for the Chase Medicine Company. He soon added other lines and became a constant conduit for U.S. and Canadian companies. He did more than anyone to get Newfoundlanders to adopt such products as Dodd's Kidney Pills, Minard's Liniment, and Chase's Nerve Food—and to make them part of the island's folklore. Doyle's promotional machine was orientated to family, community, and the island. For example, his popular publication *The Family Fireside* contained newsy notes, births and deaths, and, of course, advertisements for Doyle's products. Another enterprise was his book of collected Newfoundland songs (first edition published in 1927), which, with advertisements for Doyle's products, was distributed throughout the island. This was but one version of many song books published during the first half of the twentieth century as part of medicines promotion (e.g., *The Alka-Seltzer Song Book* and *Watkins Song Book*).

As successful as these activities were, Doyle's promotional high point was the exploitation of advertising on radio from the early 1930s. His *Doyle Bulletin,* which was to become one of the most popular radio programs throughout the island from 1932 to 1964, added a distinctive chapter to "drug advertising on the radio."[154] Although it contained news, it was designed more for weather forecasts and personal messages for those in communities without telephones. "To Scott Clancy at Humber Mouth from Irene. Had treatment Saturday afternoon, took blood test yesterday morning and special test this afternoon. Awaiting report."[155] References to Doyle products were conspicuous (Box 4.3), but beyond that the program itself constantly etched the credibility of the Doyle name in the minds of New-foundlanders, a credibility that lay behind the success of his own line of "Newfoundland" products (bottled rather than manufactured by him): the Royal Blue Line included Cod Liver Oil, Essence of Ginger Wine, Camphorated Oil, Castor Oil, Olive Oil, Spirits of Nitre, Friar's Balsam, and Essence of Peppermint.[156] Of these, the cod-liver oil became the best known partly for its elegant blue bottle, said to protect the oil from sunlight.[157]

Community Centers

Entering a Newfoundland drugstore was little different from going into many chemists' shops in Britain or drugstores elsewhere in North America. Some had a soda fountain, such as had emerged in the United States before 1900, which fostered a role as a community center. When one fountain appeared in St. John's at M. F. Wadden's Drug Store in 1914, it "made the town talk," according to a promotional report that highlighted concerns over quality.[158] Success was said to be due to the "use of products of recognized quality only [e.g., Horlick's Malted Milk, the only genuine Coca-Cola]," keeping the business "progressive and up-to-date." Professional issues relating to the venture were also hinted at:

> Having opened a new Parlour in the rear of the store, Mr. Wadden managed to keep this business altogether separate from the general Drug business, but it is a very valuable side line and keeps the crowd ever going in and out of the store.

Another St. John's drugstore, McMurdo's, became the "place to go," partly because it "had a great soda fountain where all the lawyers and business people met every morning for breakfast. And Molly serving the egg sandwiches down there and so on."[159] Other stores, even without fountains, had distinctive "events," such as the lunchtime poker games held at Parson's drugstore during the 1920s and 1930s.[160] Elsewhere, "doctors used to drop into the various pharmacies socially. Maybe have a cigar and cigarette. This was a time when

---

BOX 4.3. Advertising on Gerald Doyle's Radio "Bulletin," 1953

And now before the weather, a word about Doyle's household medicines. Doyle's blue bottle medicines have long been in brisk demand in Newfoundland for high grade household medicine in daily use in thousands of Newfoundland homes for many years. With the coming of winter, every medicine chest should be completely stocked with Doyle's first quality friar's balsam, castor oil, sweet spirits of nitre, camphorated oil, ginger wine, essence of peppermint, and olive oil. Remember the sign of good quality is the popular blue bottle, long associated with high grade Newfoundland Cod Liver Oil, prepared and bottled solely by Gerald S. Doyle Limited. The same fine quality can be found in Doyle's household medicines. These everyday remedies have been tried over the years by thousands of our people all over the island and have proven their worth time after time. The quality in Doyle's royal blue line is completely protected by the famous blue bottle which prevents light from penetrating to the contents of the bottle. Ask for Doyle's blue bottle medicines wherever you shop. They're available at leading dealers all over Newfoundland. For quality you can depend on, always insist on the royal blue line, the finest in its field.

Dr. Chase's Nerve Food can help you get natural rest night after night. Start today with Dr. Chase's Nerve Food. Dr. Chase's Nerve Food is a time tested tonic thousands use to help improve general health. Dr. Chase's Nerve Food contains blood improving iron, vitamin B, and other necessary minerals. These work together to help build up your whole system. When you take Dr. Chase's Nerve Food, you can feel better, eat better, have steadier nerves, more restful nights. Take the first step toward better general health with Dr. Chase's Nerve Food. It can help you feel better all day long, rest better all night through.

Say are you catching cold? Reach for Dr. Chase Cold Tablets now. Dr. Chase Cold Tablets with four proven cold fighting ingredients stop miserable cold symptoms in just 24 hours. Be ready for the cold season with Dr. Chase Cold Tablets.

Source: MUNFLA-NAC tapes 83B/C by kind permission of Canadian Broadcasting Corporation

---

there was a more laid-back atmosphere."[161] Recollections indicate that the Newfoundland pharmacy was more British than American in character up to the 1950s, "in style and everything," which extended beyond the shop fittings to importing British products for dispensing, and using books—the *British Pharmaceutical Codex* ("the blue one"), and the *Squire's Companion* ("the red one")—for daily reference. Drugstores contrasted sharply with other stores in the "high street" or "main street." Up to around the 1960s, drugstores in Newfoundland were distinguished by the mixed aromas of medicines permeating the air. They were often relatively small establishments with distinctive furnishings, such as show globes or carboys for windows; elegant glass-fronted, labeled, and other shop rounds on the wooden shelves of handsome cabinets; and medicine bottles bearing the embossed name of the drugstore.

Professional Services

The settings just described—informality amid a distinctive atmosphere that was different and perhaps a little intimidating—fascinated many people. "I used to love to go in the drug store. I loved the smell of it."[162] Customers were often there for counterprescribing. Although the druggist's authority was always secondary to that of the doctor, this did not apply to minor ailments, and most druggists were in demand in the early decades of the 1900s up to the 1950s.[163]

> I tell you now, you weren't always running to the doctor. The druggist would fix you. And that would be about sixty or seventy cents. When you had a bit of cold then everything was mixed. My mother would say, "Go over to Peter O'Mara." He was a druggist on Water Street West. Mr. O'Mara would say, "Have you got a sore throat? Do you find it hard to swallow?" You could be a little husky, too. Well, he'd mix up something for you and that was great.[164]

Aside from cough medicines (perhaps the one that was "lovely, a lot of licorice in it"),[165] customers well remember that druggists mixed tonics, or sold nonbrand products such as bitterchips. The latter, quassia wood, was for preparing a hairwash to keep away lice: "Mother put them in an old saucepan or something and let it simmer, and when it was simmered, take it off and let it cool, and she'd put that on our hair."[166] An alternative head-lice treatment—and a somewhat toxic one—was a mercury preparation (ammoniated mercury powder) sold as "five cents worth," which interestingly might have had side effects in children.[167]

Druggists' recollections of counterprescribing point to a wide variety of prescribed preparations which were sometimes referred to as *nostrums*. Although the term actually refers to preparations made by the druggist it was commonly used for all over-the-counter preparations. Druggists often adapted formulae gathered from elsewhere. The shop's recipe notebook of McMurdo's, for example, indicated "Dick's" Cough Mixture—a fairly complex formula of chlorodyne, compound tincture of camphor (paregoric), tinctures of squill and ipecacuanha, spirit of nitrous ether (sweet spirit of nitre), syrup of chloroform, and syrup.[168] Included in the recipe notebook was Newfoundland Fly Dope, a locally known formula created by St. John's physician Cluny Macpherson to deal with black flies; it contained quinine, wool fat, cod-liver oil, and a fragrance.

In addition to over-the-counter prescribing, druggists provided first aid: "If you cut yourself, your mother would take you to the drug store instead of to the doctor."[169] Cost was also a factor:

> There weren't many people who could afford to go to a doctor at 50 cents a visit. Someone came in with a boil, you'd cover it with a dressing to draw it. Say to them, come back the next morning and let me take it off. The core of the boil is exposed and you just take it out.[170]

Although I have suggested a "buyer beware" attitude was relevant with respect to over-the-counter remedies, reminiscences of Newfoundland pharmacists suggest that, up to the 1960s, a strong sense of moral responsibility existed toward the community and individuals and their economic circumstances, an attitude certainly not limited to Newfoundland. Obviously this was a critical aspect of professionalism, whatever legislation to "protect the public" was in place. It became, for example, an issue when opportunities arose to capitalize on public fears during an outbreak of a disease, such as promoting gargles or throat pastilles during the Spanish flu outbreak in the last months of 1918.[171] Until Britain's Dangerous Drugs Act of 1920, the only safeguard there was against the abuse of opiates in over-the-counter preparations was the integrity of individual pharmacists.[172]

Quality of Dispensed Medicines

Ethical issues are discussed in Chapter 5, but here I note some considerations about dispensing, which, had they been generally known, may well have created some concerns for Mr. Brown or Ms. Smith. One well-remembered practice follows:

> If someone came in and said, "Make me up something, I don't want anything on the shelf, boy, you know," the druggist would go in the dispensary and put up a little bottle of the same ingredients and put a label on it. Instead of putting the Diarrhoea Mixture label on it, you'd put "Take two teaspoonfuls after each loose movement," and stick a "Shake Well" label on it.[173]

The issue was that the cost of the latter (e.g., seventy-five cents) was higher than the fifty-cent version on the shelf. Another ethical matter was the sale of aspirin as "headache" tablets, "neuralgia" tablets, or "cold" tablets. "Whatever you asked for, that's what you got." Headache tablets, "neatly" wrapped and tied with "red string," commanded a higher price.[174] Keeping customers waiting, even when a medicine was taken straight out of a stock bottle, was also noted by druggists as "good" practice.

If any pangs of conscience existed over the higher charge, it could be rationalized as fostering placebo action. As one druggist said,

> You'd get a patient who was hooked on, we will say, Amytal, which is a barbiturate drug, and you fill them with sugar or lactose. But they worked. The patient got the same relief from them as from the original capsule. It didn't always work, but it did play a role.[175]

The matter of professional integrity was constantly raised by druggists themselves in repeated public announcements about their careful and accurate dispensing—announcements that changed little over time. For example, an advertisement from the 1860s stated: "Physicians' Prescriptions carefully compounded at all hours, and orders answered with care and dispatch. Our stock of Medicines is complete, warranted genuine, and of the best quality."[176] Somewhat more overt, but not atypical, was a 1900 statement:

True and Honest Dispensing

True and honest dispensing is an absolute necessity when medicines are prescribed by the physician. Our dispensing department is conducted on such perfected plans that errors are impossible. Strict attention to business, pure drugs and low prices have won for us a large measure of public confidence.[177]

And in 1928: "Our Motto:—ACCURACY, PURITY AND PROMPTNESS. All work is done by Registered Pharmacists and is re-checked before being sent out."[178]

What could the public expect from their druggists in terms of quality of medicines? How did people choose a particular drugstore? Did they take into account such promotion as "ACCURACY, PURITY and PROMPTNESS"? To what extent did choice of store depend on a druggist's authority/personality, the friendliness of the store (perhaps it offered a favorite soda during a wait for a prescription), or convenience of location? Was the price of a dispensed medicine cheaper at one store than another?

No general answers can be given to these questions; all such considerations, singly or combined, had relevance at times. At least no evidence has been found that Newfoundland physicians recommended patients to use particular drugstores, as happened elsewhere, or that they took a batch of prescriptions to their favorite store for a "commission."[179] On the other hand, the concern of many physicians with ensuring quality is reflected in their requests for specific brands to be used in the compounding of their prescriptions. Druggists were likewise mindful of the quality of products, which in Newfoundland meant "buying British":

My father told me one time about a doctor who came into the store and said, "Where do you buy your powders and salts?" Father replied, "I buy them from England, Burrough's Wellcome, and Evans Sons." And the doctor said, "Yes, I thought so. You buy quality stuff. Now, I saw a bottle of medicine made on my prescription and it was practically solid. You could hardly shake it." He guessed that someone had bought it, a cheaper brand, on this side of the water, be it American or Canadian, and the quality wasn't there. We would always be interested in buying something that had quality. Quality pays. Now, Burroughs Wellcome, the name was magic. The quality, the standards, were so high, the degree of purity.[180]

Aside from companies with good reputations, important items for dispensing generally met the standards of the *British Pharmacopoeia* or the *British Pharmaceutical Codex.*[181] However, there remained the quality of dispensing. Druggists' reminiscences from the 1990s often paint the period up to the 1950s or so as particularly "professional." In doing so, they are largely referring to the skills required in compounding medicines, especially those with multiple ingredients: "Of course the compounding wasn't simply putting them all together," as with, for example, the "cough mixture of ammonium carbonate, liquid extract of licorice and Spirits of Chloroform: . . . If you put your chloroform in that before you put your licorice you would get a curd. Now if you added the licorice to the powder first, then shook it up, you got a high foam;" on adding the chloroform to this, "the foam disappears and you get a beautiful brown mixture, like coffee."[182]

The recollection is of a time when dispensing mixtures required considerable knowledge and skills as reflected in a variety of texts addressed to physicians and druggists that highlighted constant contemporary concerns over chemical and therapeutic incompatibilities. Examples include such titles as *Essentials of Prescription Writing* (1913); *The Science and Art of Prescribing* (1919); *A Treatise on Prescription Incompatibilities and Difficulties: Including Prescription Oddities and Curiosities* (1919); and *The Students' Pocket Prescriber and Guide to Prescription Writing* (1941).[183] These are in addition to the texts directed to students and druggists, of which the many British editions of the *Art of Dispensing* was particularly popular in Newfoundland.

Although patients had no way of knowing whether a dispensed medicine met appropriate standards, appearances and taste sometimes indicated an inferior product, such as when an emulsion had been improperly prepared so that the oil separated out. Perhaps, too, their dispensed bottle of medicine came out of a "stock bottle," purchased from a manufacturer, or were solid dosage forms (tablets or capsules) increasingly popular among some physicians.

Druggists and Validation

As "second class" to doctors, druggists did not acquire authority over medicines as readily as physicians. Despite the uneasy boundary between business and professional services, Newfoundland pharmacy—a microcosm of elsewhere—suggests that the distinctiveness of drugstores, the emergence of gatekeeping roles for druggists, and the many professional services they provided gave them a social stature. If, as seemingly was happening in the United States, this declined somewhat up to the 1930s, an accepted level of professional service was maintained. With regard to the specific question whether druggists contributed to public acceptance and validation of medicines, many a Mr. Brown and Ms. Smith found authoritative help amid what was often an atmosphere of handsome furnishings and distinctive odor; even though some found this somewhat intimidating, it was nonthreatening. There was much to encourage patients' and customers' faith and confidence even if they did not ask questions: "Years ago, nobody asked questions. Nobody. They'd just come in, pick up their prescription. Never said, 'What is it for? Should I take it with water? Should I take it before or after meals?'"[184]

Chapter 5

Certainty? Maybe, Maybe Not: 1950 to 2000

Suddenly he sat bolt upright, looked piercingly at me, and cried, "Damn you, you didn't cure me," and fell back. A few minutes later he died. I went home depressed and disquieted. I asked myself, was I trying to play God. My knowledge was so limited.

Newfoundland physician[1]

THE CHALLENGES OF CHANGE

The avalanche of new medicines in the 1940s to 1950s cemented hopes of conquering disease fostered by such earlier breakthroughs as sulfonamides, penicillin, and streptomycin. The public was generally optimistic that the chemist's laboratory could offer better medicines than the plant kingdom with its "natural" products. A 1959 book about pharmaceutical companies referred to them as the "Merchants of Life" and offered an utopian prediction: "while disease has not been entirely eliminated, man in the second half of the twentieth century is closer than ever before in realizing his race-old hopes of health and long life."[2] Not appreciated at the time, however, was the lack of preparedness to meet the tensions and uncertainties that the new medicines, along with ethical dilemmas raised by technology, effected over the following decades. Such tensions ultimately did much to alter the worlds of medicine and pharmacy by forcing greater accountability to patients and the public.

If tensions were unforeseen, so was the increasing professional power of physicians as a result of their gatekeeping roles, which expanded with the growth of prescription-only medicines and new technology for diagnostic tests, as well as the extension of health considerations into lifestyles. Yet whether new gatekeeping power necessarily enhanced professional authority and social standing is questionable. After all, it has been noted that a widespread view exists that physician authority declined in the second half of the century. Clearly, it suffered challenges from various directions that undoubtedly had a cumulative impact; for example, challenges from nonphysician health care administrators, controls on medical practice by government and private medical insurance schemes, new clinical aspirations in the nursing profession, consumerism, self-help groups and increased lay knowledge of medicines, malpractice suits, the growth of complementary/alternative medicine, and antiscience and antivivisection movements.[3]

Although such considerations affected medicine on both sides of the Atlantic, challenges were often reinforced by national or regional sociopolitical factors. Sociologists pointing out considerations in Canada (by now including Newfoundland) refer to the rapid spread of government-sponsored medical insurance outside of Saskatchewan, the series of provincial and federal studies of health problems that, implicitly or explicitly, urged diminishing the overwhelming power of the medical profession to control health care, and the doctors' strikes that highlighted extra-billing as an issue, i.e., charging patients more than government insurance would pay.[4]

In short, there are reasons to believe that the second half of the 1900s saw some uncoupling of the close association of the power of the medical profession and public respect and trust (on which more is said later), that impinged on attitudes toward medicines.

Challenges to medicine raised levels of uncertainty in the public mind, beyond the inherent uncertainty that always exists about health and the outcomes of treatment.[5] A key area of uncertainty surrounded synthetic remedies—technological bullets as some saw them—and their side effects. There was always hope that medical science could bring certainty to health care. Although science continued into the 1960s to be viewed as beneficent and with the optimism that it would triumph over disease (new "wonder drugs" were thought to be just around the corner), historians and other commentators have argued that the triumphal march of medicine, particularly that driven by the pharmaceutical industry, faltered in the last decades of the twentieth century. James Le Fanu, for instance, talks of the "fall of medicine" due, in part, to a declining number of new "breakthroughs" from the early 1970s onward; in fact, discussions on enhancing innovation became a conspicuous part of the medicines story.[6]

Side effects of medicines also fueled uncertainty. Building on problems with sulfa medications (from the 1930s) and cortisone (from around 1950), and the growing concerns in the 1940s and 1950s over the misuse of and addiction to amphetamines and barbiturates, public alarm grew with the horror story of limbless children born in the early 1960s to mothers who had taken thalidomide during early pregnancy.[7] In contrast to incapacitating side effects, relatively benign lifestyle interruptions brought frustrations, such as dealing with the "cheese reaction"—hypertension induced by eating cheese when taking antidepressant monoamine oxidase inhibitors—recognized in the late 1960s.[8] New "bibles" of side effects, such as the now classic *Meyler's Side Effects of Drugs,* indexed growing worries. Continuously published since 1951, it was joined by the equally invaluable *Side Effects of Drugs Annual* in 1977.

Whatever the concerns, the century ended with a continuing commitment to synthetic medicines supported by new methods (e.g., cloned genes) to discover medicines with specific effects on receptors. This gave new meaning to the term *designer drugs*—used in the 1990s to describe recreational drugs that initially escaped legal restrictions—by extending the term to scientifically designed chemicals that might allow specific treatments for specific individuals.

Documenting at least some of the complexity of the second half of the twentieth century leaves relatively little space to consider over-the-counter medicines. However, even though the use of over-the-counter medicines remained high and even increased, prescription-only medicines became much more dominant. In the United States in 1939—as in Britain and elsewhere—over-the-counter preparations were, in value terms, more important than prescription medicines. By 1947, however, prescriptions in the United States already had a value 50 percent higher than over-the-counter products; by 1954 sales were three times higher with the relative proportion continuing to rise.[9] The ascendancy of laboratory-made, prescription-only medicines from the 1950s changed the nature of patients' choices because most were promoted to physicians only (as ethical pharmaceuticals), at least until the 1980s in the United States. Then a new U.S. policy allowed prescription medicines to be advertised directly to the public, a vexing concept for many other countries (see discussion on relationships with the pharmaceutical industry in Chapter 6).

Another major difference between the two halves of the century was an extension of the power of government and of the pharmaceutical industry as validators of medicines. Yet amid increasing controls from the state and efforts to bring greater certainty to the use of medicines, public suspicions from the 1950s and 1960s onward about safety were fed by perceptions that government testing schemes were not sufficiently independent of influences from the pharmaceutical industry. Amid this and the wider challenges to the authority of medicine, doctors, as prescribers of medicines, as researchers in clinical trials of medicines, and as key purveyors of information to patients, did retain a significant, though increasingly shared, role in the social acceptance and validation of medicines. ("You had to rely on doctors, but the druggist could help with side effects."[10]) It is no wonder, from what has just been stated, that concerns over medicines are often interwoven with questions about the professionalism of practitioners. As one senior Newfoundlander commented:

> We believe in medicines today, yes, but not as much as we did way back. Because like the feller said, it was ground into you and that was it. But now, half the people going says what the doctors is doing, and the drugstores, is just to make money and they don't care how you feel; but in them days there was no money involved at all. It was just the medicine. They'd really go after the complaint you had and give it the whole thing and you believed in them and it got better.[11]

VALIDATION, REJECTION, AMBIVALENCE, AND FOUR THEMES

It is in such settings of questioned authority that the following, according to a British psychiatrist, was all too typical of a consultation in the 1990s. A woman, in her late twenties or early thirties, depressed after the birth of her first child, is given an antidepressant after a relatively brief consultation with a primary care physician. She is further frustrated when, after referral to a psychiatrist, she is again prescribed medication; she had hoped the latter would talk with her or offer hypnotherapy.[12]

Such situations are compounded not only from the questioning of authority, but also from personal beliefs, expectations, and knowledge—for example, are medicines to be seen as "magic bullets," as less safe than "natural" remedies, or as agents to help control one's life (such as family size or freedom from anxiety)?[13] These and other considerations, especially the emphasis on science to validate medicines, point to something of a paradox, namely the widespread public acceptance and validation by the 1980s and 1990s of complementary/alternative medicine, despite castigation by physicians and the absence of scientific "proof" of efficacy.

This chapter and the next illuminate the paradox by exploring the shaping of diverse public attitudes toward medicines. I do this in the context of four overlapping themes that run throughout the fifty years. Each, however, was particularly conspicuous at one particular time, which allows them to be introduced in essentially chronological order.

The first theme, accommodating new remedies, focuses particularly on the 1950s up to around 1970. Not only does this give a sense of transition from the first half century but it also raises issues that were constantly relevant in later years. The second theme, patients' dependence on physicians, emerging at the same time as the first, takes us to the late 1960s and 1970s and centers on what can be called the "prescription-only era."

A third theme, overt public questioning of medicines, becomes evident in the 1960s. Despite dependence on prescription medicines, growing public uneasiness becomes obvious. The fourth theme, changing therapeutic relationships, covers responses to, rather than a mere questioning of, the power and authority of the medical profession and of other "experts" on medicines. New relationships between doctor and patient were arising in which treatment decisions involved negotiation, as it were—more than writing and dispensing a prescription "to be taken three times a day."

I cannot overstress that the themes ran parallel and sometimes melded into one another. Depending on their outlook and circumstances, some individuals, perhaps with great faith in medical progress, were comfortable with their dependence on physicians' decisions and medicines throughout the second half of the twentieth century; on the other hand, the questioning of side effects by others or proactive support for alternative medicine (the third theme) readily led many to negotiate treatment with their physician (the fourth theme). The themes, then, cover the diversity of people's attitudes to medicines, attitudes that might change even during the course of an illness, especially if it is chronic or life-threatening.

Catching Up: A Background

In examining the four themes existing on both sides of the Atlantic, the example of Newfoundland helps to sharpen thinking about issues facing less developed regions. Distinctive about Newfoundland was its mind-set of catching up with mainland Canada after confederation in 1949. Such a mind-set can be readily found in rural areas elsewhere. The relative buoyancy of the years following World War II was encouraged by feelings of scientific progress fueled by a host of events in the 1950s, ranging from the determination of the structure of DNA (1952) to the first kidney transplants, albeit with high failure rates and ethical questions about experimentation and expensive treatment.[14] Yet the strong optimism for a bright future was tempered in Newfoundland with concerns whether real change could happen and be sustained. Many recognized that economic advances during the previous fifty years were spread inconsistently around the world, even in countries such as the United States with its striking disparities in both rates of disease and life expectancy among different social groups.[15]

In some respects confederation with Canada replaced Newfoundland's colonial status and dependency with feelings of being a have-not province. Mitigating this, however, was a pervasive optimism for a brighter future promised by confederation. Shortly thereafter, the replacement of much boat transportation by roads in the 1950s and 1960s—to give one example—led to some blunting of rural and urban differences in health care that had long been underway in other places where the automobile replaced the horse and buggy and winter sleigh. Although this did not necessarily alter negative and condescending urban views of rural life, it meant that the heroic house calls, undertaken by doctors in horrendous winter conditions, faded into history and folklore.

Also emerging, though as a pale shadow of the universal British National Health Service (implemented in 1948), were provincial/national health programs beginning in the 1950s to be capped by far-reaching changes brought about by Canada's national Medicare system (the Federal Medical Care Act of 1966), although implemented to different levels of service by the various provinces and territories.[16] Newfoundland services, commencing April 1, 1969 (without payment for medicines), met muted comment from *The Evening Telegram:* "How far reaching can it be if the supply of doctors is inadequate?"[17] The medical profession, too, saw new horizons and felt a need to "belong" to the growing arena of global medicine. The first issue of a mimeographed *Newsletter Newfoundland Medical Association* (1958) commented that

> a subtle but significant change has been taking place in the medical profession in Newfoundland. It has become large, cosmopolitan and diverse in its makeup, and its rather parochial point of view has been giving way to awareness of its significance in the medical picture in North America.[18]

Some months later the president of the Newfoundland Pharmaceutical Association, in looking for "closer liaison with the medical profession," wrote an upbeat piece for the same newsletter. After pointing out pharmacy's contributions to "the betterment of health in the world," the president stressed that Newfoundland pharmacy "has made, and is still making, tremendous strides" with "higher standards today than ever before."[19]

If these were somewhat rosy pictures of change, as some undoubtedly felt, the medical optimism was based on the demonstrated potential of some new medicines, such as penicillin and streptomycin (specifically its use for tuberculosis). Although poliomyelitis took its toll in Newfoundland as elsewhere, the introduction of Salk (1952) and Sabin (1954) polio vaccines were among other medical "triumphs" that were tellingly highlighted on the island by a 1959 outbreak among unvaccinated children.[20] Specialist medical care, also contributing to a sense of catch-up, had an increasingly pervasive role in shaping medicine, especially in the United States during the first half of the twentieth century.[21] In Newfoundland, however, specifically trained specialists did not appear until the 1950s and 1960s (although some physicians always developed specialty areas). Their contributions soon offered a sense of advancement.[22]

Although it is impossible to measure the precise impact of the mind-set of catch-up on the acceptance of medicines, it undoubtedly fostered demands for the new ones. Change, however, was relatively slow. Conservatism on the part of physicians and patients offered some reluctance to push aside long-standing tonics. Moreover, on looking back to the 1950s and 1960s, Newfoundland seniors say that new medicines and dependence on doctors contributed to a decline in traditional values (e.g., ingenuity and self-reliance) and, as also documented in the United States, in traditional self-care, in which "you had faith," though the extent to which this was recognized at the time is unclear.[23]

If the feeling of catch-up in Newfoundland had diminished somewhat by the 1980s (even amid the constant shortage of physicians), expectations of improvements in health care continued; for example, the Canada Health Act of 1984 was interpreted as offering Canadians health care as a "right" rather than a "privilege."[24] At home, Memorial University of Newfoundland, opened in 1969, also added to a sense of health as a right in so far as it was seen by the public to serve the province rather than Canadian medicine as a whole. It was just one of some thirty medical schools that opened in North America in the 1960s and 1970s.[25] One impetus, as in Newfoundland, was concern over shortages of general practitioners—forecasts of their "extinction" existed in the United States—especially in rural areas. The Newfoundland school, also a catalyst to improve quality of care in general, challenged Newfoundland's "inferiority complex," which felt a successful Newfoundland school was impossible.[26] Matching at least the standards of the mainland was as important for the island as it was for accreditation of the school.

In the 1970s, the school moved with The General Hospital to a brand-new building designated as "The Health Sciences Centre"—the language of "modern" medicine.[27] The school also linked Newfoundland with the research thrust characterizing medicine elsewhere. One notable area was hypertension. Both the 1950s' concern about the amount of salt fish and salt meat eaten (the substantial salt intake was thought to lie behind the high incidence of the condition) and a 1960s' survey to see whether Newfoundlanders were particularly prone to hypertension were premedical school skirmishes with the problem; subsequent research activity in the school indicated that "high blood pressure was more prevalent [in Newfoundland] than in other areas of North America, Great Britain or Ireland."[28]

Although the measurement of blood pressure was a "universal desire" among patients in some Newfoundland communities in the 1960s, such that it made the doctor's "rounds of house calls slow,"[29] the research program helped to heighten public awareness and the need for treatment, of which a wide range of vigorously promoted medications had appeared since the 1950s. On looking back, some critics consider that, generally speaking, treatment for hypertension initially overemphasized medication rather than lifestyle and diet.[30] The high salt content in Newfoundland diet, however, was well appreciated, and appropriate advice was given. Nevertheless, as with the brown flour story, changing lifestyles was easier to talk about than to accomplish; noncompliance, to be discussed in Chapter 6, extended beyond medicines to other aspects of health care. In short, this characterizes much of the catching-up period in Newfoundland, namely looking for and hoping for parity with elsewhere, only to face stumbling blocks intrinsic and extrinsic to the island, but not unique to it.

THEME 1: ACCOMMODATING NEW MEDICINES

Dear Doc, please send me some hopping pills for my wife. They made her hop all around and she was able to work again. [She] draws the water, tends the garden and cuts the wood.

From a letter to a Newfoundland physician[31]

Although new medicines were often received enthusiastically by physicians and the public alike, the majority entered without public fanfare. In endeavoring to understand the diversity of medicines—over the counter and prescription—in use at the time, it cannot be overemphasized that the lengthy list of new medicines marketed in the 1950s and 1960s did not sweep aside the old ones as quickly as often supposed. Although marketing strategies were key issues, much depended on the conservatism and prudence of physicians in their choice of a new medication over an existing product. Relevant, too, was whether patients were aware of new medicines advertised to physicians only, asked for them, and could afford them. The persistence and continued popularity of many "old" medicines depended on local conditions; many perhaps fared less well in, say, Britain when the National Health Service allowed ready access to new prescription medicines.[32]

In discussing here the acceptance of new medicines, I begin with the 1950s, a transition period before serious public questioning of new medicines had emerged. In looking at three broad topics—existing popular medicines, conservative or prudent doctors, and costs—the primary issue is curtailment of choice in physician prescribing.

Existing Medicines: Easy to Replace?

At the end of the 1950s and into the 1960s, Mr. Brown or Ms. Smith, sensing the end of a visit with his or her Newfoundland doctor, commonly said, "I'd like a tonic, doctor," a request that had commonly faded elsewhere. In response, a bottle of Maltlevol—an iron-vitamin preparation of ferric ammonium citrate, liver extract, malt and vitamins, popular on the island at the time as an over-the-counter remedy—was often prescribed by Newfoundland doctors, especially for female patients.[33] The complaints of one such patient, "run down, loss of energy, worse in morning," were typical of many.[34] Around 1960, the doctor of this patient still prescribed many other "bottles" of medicine increasingly viewed as old fashioned, for example, Mist. Alk. Kidney, Mist. Benylin Expect, Mist. Rheum, and, occasionally, laudanum.

Maltlevol offers an interesting illustration of the transition from general tonics (for improving appetite and strengthening the body as a whole) to vitamins, although the latter were also promoted as tonics for many years as part of what one author has called "vitamania."[35] A commentator on the British vitamin scene in 1959 would surely have seen Newfoundland practices in the same light; he noted that multivitamin preparations were abused by being taken "when there is no recognizable indication for them. The public wrongly believes them to be tonics [as they continued to do] and demand their prescription."[36] In fact, liquid tonics, with their distinctive tastes, retained a strong following in Newfoundland relative to solid-dose vitamin preparations throughout the 1960s. One indication is the local success of one Newfoundland physician who, in the 1960s, developed his own formula for his elderly patients, one that completed the "family" of tonic/vitamin preparations (i.e., in addition to Maltlevol and Infantol). He called his preparation—which was a "beautiful orange color" mixture of Infantol, Benylin, and Dexedrine—"Granitol."[37] This is not to say that numerous Newfoundlanders—perhaps influenced by the marketing success of Gerald Doyle (Chapter 4)—like millions of people elsewhere, had not already made the transition to solid-dose "vitamin" preparations by this time.

Anyone asking doctors for tonics in the 1950s and 1960s was continuing a long-established tradition. Aside from antibiotics and some prescribing of new hypertensive and other treatments, most patients in the 1950s did not feel any radical change in the overall character of medicines from earlier decades. The sense of continuity was also fostered by favorite over-the-counter medicines that survived World War II. For instance, competing with such tonic wines as Wincarnis and Beef Iron Wine was the well-advertised Buckfast Tonic Wine (containing potassium and sodium phosphates, sodium glycerophosphate, and caffeine).[38] Prepared by the Benedictine Monks of Buckfast Abbey in Devon, England (and "obtainable at all Druggists and Grocers"), this preparation proclaimed that it restored "lost vigour and jaded nerves."[39]

While Maltlevol and tonic wines were popular, they were still competing with cod-liver oil, the perennial favorite for maintaining health. When it looked as though its popularity was beginning to fade in Newfoundland, never mind elsewhere, Gerald Doyle responded with one of his advertising blitzes in 1954 with such headline copy for Brick's Tasteless Cod Liver Oil as: "Will Help People in Getting Over the 'Flu,'"[40] "Gives Good Appetite After Taking it a Few Days,"[41] and "Will Help You Make Rapid Recovery After Sickness." The "tonic" value was still being stressed: "Sometimes it takes a long while to recover from the effects of even an ordinary cold, and at such times Brick's Tasteless—the tonic that gives a good appetite for wholesome food—is very helpful as it restores strength and thus hastens recovery."[42] Brick's competition included Doyle's own brand promoted as a "great resistance-builder now that the season is here when something extra is needed to build resistance."[43]

An equally strong 1950s' sense of continuity with the past came from the still-popular kidney medicines, Chase's Liver and Kidney Pills, Dodd's Pills, Gin Pills and, as a "runner-up" in Newfoundland, Cystex Pills (Chapter 3). Although, as noted already, the character of advertising over-the-counter medicines had changed in the 1930s, particularly through prohibitions on mentioning treatments for certain diseases, many old concepts and claims continued into the 1950s and beyond. If Chase's Kidney-Liver Pills advertisements (e.g., "Lost Your Bounce Because of Backache?") merely implied such concepts as autointoxication,[44] Dodd's Kidney Pills—more intensely promoted on the island at the time—continued to focus on tiredness due to "excess acids and wastes" in the bloodstream. For example, "When kidneys fail to remove excess acids and wastes, backache, tired feeling, disturbed rest often follow."[45] If Newfoundlanders wanted medical confirmation that acidosis was still an issue, they had only to be patients of physician Cluny Macpherson, who was still prescribing "acidosis" mixtures in the 1950s.[46]

Another kidney medicine, Cystex Pills, was promoted for controlling germs; however, as good, persuasive advertising copy for the time, it also referred to "acid." Specifically it was claimed that Cystex: "1. Helps nature remove certain irritating non-specific germs in acid conditions. 2. Relieves Rheumatic Pains and tired, achy feeling due to colds. 3. By relieving and calming irritated Bladder tissues it helps reduce frequent or smarting passages day and night."[47]

Other international favorites, as popular in Britain, the United States, and mainland Canada as in Newfoundland, to survive with little change in promotional language through the 1950s and after, included "health foods" such as OXO (to avoid weakness and illness, "the vital properties of fresh lean Beef fortify and stimulate the body"[48]), Ovaltine (to help relieve "nervous tension," and to aid "relaxation for complete sleep"[49]), Ironized Yeast (to build "strength fast!"), and Virol (for "strong and healthy children"). There were, too, "gentle" laxatives such as Andrew's Sparkling Effervescent Salt for "upset stomach, biliousness, irregularity," and Eno's Fruit Salt (also a mild antacid) taken for a "bad stomach."[50]

Despite the continuing presence of the remedies just discussed, the writing was on the wall for countless others by around 1960. Some were becoming old fashioned partly from the fading of popular concepts, thus weakening validation. *Time* (1960) noted that in the United States such favorites as Hill's Cascara Quinine and Bromo Quinine "retain a faithful but shrinking following." Such preparations were said to have been "crowded to the side of druggists' counters by supposedly more sophisticated products of the antibiotic, antihistamine age," such as Coricidin, "combining APC [aspirin, phenacetin, and caffeine] with a small enough dose of the anti-histamine Chlor-Trimeton."[51] In succeeding years other old favorites were subject to additional regulatory pressures. For example, in the wake of the U.S. Federal Trade Commission's truth-in-advertising campaign, Dr. Chase's Nerve Food removed "nerve," Dodd's Kidney Pills, "kidney," Carter's Little Liver Pills, "liver," and, from the promotion of analgesics all references to "nervous tension"—the words being viewed as misleading.[52]

Local or regional remedies were often at the forefront of casualties from new regulations. This happened to those manufactured in Newfoundland, in part through new Canadian federal regulations in 1953 mandating inspection of manufacturing as well as the catch-up mindset in Newfoundland encouraging the use of new products.[53] The situation was in some ways reminiscent of the time when the convenience of commercial over-the-counter preparations displaced many "folk medicine" practices, even though many lingered in memory for decades. Such lingering was often called upon to underscore progress by stressing the "primitiveness" of medicines of the past. Long remembered is the regimen of heating salt fish in a sock and then tying the sock around the neck to treat a sore throat: "The steam from it, the vapour from the hot salt around your neck in no time would take it off you."[54]

Selective Welcome for New Medicines, Costs, and Retiring the Old

Conservative or Prudent Doctors

A 1959 U.S. study on the "Social Processes in Physicians' Adoption of a New Drug" indicated that sixteen and seventeen months after the introduction of a new medicine that competed with two older drugs of the same general type, only 22 percent of the doctors were prescribing the new one exclusively, and 20 percent were prescribing all three.[55] Clearly, the acceptance of many new medicines is far from straightforward.

Just as the existing popular medicines established an aura of continuity into the 1950s, even to the 1960s, many patients found little change in prescription medicines from the old days. Although in some instances this might be viewed as physician resistance to change, in many cases it was conservatism or more often, according to physician's recollections of the period, "prudence." Experiences with, for example, the side effects of sulfonamides and allergic responses to penicillin had had a salutary effect.[56] It is noteworthy that, although cost was a consideration, the new medicine cortisone was not prescribed for rheumatoid arthritis by some Newfoundland physicians up to around 1960 (neither were many other new medicines).[57]

Conservative or prudent prescribers were constantly contrasted during the rest of the century with liberal prescribers. In 1984, British physician Michael Rawlins said that some pharmaceutical companies categorized general practitioners as "conservatives" or "risk-takers" and used different marketing strategies for the two groups. "Risk-takers" were much more prepared to try new lines, and sales representatives "will try to obtain a commitment from them to use their new products on a few patients in the first place."[58] An ongoing issue was the strong sense that physicians in general were not prepared or did not have the knowledge base to deal critically with the avalanche of new information. In the 1950s, sales representatives with vested interests were even reaching remote parts of Newfoundland; moreover, the new medicines could not be ignored as they were often promoted as having no existing counterpart, for conditions ranging from infections to hypertension. Criticisms that physicians capitulated to drug companies had validity, but the pressures on physicians were substantial.

It must also be recognized that conservative physicians were not always slow to respond to new medications. Some, for instance, soon welcomed minor tranquilizers to replace barbiturates with the hope of reducing abuse and suicide. One respected and influential British practitioner noted that the new medications

promised to cause less dependence. I looked after many patients who were chronically anxious and I had reason to give relatively high importance to mental as opposed to physical suffering. Experience with depressed patients taught me that psychotropic drugs must sometimes be taken. . . . The idea of long-term medication, certainly for depression, possibly for anxiety, seemed in principle to be reasonable. The problem of dependence on tranquillisers was not so obvious in the 1970s as it was to become in the 1980s.[59]

This physician seemingly acknowledges the importance of clinical judgment, a commonplace term in medicine, albeit not easy to define. Some see it as almost intuitive decision making that rests, in large part, on considerable knowledge and experience. At issue, however, especially with new medications, was the involvement of other factors in decision making. For example, outside pressures (e.g., from governments, patients' worries over side effects) led perhaps to the therapeutic conservatism said to exist in Britain in the 1990s.[60] A physician's personal values could also shape decisions. As was said in 1973, physicians were not immune from "irrational attitudes to the remarkable benefits of the current revolution in pharmacology." Patients could suffer unnecessary pain due to "an unholy combination of neurotic fear of addiction with the traditional Christian glorification of suffering [that] leads to a minority of physicians to practise unjustifiable parsimony in the dispensation of pain-relieving drugs."[61]

Costs

Regardless of how well-intentioned the physician may be, another party can never be expected to be as interested in price as the individual who has to spend his own money.[62]

Any discussion on conservative/prudent prescribing and its effects on the treatment of Mr. Brown and Ms. Smith has to consider how much of it was driven by costs. Even before government and private insurance schemes made this an increasingly "hot topic" by the 1950s, edical practice was invariably undertaken with due consideration to what a patient could afford.[63] However, it seems fairly clear that, as with the explosion of knowledge on medicines, no one—from government officials to rural general practitioners—was prepared for the massive increase in costs associated with new treatments.

In Britain, the National Health Service (implemented in 1948) soon broadcast worldwide the problems of rapidly increasing prices. For example, costs to the Exchequer rose in real terms from £6.8 million to £55.6 million between 1948 and 1955-1956. Various unsuccessful efforts attempted to control costs through both patient education and educating or disciplining the prescribers. By 1951, however, the British government was already attaching much of the blame on the "wholly improper pressure put upon doctors by patients on the one hand and more seriously by manufacturers on the other."[64]

In 1953, the minister of health admitted that expenditure on pharmaceutical products caused him more "concern than any other item, even including the hospitals."[65] Government efforts at cost control shifted to manufacturers' prices and profit margins, but all that emerged was the Voluntary Price Regulation Scheme, which saved the government relatively little money. This was one of ten different cost-cutting measures that the British government introduced up to the 1990s with various shades of success.[66]

There were, of course, local ad hoc efforts at economies, also a reflection of initial unpreparedness in dealing with new costs. Early local initiatives have been little studied in Britain or elsewhere, which makes Newfoundland's efforts—using a "one-physician" committee as it were—of particular interest. In the 1950s, Ian Rusted, prior to becoming dean of Newfoundland's medical school, was given a significant role in reviewing new medicines; the province's health and welfare programs were already demanding attention, well before the escalation of costs deepened problems from the 1970s onward.[67] As part of his responsibilities, Rusted offered advice on new medications to medical officers of health throughout the province and on purchases for use in cottage hospitals. His advice was always based on careful clinical assessment but within a framework of economic considerations. He told one doctor in 1955 that a chief drawback to Banthine was the cost—"four or five times as much as Belladonna" and without any certainty that it was any better.[68]

Cortisone, one of the most far-reaching drugs introduced in the twentieth century, was even more problematic. In its early years, Britain introduced protocols for its use, as did Newfoundland.[69] On October 26, 1953, when responding to a physician's request to prescribe cortisone for a patient with rheumatoid arthritis, Rusted wrote: "the problem, of course, is the excessive cost of cortisone treatment plus the difficulty in avoiding unavoidable side-effects." He indicated that a very limited supply of the drug was available and that detailed requirements had to be met before usage. Aside from noting medical conditions that might prohibit or complicate the use of the drug, he stated, "before starting cortisone we would like [rheumatism] patients with chief involvement in distal extremities to have tried physiotherapy and exercises of the hands so as to prevent deformities."

Cortisone, extracted from adrenal glands, created a particular dilemma for Rusted and the Newfoundland Department of Health as it

did everywhere else, if only because of the initial high cost and conflicting medical opinions. As a "miracle" treatment for rheumatoid
arthritis, when introduced in 1949, the trumpeted enthusiasm within
the medical profession spread quickly to the public. Physician enthusiasm, however, was soon embroiled in disagreements over whether
side effects were serious or overstated. Historian David Cantor has
hinted at the existence of professional self-serving following the
medical enthusiasm over cortisone in 1949-1950: "Rheumatologists
would turn the dangers of cortisone to their own professional advantage, arguing that such hazards required specialist use of the drug."
Cantor, however, does concede that it remained "unclear how far
rheumatologists themselves were exaggerating the harmful side-effects of the hormone, to limit demand."[70] Certainly, with hindsight of
horrendous side effects, many senior rheumatologists now believe
strongly that their early prudence over cortisone was amply justified.[71] Additional issues were the high cost —around U.S. $250 per
gram in 1952—and a seemingly authoritative British research announcement in 1954 that there was "little to choose between aspirin
and cortisone in the treatment of rheumatoid arthritis."[72] Ultimately,
however, clinical experience did not tally with this, and cortisone became generally available in Newfoundland by prescription only around
1955.

Retirement of the "Old": Questions of Clinical Freedom

The new medicines of the 1940s and 1950s plus rising costs added
impetus to the reform of older medicines; after all, many prescription
medicines (like over-the-counter preparations) had long been subjected to contemporary criticism. Limiting physicians' prescribing
choices, however, raised what was to become a substantial issue
through the second half of the century, namely the curtailment of
physicians' "clinical freedom" to prescribe what they felt to be the
most suitable or the "best" medication for a patient. Clearly, too, this
was an important issue for patients, perhaps when they felt that one
medicine was more agreeable, even if no more effective, than another.

Although the earlier control of narcotics and a few other medicines
had limited the clinical freedom of physicians, especially in the treatment of addicts in the United States and Canada (see Chapter 4), none

could argue seriously that it compromised his or her practice in ways that happened after the 1950s due to the pressure of rising costs.[73] Typical physicians' comments of the 1960s to 1980s expressed strong disapproval of limitations to prescribe: "Doctors should always be allowed to prescribe whatever particular preparation they deem the most appropriate in the case of any given patient."[74] The mind-set of clinical freedom was pervasive. For instance, a study on the 1975 withdrawal of Practalol from the British market (it had been introduced in 1970) came to the conclusion that the British deference to clinical freedom was undoubtedly one of the main reasons for the tentative nature of warnings sent to doctors by the Committee on the Safety of Medicines.[75] Although, in 1983, clinical freedom was said to be "dead," others held this was a premature opinion.[76] Increasingly, however, economic pressures further limited choices for those under public and private insurance. Ethical/legal issues came to the forefront against a background of the allocation of scarce resources. Thus a 2002 discussion in noting Alberta's eligibility guidelines for patients to receive certain treatments for osteoporosis concluded that they violate the tenets of evidence-based medicine because "health reform programs often ask (or force) physicians to curtail costs for the good of other members of society, [the existing] patient-focused ethic is strained to the point of becoming a liability issue."[77]

That Newfoundland's retrenchment of older remedies—again an illustration of local initiatives—is not remembered to have aroused concerns over clinical freedom does not mean no minor frustrations existed. Aside from the advice Rusted gave to physicians on medications, he helped with the 1950s' reform of medicines at the central pharmacy situated in St. John's. It supplied stock medicines (some produced at the pharmacy) to the cottage hospitals and medical officers of health (and their general practice patients).[78] Reform of compound mixtures (e.g., for coughs), in line with that already discussed in Chapter 4, reduced the number with similar basic formulae. Although there is no reason to suggest this had any negative impact on patient care, it did limit a physician's ability to prescribe a patient's "favorite" medicine.

Such a reform paralleled changes in hospital formularies. Although the purposes of formularies over their long history varied depending on the needs of particular institutions, key features were standardization of therapeutic agents, use as teaching aids, and control of costs.[79] While I am not concerned with hospital care, it impinged on everyday practice if only because general practitioners, as in St. John's, commonly looked after their own patients within the hospital. The *Canadian Formulary,* with a history from 1905 to 1949, certainly known in Newfoundland, was promoted as a "list of formulae suitable to meet many of the ordinary needs of a hospital."[80] However, by the 1950s, formularies for single hospitals were fading in favor of national works such as the *British National Formulary* (1949) and the *American Hospital Formulary Service* in the United States (first publication in 1959).[81]

Despite such trends, many institutions continued to use their own formularies, as was the case with St. John's General Hospital. The 1955 edition of its *Formulary* was clearly created to control costs through standardization of treatment. According to the introduction, nonpaying patients, as a general principle, were to be restricted to listed drugs:

If a special drug is required, for a non-paying patient, a prescription with the diagnosis and the indication for the drug requested should be forwarded to the Dispensary and if the diagnosis and indication are accepted, the drug will be supplied.

It is noteworthy that the next edition (1965), in stating that the intention was not to restrict the physicians in their choice of drugs—it was to assist them "while prescribing in the hospital"—seemingly acknowledged the physician's authority and clinical freedom.[82] In fact, it might have been merely acknowledging the status quo. The authority of physicians was such that they were able to insist on being able to prescribe whatever they wanted, perhaps even an "old-time" mixture not in the *Formulary.*[83]

A many-pronged assault on clinical freedom by controlling costs came in the last two decades of the twentieth century. Various policies tried to ensure that physicians followed prescribing guidelines, if not on a voluntary basis, then increasingly on an involuntary basis. For example, the British government mandated in 1984 that certain groups of medicines were no longer available on National Health Service prescriptions; similar policies were established by health maintenance organizations (HMOs) in the United States during the 1990s. One consequence was a revitalized formulary movement. In Britain, interest in formularies has extended beyond hospitals into primary care, with a limited number of medicines being agreed to by general practitioners to cover most patients.[84] Back across the Atlantic, pharmacy benefit management companies (commonly referred to as PBMs), which managed pharmaceutical services for HMOs, were emerging in the United States. Their policies of limiting the size of formularies was soon noted as were other trends affecting clinical freedom.[85]

Revising Formulae

Another aspect of medicines reform driven partly by costs was revision of formulae within hospitals, in standard national formularies, and so on. Although formula revision has been a long-standing and constant part of pharmacy, in the 1950s and 1960s it became part of an increasingly critical approach to new and existing medicines. The traditional mixture became the "mixture problem."[86]

Changes in the formula of the tonic Maltlevol, already mentioned as a Newfoundland favorite, is of special interest in offering some "small-print" detail of a general trend, although not an economic issue. Although the product's name was unchanged and continued to suggest that it contained malt, this was omitted from the formula at around the same time (1964) that liver extract was deleted. Ian Rusted, in his role as consultant to the Newfoundland Department of Health, had written to the Horner company in 1955 asking for information on the "actual amount of liver extract, if measurable, in [Maltlevol]," He said:

Maltlevol remains on our drug list and I myself am satisfied about prescribing it, but we have deleted similar preparations with significant amounts of liver or B_{12} and I wanted to be prepared to quote figures if anyone questioned the liver content of [Maltlevol].[87]

Rusted was concerned about the presence of liver masking a diagnosis of pernicious anemia. He was uncertain about an earlier statement from the company that the liver extract contained in Maltlevol was included as a supplementary source of natural B-complex vitamins and had no antipernicious anemia activity.[88] There is no evidence that Rusted's letter had any influence, for a switch to pure B_{12} rather than liver extract reflects the long-standing, continuing trend to use "pure" substances that could be standardized precisely.

Accommodating new medicines brought many challenges. Physicians commonly recollect the dilemma of relying heavily on pharmaceutical company representatives for new medicines information. For many, it challenged their conservatism or prudence. It put pressure on such attitudes as: "If a patient was doing reasonably well, you'd leave them rather than trying something you did not know."[89] Yet the 1950s to early 1960s were clearly a watershed. Bolstered by a mind-set of catch-up (at least in places such as Newfoundland) and of progress, slowly but surely new products were being accommodated and countless old preparations marginalized. The self-care of the past—the world of tonics, medicines that treated cascades of symptoms, and legacies of the old humoral theory and purification ("Look for Blood Humors. They Crop out Constantly, Showing the System Needs Purifying"[90])—was disappearing. Senior Newfoundlanders, on looking back to the 1950s and 1960s, generally remember that many of the old self-care practices were being used less and less frequently. Confidence in the authority of doctors and hence of new medicines was still widespread, but, if necessary, Mr. Brown or Ms. Smith could fall back on the old favorites.

THEME 2: PATIENTS' DEPENDENCE AND PROFESSIONAL GATEKEEPING

In one very real sense sick people have always been dependent on doctors or other people, but here I look at the emergence of a new level of dependence in the 1950s and 1960s in consequence of a confluence of major developments in health care. These included greater accessibility to physicians for many people under government and private insurance schemes, new legislation controlling medicines, physician authority, and a growing number of prescription-only medicines, for example, antibiotics, antihypertensive medicines (e.g., hydrallazine, beta-blocking drugs, reserpine, chlorothiazide, and other diuretics), major tranquilizers (e.g., phenothiazine derivatives and rauwolfia alkaloids), minor tranquilizers (e.g., benzodiazepines), antihistamines, and anticoagulants (warfarin). As said at the beginning of this chapter, the increased power of the medical profession that came with these prescription-only medicines did not necessarily translate into greater social authority.

Prescription-Only Medicines

Specificity

Before looking specifically at new patient dependence, a particular mind-set surrounding prescription products needs comment. This mind-set, an emphasis on specificity or that effective medicines had specific physiological actions, drove much of the thinking about medicines throughout the century. Well before the concept reached its heyday after the 1960s, it had been reshaping ideas in therapy and was certainly a backdrop to the simplification of therapies in the first half of the century. Although not a new idea at the end of the nineteenth century, two factors accelerated interest: the recognition that newly discovered germs could be attacked by specific substances (e.g., antitoxins), and studies that suggested certain chemical structures accounted for particular physiological actions. The idea of a "rational" or scientific system of therapeutics was being aired by the 1880s. Roberts Bartholow, for example, made clear that studying antagonism between two medicines would reveal treatments targeted to a specific abnormal physiological lesion.[91] Such a concept was vastly different from existing notions of specificity, such as claims, often viewed as quackery, that an over-the-counter medicine was specific treatment for a particular condition. This was problematic for the marketing of "specific" medications of the Eclectic School of Medicine, which were promoted as a reform in the preparation of active medicines.[92] Confusingly, the concept of specificity also covered physicians' efforts to tailor treatment to the needs and constitution of a patient.[93]

Development of the concept of specificity of action due to particular chemical structures was encouraged by new synthetic medicines from the laboratories of chemists during the last decades of the 1800s and the early 1900s; far-reaching was Paul Ehrlich's chemotherapy and concept of the magic bullet through the introduction (1910) of an organic arsenical (Salvarsan) for treating syphilis. The next few decades witnessed mounting interest in specificity through a better understanding of many diseases, the identification of new disease entities, and new treatments such as vitamins (D for rickets, B_1 for beriberi, and C for scurvy) and hormones (e.g., thyroxine, insulin, estrone, testosterone). However, by the 1950s successes with sulfonamides and antibiotics cemented the ideal of one medicine for one condition (rather than for a cascade or array of symptoms) in the minds of not only general practitioners and druggists but also the general public. The 1950 *Annual Review of Medicine* stated that an "extraordinary feature of recent progress is a marked tendency toward genuine or apparent specificity."[94]

The growth in popularity from the 1950s onward of the receptor theory of drug action—postulating that medicines acted on cells or enzymes as if they were a key fitting only one specific lock—further encouraged the concept of magic bullets and specificity. Media support could also be enthusiastic, as was the upbeat syndicated U.S. column "How We Get New Drugs." Written by American physician Walter Alvarez—a well-known popularizer of medicine—one particular editorial, published in Newfoundland's *Daily Telegram* in 1959, gave an accolade to "brilliant chemists who, in recent years, have given us our wonderful new drugs." The chemists, Alvarez said, take a drug apart and rebuild it "in perhaps a hundred ways" hoping always to strengthen its good qualities and, at the same time, "get rid of its few bad ones." With drug making an "exact" science, Alvarez suggested that one of the difficult problems was acquainting doctors with all the information, in "view of the fact that last year [1958] 350 new drugs were put on the market."[95]

One commentator, psychiatrist-historian David Healy, has suggested that the 1962 U.S. policy to allow the federal Food and Drug Administration (FDA) to continue to designate certain drugs as prescription only had far-reaching implications. In giving the FDA much more control over the introduction of new medicines (they had a mandate to ensure they were efficacious), it ensured that the research agenda of the pharmaceutical industry would be to search for drugs with specific actions. Marketing approval came only when a specific diagnostic indication was demonstrated, with the consequent focus on finding compounds that targeted the presumed mechanism of the disease process. Clearly this left no place for tonics and drugs having only placebo action.[96]

The receptor theory continued as a key research concept into the 2000s, but not without some physicians questioning the view that "cure by specific therapy is the only really proper sphere for the physician."[97] Concerns have been expressed that the receptor concept is overly reductionist and tends to ignore an individual's personality and response to a disease; encourages the view that, if a small number of "magic bullets" fail to act, more should be given; and discourages individual treatment and asking patients about unexpected side effects, e.g., effects on libido, which patients are often reluctant to raise with doctors.[98] As was said, "We need to look at how this form of drug reputation has come about and whether it's done a disservice to the area."[99]

Gatekeeping

Here I pick up on the account of legislation and gatekeeping from Chapter 4. It is not my purpose to detail the increasing legislative controls that gave medicines prescription-only status in the second half of the twentieth century; rather, it is to notice: (1) the consolidation of patients' dependence on physicians or, as some see it, the pharmaceutical industry; (2) the limits legislation puts on patients' choices; and (3) the professional responsibilities placed on practitioners.

In fact, a full historical account of the inexorable trend toward more and more medicines legislation in Britain, the United States, and Canada in the new situations of the post-1950s remains to be told. Until then we can only partially understand the reasons for the differences, some significant, that existed between countries. For example, as will be discussed later, although the British government decided immediately to phase out high-dose estrogen contraceptive pills in 1969 following new information on a link with thrombotic disease, the United States felt, until the 1980s, that so long as the woman was well aware of the issues, it was a decision between her and her practitioner.[100] And, in Canada, although the Food and Drug Directorate soon issued advice that "whenever possible, physicians should be advised to prescribe a preparation containing not more than 50 micrograms of estrogen," no effort was made to actually remove higher-dose preparations from the market or inform women directly about safety issues.[101]

The 1950s and 1960s were decades of constant and widespread change. Of particular significance in consolidating patients' dependence on physicians was that more and more patients had ready access to physicians through insurance schemes such as the National Health Service in Britain (1948), Medicare and Medicaid in the United States (1965), and Canadian Medicare (1969 in Newfoundland). The level of reimbursement for prescriptions varied (in Newfoundland, for example, it was available only to the needy), but manufacturers' samples were commonly available to help those who could not afford the prescriptions.[102] Further, trends to standardize state and provincial regulations occurred in the United States and Canada. When Newfoundland shifted to Canadian legislation in 1949, it faced the relative stringency of the federal regulations for prescription-only medications. A change in attitude was needed to accommodate both federal and provincial regulations.[103] Some sense of this is perhaps reflected in the first prosecution of a Newfoundland druggist for a breach of the federal Food and Drugs Act by selling penicillin ointment without a doctor's prescription. "The accused," it was reported, "said he thought other druggists were selling the ointment and did not think it was being classed as a prescription drug. He admitted that he never troubled to look at the Act, though he had had a copy for four years."[104]

The thalidomide tragedy of the early 1960s precipitated new controls by governments around the world regarding not only safety but also efficacy; as such, it encouraged a mind-set of banning the sale "except on medical advice and prescription, of drugs that might otherwise be harmful."[105] In the United States, this was enshrined in the 1962 Kefauver-Harris Amendments to the 1938 Food, Drug, and Cosmetic Act; in Britain, in the Committee on the Safety of Drugs (1964) and the 1968 Medicines Act; and in Canada, in 1962 amendments to the Food and Drugs Act. The reason thalidomide was not available in the United States, unlike in Britain and Canada, has often been told as an instructive story to encourage stringent controls. It centers on an FDA official, Frances Kelsey, who judged that the data provided by Richardson-Merrell—the pharmaceutical company licensed to market the German product in the United States—were of inadequate quality.[106] The effects of the tragedy rippled in many directions, particularly in raising public concerns that contributed to the development of organized consumerism. Newfoundland physicians remember that, for a number of years afterward, pregnant women were very fearful of taking any medication, even vitamins, during pregnancy. Certainly an overlay of angst existed in Canada, not only because the United States had prevented its use and that Frances Kelsey was Canadian born, but also due to the Canadian delay in taking it off the market. As was said in the Canadian House of Commons' debate on the 1962 amendments to the Food and Drugs Act, the drug was withdrawn from the market in Germany, where it was first made, on November 26, 1961, from England on December 2, 1961, and only from the Canadian market on March 2, 1962—"three months of wasted time during which it might have been the source of further suffering."[107]

Some comments on the new standards of controls—interpreted to include rigorous clinical trials—that included efficacy are important, for this had a radical impact on availability and choices of medicines. It is also useful to distinguish efficacy (information obtained via rigorously controlled clinical trials) from effectiveness (evidence obtained when the product is in general use and subject to many more variables)—a distinction that became widely accepted in the 1990s. Aspirations to ensure efficacy, but really effectiveness, of medicines was not new to the Kefauver-Harris Amendments, as has been shown for the United States.[108] In Britain, too, following the introduction of the National Health Service, a Joint Committee on Prescribing was established in 1949 to consider whether it was desirable to restrict or discourage NHS doctors from prescribing "drugs of doubtful value" or "unnecessarily expensive brands of standard drugs." The committee reported on products of new and proven therapeutic value and those that lacked any proof.[109] The proposed "reforms," or cost-cutting measures, were challenged by the pharmaceutical industry; it argued that "banning" certain products would handicap the nation's pharmaceutical exports. That the government ultimately accepted this reasoning, as happened on later occasions, raises questions whether public safety was jeopardized. A Voluntary Price Regulation Scheme in 1957 was put in place rather than regulation.[110]

The Kefauver-Harris Amendments, however, were to be the first jurisdictional mandate for efficacy, albeit not without opposition from the pharmaceutical industry and the American Medical Association.[111] Before 1962, the FDA could ban a drug only by proving that the therapeutic claims made in labeling were false or misleading. Under the new amendments, the FDA could ban the marketing of a new drug or force the withdrawal of an old drug in the absence of evidence showing efficacy.[112]

The problem of measuring efficacy was being solved, or so it seemed, with the maturing of the clinical trial to become the "gold standard" for testing new drugs. This marked a change in approach to evaluating new remedies and contributed to repeated claims from proponents of "rational therapeutics" that the "ordinary" practitioner was incapable of evaluating a remedy. As was said in 1964, some people cast "serious doubt on the capability of the average physician to contribute significantly to the clinical judgment essential to the wise use of a new drug."[113] Such a view pitched trials and statistics against practitioner experience, one further example of different mind-sets between academic/scientific researchers and clinicians. In an age of growing specialization, this fostered further fragmentation of medical authority such that it became easy to find an expert to contest almost any aspect of medical knowledge.[114]

Issues over clinical trials, especially their quality, led in the last two decades or so of the twentieth century to the emergence of "evidence-based medicine." This is the philosophy—at least as widely interpreted—that all treatments should be based on clinical trial data that have been subjected to critical and systematic review, including meta-analysis (where possible). However, the emphasis placed on this worries many; although the clinical trials provide data on selected populations, physicians treat individuals, and thus the nuances and idiosyncrasies involved in individual patient treatment are an important factor that may not always be considered in the new evidence-based medicine era.[115]

Ethical Considerations

Overall, increasing regulations suggest that the public was being adequately protected from dangerous products. However, many issues remained. One was whether Mr. Brown or Ms. Smith faced physicians and pharmacists who responded ethically to the legislated responsibility placed on them. "Protecting" the public through legislation always leaves a high level of responsibility for practitioners. Irresponsibility on the part of even a minority can have major repercussions, as happened in Britain during the 1960s when, as noted in Chapter 4, the actions of a small number of physicians, infamous for overprescribing narcotics, led to changes in the law.[116]

·

It is not difficult to find complaints in the literature; indeed, charges were made against both physicians and druggists for irresponsible, if not illegal, prescribing or sale of narcotics or medicines well before the 1950s. For example, a Canadian physician, complaining in 1939 on how patients failed to comply with a sulfanilamide regimen for gonorrhea, said that a great share in the responsibility for the incidence of chronic gonorrhea is due to unethical druggists who, "regardless of the new regulations requiring a doctor's prescription, still occasionally dispense this 'sure cure.' "[117] In 1951, many issues surrounded the enactment of the Durham-Humphrey Amendment to the 1938 U.S. Food, Drug, and Cosmetic Act, which established precise boundaries for prescription and over-the-counter medicines. One was the belief of many druggists that they could use professional judgment in refilling a physician's prescription. Physicians, in general, found this a particularly contentious issue. Patients naturally not only found a refill at a drugstore convenient, but also a way to avoid a physician's fee.[118] One U.S. editorial condemned the unprofessional behavior by druggists as a factor behind the need for the amendment:

> At the very outset it should have been evident to all honest pharmacists that no prescription should be refilled unless it were almost certain that the physician would endorse such action. Yet pharmacists, by and large, refilled prescriptions *ad libitum* with little or no regard for the patient's welfare or the physician's wishes.[119]

The 1940s' controversies over the addiction/habituation potential of barbiturates (see Chapter 4) added weight to these remarks. An FDA official recollected that twenty drugstores in Cincinnati were assisting those addicted to barbiturates/amphetamines be either illegally refilling or selling directly over the counter.

> We did the close out on all twenty stores on the same day. . . . At the time this attracted a great deal of attention and caused the state of Ohio to enact a rather strict law for those days on the sale of barbiturates.[120]

By the 1950s worries over new medicines meant that the health professions had to pay closer attention to ethical transgressions by their members. A mind-set of guardianship—reinforcing legislative gatekeeping—was being cemented into place, adding to the mind-set of quality control that characterized pharmacy during the heyday of extemporaneous dispensing. This is well illustrated by a succession of relatively minor matters arising in Newfoundland in the late 1940s and 1950s, which began to receive attention as the Newfoundland Pharmaceutical Association found that, for the first time, it was obliged to look at professional standards elsewhere, especially in other Canadian provinces.[121] The association first had to deal with 1948 reports of the sale of antibiotics ("not permitted in Canada") by wholesalers who were not druggists. Nothing could be done under the existing Pharmacy Act, but the association decided to request that all "antibiotics such as streptomycin and penicillin" be included in the Health and Public Welfare Act.[122] Some years later, in 1954, the indiscriminate use of barbiturates finally became an issue in St. John's.[123]

Specific problems with pharmacists were raised in 1958 about "unethical practices" on the west coast of Newfoundland, but were not limited to that area. The general public and the medical profession raised concerns about substitutions in prescriptions (presumably by cheaper brands), a problem being dealt with in the United States through antisubstitution laws (see account of generic medicines in Chapter 6). Two years later the president of the Newfoundland Pharmaceutical Association stated that he "deplored the necessity of having to advise members that the practice of unauthorized persons dispensing prescriptions was to be dealt with severely."[124] The same applied to prescription items being sold over the counter.

Ongoing interprofessional issues were also raised from time to time, such as doctors selling manufacturers' samples to the public (July 24, 1961); and doctor-owned drugstores in Corner Brook price-cutting over-the-counter medicines by prescribing them at a lower cost.[125] Another matter spotlighted concerns about the pharmaceutical industry. The St. John's Clinical Society deplored that "certain detail men representing various pharmaceutical companies had gained access to prescription files and were using the information so obtained to promote their own products."[126]

Gatekeeping roles of druggists were ripe for strengthening in Newfoundland. Arguments for this, as elsewhere, came from within the profession, but by the 1960s societal pressures were increasing, if only because of rising costs. Eventually, by the 1990s, pharmacy had to respond to one characteristic of health care—evident more in the United States than elsewhere—the increasing influence of "bioethics," which emerged as a discipline in the 1970s. Aside from growing public challenges (malpractice litigation in the United States in the 1970s, for instance), philosophers, in particular, had helped to create a new discipline of bioethics.[127] A central tenet in much of this discipline—with perhaps more emphasis on individualistic culture in the United States than elsewhere—is respect for the autonomy of the patient, a thrust behind the patients' rights movement.

Ethics and "drug lag." One national, indeed international, issue with ethical overtones arose from the new assessments required to license a new medicine, namely what came to be known as the "drug lag." This became a particularly vexing issue in the United States in consequence of the way the FDA implemented its authorization under the Kefauver-Harris Amendment to set standards for every stage of testing a new medicine. By the 1970s representatives of the pharmaceutical industry, economists, policymakers, physicians, and scientists all weighed into a vigorous debate on whether Americans were being deprived of new drugs which were invariably said to be lifesaving.[128] One of the big issues was that fewer new products were approved in the United States than elsewhere. For example, it was stated in 1973 that "nearly four times as many new drugs became exclusively available in Great Britain as in the United States." Moreover, "where differences occurred in the introduction dates of mutually introduced drugs, about twice as many were introduced first in Great Britain as introduced first in the United States."[129] This oft-repeated message raised intense debate about the reasons for this disparity and whether the American public was seriously disadvantaged. The consequent speeding up of the process in the 1990s, in large measure due to activism from HIV/AIDS patients, still leave concerns about whether public safety is being balanced appropriately with the need to introduce new medicines.[130]

New Medications

I continue the subject of patients' dependence on physicians and the medicines they prescribed or administered by looking at three categories of medications—antimicrobials, psychopharmacologicals (tranquilizers and antidepressants), and hormones in women's health.

Although their stories have often been told, the discussion here not only provides a sense of issues facing physicians and patients but also illustrates that growing patient dependence on physicians was linked to public acceptance of, and often enthusiasm for, scientifically based remedies. Sulfonamides, the first to be discussed, followed relatively quickly on the heels of the important new medications of the 1920s (insulin; a toxoid for immunizing against the scourge of diphtheria; and liver (ultimately vitamin B_{12}) for pernicious anemia), and it added to the public's growing confidence in science and medicine. Particularly noteworthy is the extraordinary amount of antimicrobials and psychopharmacologicals prescribed in the second half of the century. By the 1960s they accounted for 44 percent of worldwide drug sales and thereby already had a special place in the relations between the public and the medical profession.[131] Even in the 1930s, according to one recent review of sulfonamides in the United States, they "proved invaluable to ongoing attempts within the profession to secure status within American society."[132]

Sulfonamides, Penicillin, and Syphilis

Although the history of antimicrobials[133] starts well before the 1950s, even before the first investigations in 1935 on a sulfa medicine (Prontosil), the relative success of the latter, with demonstrations of its value for treating puerperal fever, opened the door to a new era.[134] A flood of articles in medical journals soon showed its potential for treating life-threatening blood infections and chronic conditions (notably gonorrhea); public enthusiasm was raised.[135] However, an article in a 1936 issue of *The Practitioner* hinted at caution when acknowledging that the "enthusiasm of this group of compounds in Germany and France is little short of astonishing." The article noted that

> a great deal of work will have to be done to investigate the mode of action and the chemical constitution associated with the maximum degree of activity. The whole field is one of the most fascinating that has been presented for some considerable time alike to the clinician, the chemist, and the bacteriologist.[136]

By early 1937 the new sulfa medicines were well publicized (at least five proprietary brands were available for general use by the spring), and seemingly generally widely used, including in Newfoundland.[137] This was before the earth-shattering news reached the island of a major tragedy in the United States. In September 1937, the Massengill Company marketed an Elixir Sulfanilamide (the latter was the active breakdown product of the first sulfa medicine, Prontosil), which led to the deaths of more than one hundred people.[138] The horror—due to the toxicity of the solvent used for the sulfanilamide, not the sulfa drug itself—quickened drug regulatory controls in the United States and sent a message to all other governments about the need to control the safety of medicines, albeit said to have been ignored in Britain.[139]

Newfoundland's contribution to the sulfonamide story, as it relates to physicians, illustrates what is said to have characterized the United States—namely a generally cautious, perhaps skeptical, attitude on the part of physicians; there is, however, no evidence that this was because Newfoundland physicians, perhaps unlike their U.S. counterparts, viewed the introduction of sulfa medicines as if they were merely more questionable over-the-counter preparations.[140]

The Newfoundland record suggests a physician's need for personal experience, or that of close colleagues, before validating claims, despite questions raised elsewhere about the validity of personal experiences and the need for independent studies.[141] This is suggested by two talks delivered (in May and June 1939) to the small St. John's Clinical Society on a new sulfa medicine, M&B 693 (sulfapyridine). Introduced in 1938 by British pharmaceutical company May and Baker, it aroused excitement because of its value in treating pneumococcal pneumonia—for a long time dubbed "Captain of the Men of Death"—a condition untouched by the earlier sulfonamides.[142] The first of the St. John's talks noted two months of "work" in cases of pneumonia, "although we used it in one case of vaginal discharge which it cleared up." Local findings were said to "correspond" with those reported in the English journals.[143] Two noteworthy comments in the talk signaled the particular impact to the island. One referred to the lack of medical services in rural Newfoundland, an issue, of course, that existed elsewhere: "the advantage of this drug to us in Newfoundland where hospital accommodation is so inadequate, is easily seen, especially to the men in the outports where no accommodation is available at all." The second comment reflected the particular popularity of poultices among Newfoundlanders: "We have used no poultices [as an adjunct treatment to sulfapyridine] which, we think, has been a great boon. The patients have not been nearly so distressed." To put this comment in perspective and to indicate the dramatic change ultimately brought about by sulfonamides (and, soon, penicillin and other antibiotics), the extensive use and popularity of poultices in the island needs appreciating.[144]

Physicians at the second sulfonamide presentation heard a comprehensive review of the chemistry, microbiological properties, and side effects of M&B 693. The speaker added to calls for caution and prudence:

> The danger with drugs which have such a wide scope as . . . sulfapyridine is its indiscriminate use [a complaint also made about sulfanilamide]. One is tempted to use it in cases of obscure infection and in febrile illness of unknown origin, i.e., depending on the drug not only to cure a case but also to diagnose one, such use only tends to discredit a drug. Sound clinical judgement and adequate bacteriological control is essential.[145]

In concluding on a positive note—the "future is bright with hope in the battle against the bacterial diseases that plague mankind"—the speaker reflected the mind-set of thoughtful doctors, namely caution over new treatments that should be approached on the basis of scientific knowledge and, more important, experience and sound clinical judgment.

Not all Newfoundland physicians were as prudent, perhaps contributing to sulfonamides being viewed as panaceas (see Box 5.1).[146] Perhaps this tallies with Newfoundland recollections of doctors in one community as not "amounting to much." Undoubtedly, some were "casualties" of the constant toil in isolated situations; as with rural physicians elsewhere, they faced not only travel difficulties and insurmountable medical problems without the advice of colleagues but also difficulty in building up necessary experience with prescribing new medications.

New challenges came with an exacerbation of venereal disease during World War II. In Britain, the chief medical officer hardly used British understatement in saying that during the war, "Sexual promiscuity must have been practised on a scale never previously attained in this country." Newfoundland, where members of the U.S. military were stationed, faced the same problem.[147] Although, by 1937, treatment of venereal disease was free to all Newfoundlanders, U.S. ob-

---

BOX 5.1. Sulfonamides As Panaceas

Sulfonamides, like many medicines, went through a panacea stage of indiscriminate use before studies and controls established appropriate usage. The St. John's Clinical Society heard the following verses in May 1939:

If your patient has G.C,
Use sulfanilamide,
If he's water on his knee,
Use sulfanilamide.
If he's bothered by the hives,
Or echinoccus thrives,
Don't you fret about these guys,
Use sulfanilamide.

If little Johnny has a spell,
Use sulfanilamide,
If it's just his feet that smell,
Use sulfanilamide.
If his liver seems to quit,
There's no need to have a fit,
What you need to make a hit,
Use sulfanilamide.

If you want her to conceive,
Use sulfanilamide,
If it's piles you would relieve,
Use sulfanilamide,
If you've fallen down on knowledge,
You don't need to go to college,
For all ills you'll now abolish,
Use sulfanilamide.

Source: E. F. Moores, "Treatment of Urinary Infections," unpublished lecture to St. John's Clinical Society, May 4, 1939.

---

servers questioned whether Newfoundland was taking relevant public health issues seriously.[148] Sulfa medications were used for treating gonorrhea on the island in 1937, although this was not widespread. Disputes existed over their effectiveness compared with existing treatment regimens. An early discussion on treating gonorrhea in the *Canadian Medical Association Journal* (1939) counseled against sulfanilamide on grounds of doubtful value compared with the existing regimens and because of toxicity and the dangers of inadequate dosages masking symptoms; thus patients might fail to complete treatment. Seemingly, the writer felt that the patient needed to "feel himself a sick man" in order to comply with recommendations.[149]

Syphilis was a far more worrisome problem, and it is clear that U.S. military concerns pushed along appropriate public health reforms on the island which were already advocated by local physicians. A speaker noted that doctors must "do our part in inhibiting the gonococci of our waterfront, the spirochaete of our secluded corners, as well as our ubiquitous tubercle bacillus."[150] However, penicillin brought dramatic change.[151] Its potential as an antimicrobial became clear in 1941, but its value for treating syphilis (at least from initial studies on four patients) was announced at an American Public Health Association meeting in October 1943.[152] Follow-up studies paved the way for the U.S. armed services to adopt penicillin as the routine treatment of syphilis toward the end of June 1944. A few Newfoundlanders benefited from military-supply penicillin without any hint of the black-market activity that happened elsewhere.[153] "Official" treatment of Newfoundlanders began in St. John's hospitals toward the end of 1944, by which time the supply problem was largely overcome. The first "official" case was a three-year-old child with gonorrhea, not syphilis, who had been treated previously with sulfonamides. Treatment was successful, and it was noted that adult venereal disease treatment with penicillin was to start on December 13.[154]

Ironically, perhaps, Newfoundland's Venereal Disease Prevention Act of 1944 appeared at the same time as penicillin was becoming available. The five methods (in addition to penicillin) for the "treatment, alleviation and cure" of syphilis that were approved—a belated effort to standardize care and hence control the condition—are worthy of note to underscore the sense of change which came with penicillin: (1) organic arsenicals given intravenously; (2) bismuth administered intramuscularly; (3) mercury orally, intramuscularly, or by inunction; (4) iodides orally or intravenously; and (5) induced fever therapy.[155]

By 1945 expectations among physicians and the public about penicillin's ability to cure infections was high.[156] It was in fact public enthusiasm, with the presumption of misuse, that contributed to making penicillin prescription only. For example, in the Canadian House of Commons' debate in 1946, the government stated that some people have the idea that if they go to a druggist and buy some penicillin they are almost certain to be cured of any one of a number of diseases, including particularly gonorrhea and syphilis. Penicillin, used in the right doses and the right way and at the right time, is a cure for gonorrhea and has a powerful effect on syphilis; but used in the wrong doses or in the wrong way or at the wrong time, it not only does not cure the disease but may itself set up immunity against the proper use of penicillin.[157]

The subsequent story of penicillin and antibiotics in Newfoundland illustrates a general pattern elsewhere, namely, the public demand and rapid increase in usage of antibiotics, despite warnings over antibiotic resistance common enough by the 1950s. Following this, as considered in Chapter 6, there were constant charges of overprescribing and a lengthy time lag before resistance was taken seriously by countless practitioners and by the public.

A variety of factors built up the publicity of penicillin. Liberal prescribing in Britain and the United States—fostering widespread use and patient dependence—was particularly significant, as noted by medical journals and from recollections of senior citizens on both sides of the Atlantic. One British patient recalled in 1991: "In the old days it was penicillin for everything. Penicillin was the golden spoonful that answered everything."[158] Experience in Newfoundland, even in rural areas, was little different where the cottage hospitals, like insurance schemes, allowed patients more access to physicians. Although payment was expected in Newfoundland, it was overlooked if patients could not afford to pay. Little doubt exists that by the late 1950s many Newfoundlanders, rather than visiting the druggist for treatments for coughs, colds, and sore throats, went "to the doctor's" for antibiotics. The case notes (1958-1960) of one general practitioner working in a cottage hospital make this clear with such annotations as "req [requested] penicillin" for, say, coughs and sore throats. In fact, patients often got an injection ("shot") of penicillin (600,000 units) in the office, along with Trulfacillin, a combination of three sulfa drugs and penicillin that was a common prescription by this physician, especially, it seems, if a sore throat was present. Indeed, in almost 50 percent of cases of "coughs, coryza, [and] sore throats" treated by the physician, an antibiotic or triple sulfa drug was prescribed often along with the expectorant Benylin.[159]

One must wonder, too, whether the over-the-counter availability of penicillin lozenges for sore throats in the 1950s and 1960s contributed to the demand for "stronger penicillin." "In the 1950s," remembered one senior Newfoundland pharmacist, "we used to sell thousands and thousands of packages."[160]

Streptomycin and Tuberculosis

Although penicillin steals most of the limelight in the history of antibiotics, streptomycin (announced in 1944 and available in general practice, although still in limited supplies, in 1947) may well have done as much as penicillin to instill confidence in and raise Newfoundlanders' expectations of the new "scientific" medicine.[161] On the human level, the desperate search for streptomycin by patients and physicians at the time is illustrated in recollections of an event at Newfoundland's International Grenfell Association hospital. There, a memorial fund established for a patient was used to purchase expensive streptomycin, which demonstrated its value in inoperable tuberculous meningitis.[162] In other places, demands for streptomycin led to heart-rending appeals for a supply from seriously ill patients occasionally broadcast, for example, by the BBC in Britain.[163]

By the 1940s, tuberculosis on the island had hardly been tamed. Unfortunately, because the Newfoundland scourge has not been studied in detail, it cannot be compared with elsewhere and cannot add to the debate among historians over the relative roles of improved lifestyles and of medical/surgical/sanatoria treatment in the pre-streptomycin decline of the disease.[164] However, unlike many places, improvements in lifestyles were of questionable significance until the 1960s, if only because overcrowded homes and questionable diets persisted.[165] Moreover, it cannot be doubted that physicians and the public alike saw Bacillus Calmette-Guérin (BCG) vaccinations for children (started in Newfoundland in 1951), streptomycin, and improvements in diagnosis (modern X-ray equipment) to be the ultimate victors over the disease.

In St. John's, streptomycin was taken up with alacrity, and two resident physicians at the Newfoundland Government Sanatorium published a series of eleven cases. The earliest date for commencement of treatment was April 1947, when streptomycin was still in short supply and expensive, as reflected in the physicians' comments on patient selection:

the selection [of patients] was in the nature of an economic one. The high cost and the large quantity required made the drug available only to those patients who could afford to provide it themselves, and proved a barrier to many who would presumably have responded favourably.[166]

The cautious conclusion to the report—that the future of antibiotics in the treatment of pulmonary tuberculosis was "promising"—was soon confirmed in part by a celebrated British Medical Council trial (1948), which had a seminal influence in the development of randomized clinical trials that came to dominate the testing of medicines for the rest of the century.

Nerves, Tranquilizers, and Antidepressants

"Nerves" has long been a common lay diagnosis in Newfoundland that contains multiple meanings (Chapter 3). The recent history of the condition is of particular interest, for it suggests that new therapies can be partly validated by reshaping physicians' diagnoses—for example, with respect to anxiety and depression. As one historian put it:

As the highly competitive drug companies rushed into psychopharmaceuticals, they began to distort psychiatry's own diagnostic sense. In trying to create for themselves market niches, drug companies would balloon illness categories. A given disorder might have been scarcely noticed until a drug company claimed to have a remedy for it, after which it became epidemic.[167]

Around the late 1950s, Newfoundland general practitioners (in community, not mental institution, settings) often diagnosed complaints of "nerves" as nervousness or anxiety. Well-known sedatives in the first half of the century—e.g., mixture of potassium bromide and valerian, or the "Green Medicine" containing hyoscine and phenobarbitone in peppermint water for "mild or moderate emotional disorders"[168]—were still being prescribed, though most physicians favored barbiturates (notably phenobarbitone tablets) as more convenient to take.[169] Prescribing patterns began to change around 1955 (slowly in places) with the marketing of meprobamate (known by the brand names Equanil and Miltown), the front-runner of what was to become an avalanche of new minor tranquilizers (also called anxiolytics).[170] Through a successful U.S. marketing policy, early demand at times could outstrip supply with American drugstores posting window notices: "Out of Miltown" or "Miltown available tomorrow."[171] Yet only ten years later, *Time* magazine was telling readers about a growing disillusionment with Miltown, with some doctors doubting that it had "any more tranquilizing effect than a dummy sugar pill."[172] In Newfoundland, excitement had been muted, with many patients continuing on the old regimens, at least until well into the 1960s; some doctors seemingly tried the new treatments only on difficult patients who perhaps worried "easily" or had intractable "insomnia."[173]

That rapid popularity of a new class of minor tranquilizers, benzodiazepines (Librium, the first, was marketed in 1960, soon followed by Valium), had an additional factor going for it—growing concerns over the addictive properties of barbiturates. A new era was well under way. Writing on the new tranquilizers in 1962, a British physician reminded readers of the newness of the term *tranquilizer* ("rather less than ten years") and confirmed that, aside from their value for institutionalized patients (referring particularly to such major tranquilizers as chlorpromazine, marketed as Largactil in the United Kingdom or Thorazine in the United States), they were being used for "troublesome patients in general practice."[174] Such a reference to "troublesome patients"—hypochondriacs, demanding patients, constant sufferers from nerves, and many others who defied precise diagnoses—is noteworthy, for a sense exists that physicians were soon finding minor tranquilizers useful for such patients. As the "popularity" of minor tranquilizers grew, so did fears that they squashed creativity and opened the door for society to enter Aldous Huxley's *Brave New World* or George Orwell's *1984*.[175]

Not all patients in the 1950s with nerves were diagnosed with anxiety. After all, physicians had to recognize a patient's self-diagnosis of a "run-down feeling," "the blues," and their demands for the ubiquitous tonic, if not the stimulant amphetamine (as Benzedrine). Thus the door was open for pushing aside tonics by the growing numbers of new antidepressants from the 1950s to the end of the century, the tricyclics, e.g., Tofranil (imipramine), the monoamine oxidase inhibitors, e.g., Marsilid (iproniazid), and the selective serotonin reuptake inhibitors or SSRIs, e.g., Prozac (fluoxetine), which aroused almost unprecedented enthusiasm and demand.[176] In fact, the 1980s saw the ascendancy of antidepressives over minor tranquilizers (but certainly not their eclipse), partly a reaction to concerns over the addictive properties of the latter, especially Valium, though other concerns such as cancer were raised.[177]

A dilemma for many physicians in the 1950s and 1960s (and after) was deciding whether a patient's self-diagnosis of nerves constituted anxiety *or* depression (or a mixed anxiety-depression). Differentiating the two often required very careful history taking and sound clinical acumen.[178] One reason for the relative popularity of Drinamyl (a combination preparation of amphetamine and amylobarbitone) was that it could be prescribed when a general practitioner was unsure whether depression, anxiety, or a combination was the issue.[179]

Such combination preparations lost favor not only because of widespread abuse in the 1960s but also because "half-way" diagnoses between anxiety and depression became less acceptable.[180] A vigorous exponent of the view that the availability of certain therapies reshaped diagnoses within mental health is David Healy, who joins others concerned over what has been called "disease mongering."[181] Healy argues that when antidepressants were introduced, widespread depression in the community (as distinct from serious, self-evident mental health problems) did not exist, and that "although epidemiological studies from the mid-1960s onward have pointed to widespread levels of nervous conditions in the community, the assumption that they are in the main depressive disorders only began to take root in the 1980s." According to Healy, contributing to this was pharmaceutical company promotion that coincided with worries over patient dependence on the benzodiazepine tranquilizers such as Valium, just as in the 1960s minor tranquilizers had offered an alternative to the barbiturates.[182]

The Newfoundland scene offers some documentary support for Healy's claim for a shift in diagnostic labels from anxiety to depression, just as it indicates miscommunication on the subject of nerves. In an ethnographical study on nerves in Newfoundland in the late 1970s, D. L. Davis, in highlighting the variable meanings given to nerves—from a range of symptoms to expressions of "feelings"—revealed problems between doctors and Newfoundland women.[183] She relates the story of a patient named Ruth Bunt, who goes to the "Monday" clinic in a small Newfoundland fishing village. The attending physician asks Ruth what is wrong and she responds, doctor, my nerves are "acting-up some awful." Without further ado the doctor writes a prescription and informs Ruth that it is for nerve pills, which will help her to relax. Davis makes clear that because the physician did not explore the meaning of nerves, Ruth Bunt received inappropriate treatment—in all likelihood Valium for anxiety—as did other women.[184] It was said that most doctors "rode roughshod over nerves." They failed to recognize that "nerves" might have referred to menopause and that nerves and headaches (or a "wonderful bad head") were often one and the same for many Newfoundlanders.[185] That physicians in Newfoundland interpreted a self-diagnosis of nerves— at least at times—as depression is tellingly reflected in the comments of one Newfoundlander in the late 1970s: "Now nerves is depression, not really nerves."[186]

A notable feature of the psychoactive medication story is the continued rise in the use of antidepressants in the last years of the twentieth century. For example, throughout Canada patients' visits for depressive disorders showed the largest increase (36 percent) from 1995 to 2000 among Canada's leading diagnoses.[187] One professor of psychiatry said that he was not "surprised by the increase in visits for depression. . . . The disorder is now better understood by physicians and the population in general. People tend to consult more as it does not carry the same stigma seen 10 or 15 years ago."[188] It is too early to say whether this means dependence has increased, whether the countless concerns raised about psychoactive medications in popular articles and books have been recognized as somewhat inflated, or whether these concerns are being dealt with by physicians.[189]

Hormones in Women's Health

Although this chapter has made clear the existence of disquiet and uncertainty, much of the account has noted optimism and a sense that certainty was just around the corner despite setbacks such as the thalidomide tragedy and other ongoing issues over side effects. However, in turning to hormones and women's health care, uncertainty becomes more of a public issue rather than a professional issue, and one that won't go away, as Renée Fox makes abundantly clear.[190]

Administering hormones to healthy women—the oral contraceptive "Pill," DES (diethylstilbestrol) during pregnancy, and hormone replacement therapy—opened a host of new issues. One was significantly increased dependence on physicians (often viewed as the medicalization of contraception, menstrual health, and menopause), as well as causing countless women to ponder carefully the safety of what they were placing in their bodies. For the first time, medications were prescribed for *healthy* women for use over *long periods of time;* clearly, possible long-term effects demanded special attention to evaluating safety that raised questions about medicines and side effects in general.

Unending debates and controversies—far more than can be mentioned here—have centered on the safety of and social issues surrounding oral contraceptives, first available in the United States and Canada as Enovid (1960), and in Britain as Enavid/Conovid (1961). It is certainly noteworthy that the Pill arrived when various jurisdictions in the United States and Canada still banned the advertising and selling of contraceptives. Mocking the Canadian Criminal Code, a poem, "The Pill," published in the *Canadian Medical Association Journal* in 1966, opened with the verses:

> To Annie Besant, Marie Stopes
> And later Margaret Sanger,
> An unrestricted birth-rate was
> A cause of righteous anger.
>
> Yet Contraception's remedy
> The Law would not allow,
> Nor will it yet, unless one can
> The Public Good avow.[191]

Mention of the "public good" referred to a defense under the Criminal Code, namely whether the public good was being served by selling a contraceptive.[192] By the mid-1960s, although the Canadian law was still not repealed, such euphemisms as prescribing the Pill to "regulate the menstrual cycle" were no longer necessary.[193]

Despite the rapidity of widespread use of the Pill, the constant, mixed messages (continuing into the twenty-first century) about safety created dilemmas for women; they had to balance the freedom that went with generally secure control over unwanted pregnancy with the possibility of endangering their health.[194] Although side effects were recognized early—e.g., thromboembolism (sometimes fatal) and thrombophlebitis—some reassuring voices suggested that, because hormones were natural, these problems were no greater than their normal incidence in women. Similar arguments—that hormones were natural—allowed some influential voices to suggest that the Pill was acceptable birth control for Roman Catholics.[195] If concerns during the early years of the Pill about serious side effects were pushed to the background amid demands for it, the late 1960s witnessed a dramatic reevaluation. Media publicity on both sides of the Atlantic about a British report linking the Pill with thromboembolic side effects restored concerns about safety, leading to a 1970 U.S. National Fertility Study that stated the obvious:

> it seems plausible that the sustained rise in the dropout rate [of women using the Pill] that occurred in the late 1960s despite improvements in the product which reduced side effects was due to the anxiety about serious health implications generated by responsible medical reports and sometimes exaggerated publicity.[196]

The "improvements" noted were nonestrogen or low-dose estrogen products—the latter in fact having been used more widely in Britain than in the United States and Canada in the 1960s.[197] Uncertainties, however, remained, as reflected in 1970 when *Time* magazine told readers about a new progestogen-only product:

> Chlormadinone differs from conventional forms of the Pill in two vital respects: 1) it consists simply of a synthetic analogue of the hormone progesterone and contains none of the estrogen that has been implicated in clotting disorders among Pill users . . . 2) it is taken every day of the year, and not on the 21-days-on, seven-days-off schedule of other forms of the Pill. Like the other versions—and, in fact like all other potent medications—chlormadinone has its drawbacks. The failure rate, judged by unwanted pregnancies, is slightly higher than with other pills, and some women complain of irregular menstrual bleeding.[198]

This cautious optimism, reflecting authoritative medical opinion at the time, was fair comment given the existing state of knowledge.[199]

If the Pill was an important learning experience for the public about the uncertainties of medications and of safety, it also contributed significantly to the growth of consumerism in medicine. Although the Pill was prescription only, with consequent dependence on physicians, women went to physicians with the expectation of receiving the Pill, perhaps even to *demand* it.[200] It meant, too, that physicians were obliged to expand their services beyond "healing" (in 1962 prescribing oral contraceptives was described as "not a medical practice") to offering family planning advice, a service demanding new skills and knowledge of side effects.[201] When the Family Planning Association of Newfoundland and Labrador was first organized in 1972, somewhat later than in many other regions, physicians, as elsewhere, were reported to be the primary source of information on birth control.[202]

That does not mean to say there was evenness in advice—contraception was an area in which personal values (e.g., regarding abortion) could readily enter, sometimes creating an upsetting situation for Ms. Smith. There was, too, a tendency for many to fall back on the statement that the risks were no greater, indeed less, than having a pregnancy but to leave decisions about risk to the user. An article in the *Canadian Medical Association Journal* in 1968 on oral contraception and thromboembolic disease concluded with comments that may or may not have helped Ms. Smith. The article stressed that "practically all human activities involve a risk of some degree to life," but that the risk of thrombosis from oral contraceptives was not so high as lung cancer from smoking and that the "appalling number of fatal road accidents does not reduce the volume of motor traffic; [and] the deaths from drowning, from hunting accidents and so on do not persuade the public to give up sports."[203]

Those who followed Pill issues closely may well have had their level of uncertainty increased by knowing about different government responses to safety questions at the end of the 1960s. Britain's policy was to phase out high-dose estrogen pills, in sharp contrast to the United States, where a policy of package inserts for patients (they were already available for physicians) was developed to inform women of side effects, risks, and contraindications of oral contraceptive use.

The patient package insert is of more than passing interest because of the widespread debate it created both with the Pill and, later in the

United States, when efforts were made to include inserts with other products. Both the medical profession and the pharmaceutical industry vigorously asserted that the inserts would unnecessarily frighten women, encourage patients to develop imagined side effects, increase costs, and violate physicians' authority and their role in giving information appropriate for an individual patient. Patient anxiety, it was argued, would be reduced by withholding information. The strength of the opposition led the FDA to introduce abbreviated inserts for the Pill in 1970 (rather than the detailed ones planned). In 1978, however, new regulations mandated "significantly more detailed information, some of which reflected newly discovered hazards," such as gynecological cancers, an issue already recognized as resulting from cases in which diethylstilbestrol (DES) was administered to reduce the risk of miscarriage.[204] Patient package inserts had, in fact, been extended to cover the use of all estrogens (e.g., for menopause and hormone replacement therapy), such that from 1977 the FDA mandated that every package of estrogen include printed information about the medication and potential side effects.[205] The rationale, according to the FDA, was to use package insert requirements for largely elective drug products that present significant risks to patients. One rationale was to help patients participate with physicians in choosing whether to use the products.

The Canadian response to the new British information on the dangers of side effects of the Pill, at least as physicians and the public saw it, was low key. As the Canadian Medical Association stated, "the [Drug Advisory Bureau of the Food and Drug Directorate] takes the position that the Pill is not without danger, but that the Pill is less dangerous than being without it."[206] This was in line with a widespread sentiment at the time that the medical profession was becoming aware that more care should be taken in patient selection before the Pill is prescribed. No policy of phasing out high-dose estrogen pills or introducing patient inserts was developed, basically leaving the issue to physicians. In fact, a committee of the Canadian Medical Association, although accepting the general advisability of the lowest possible dose, decided that "it remains responsible practice to prescribe, when indicated, oral contraceptives containing more than 50 or 80 micrograms of estrogen."[207] Fifteen years later a Canadian oral contraceptive report approved the *move* to low-dose estrogen pills.[208]

Although it is perhaps unnecessary to belabor further the many safety concerns that have arisen over the Pill and female hormone therapies, a later example, from the 1990s, is salutary. In 1995, the British Committee on the Safety of Medicines announced that "third generation" oral contraceptives containing the progestins desogestrel or gestodene had a higher risk for producing venous thromboembolism.[209] Problematic, however, were differences in reported figures on the extent of the increased risk compared with second generation pills (i.e., those with lower estrogenic doses of 50 µg or less). A meta-analysis published in 2001 concluded that the increased risk was 1.7 times greater, but problems existed with distorted data depending on whether it was funded by manufacturers of the Pill (producing more favorable results than independent studies).[210]

Adding to the difficulty for women in assessing risks/benefits and making decisions was the emergence of promoting the Pill for noncontraceptive health benefits. Thus in a 1999 review, written for *fellow* professionals, one authority concluded that it is important to view its benefits for the individual woman, both from the perspective of contraceptive effectiveness and from that of supplemental health benefits. "It is here where one can fully appreciate the significant contribution the pill has made in so many areas of modern life."[211]

I close this section by noting the saga of mothers taking DES in pregnancy and the long-term cancer risk they developed from this therapy. This higher risk of cancer was also passed on to the female babies they gave birth to (known as DES daughters).[212] I also comment on hormone replacement therapy (HRT) for menopausal and postmenopausal women. Since the 1960s HRT has been recommended to treat not only the hot flashes and mood swings of menopause but also such diseases of old age as hypertension and coronary heart disease.[213] But as with the Pill, the subsequent history was and continues to be a roller coaster. When users of estrogen (for purposes of contraception or otherwise) were found in 1985 to be five to fourteen times more likely to develop endometrial cancer than nonusers, all estrogen products became villains. The reputation of HRT (in newly formulated doses) recovered, however, in large part because of the reaffirmation of its positive medical benefits, ranging from quality of life in general to osteoporosis, albeit in the context of targeted promotion by pharmaceutical companies that, according to one academic publication, seemed intent on creating a "collective consciousness that women over 40 need medical and pharmacological treatment."[214] Thus "refraining from prescribing HRT seems to necessitate specific justification" on the part of a woman and her practitioner.

Such promotion was faced with further uncertainty in 2002 with a suggested long-term association between HRT and increased incidence of ovarian cancer. These new research results offer an ironic twist: Just as individuals are becoming more proactive and personally responsible for their own preventive health care, it appears that one of the mainstays of older women's preventive care is actually a danger to them. Such contradictions ultimately create more uncertainty.[215]

Chapter 6

Hope Amid Uncertainty: 1950 to 2000

"Hope, like sleep, food, and smiles, is among the most potent of all therapeutic measures."

Physician Tinsley Harrison, 1973[1]

Many issues raised in Chapter 5 continue directly in this chapter, albeit shifting into more open questioning about medicine and health care as a whole. In the following discussions on public confidence in medicines and changing therapeutic relationships, it is suggested that many Mr. Browns and Ms. Smiths had substantial difficulty in validating, in their own minds, new prescription medicines. Perhaps, too, they had questions about the safety of the transference, from the 1980s onward, of many prescription medicines to over-the-counter status.

There are small, but important style changes in this chapter. I sometimes move from the past into the present tense because many issues raised continue to vex health care in the early twenty-first century and are likely to do so for some time. Further, the term *pharmacist* rather than *druggist* (or *chemist* in Britain) is used in recognition not only of its wider public usage but also the efforts of the pharmaceutical profession to develop new roles.

THEME 3: PUBLIC CONFIDENCE: CHALLENGES AND RESPONSES

Although public questioning of and concerns over medicines, especially side effects, have already been made abundantly clear, they reached new levels of public awareness by the late 1960s.[2] One anomaly became more obvious: as patients' reliance on prescription-only medicines continued, more and more uncertainties arose over their use. This set the stage for an increasingly vigorous debate (some might say "war") among the experts of science and medicine and laypeople who held a range of attitudes, from being suspicious of authoritative claims to being downright critical of conventional medicine.[3] Indeed, in looking at various aspects of the debates on medications in the last three decades of the twentieth century, it is evident that they were very much part and parcel of challenges to the authority of medicine as a whole.

The collective influence of many critiques of the 1960s and 1970s was led by Ivan Illich's fully referenced *Limits to Medicine—Medical Nemesis: The Expropriation of Health* (1976), whose impact lasted for years.[4] Illich, an academic, in maintaining that the medical establishment was a threat to health, captured many readers with such evocative statements as, "Physicians are those [experts] trained to the highest level of specialized incompetence."[5] Specifically, Illich critiqued the pharmaceutical industry for its role in the worldwide "medicalization of life," a theme that continued to be raised with respect to medicine as a whole and medicines in particular.[6] His targets ranged from the misuse of the antibiotic chloramphenicol (which was part of that well-known medical "horror story") to overconsumption of medicine that, he admitted, reflected a "socially sanctioned, sentimental hankering for yesterday's progress."[7]

Joining Illich's work was a torrent of avowedly popular writings that challenged the quality and safety of many aspects of health care, especially medicines. Some focused on what can be called the "theater of malpractice," situated mostly in the United States. For example, Louise Lander's (1978) *Defective Medicine: Risk, Anger, and the Malpractice Crisis* added to the media coverage that was encouraging discomfort with the health care system. Amid many issues, Lander focused on medication errors, noting that 11 percent of successful malpractice claims involved treatment with medicines.[8] Much of this was ammunition for the consumer movement, especially prominent in the United States; it ranged from Ralph Nader's attacks on the FDA (e.g., that it was in bed with industry) to public pressure that killed the FDA's efforts to control vitamins as drugs rather than food supplements.[9]

Members of the medical profession often publicized, wittingly and unwittingly, their own uncertainty, if not disquiet. For instance, books such as *Controversy in Internal Medicine I* and *II* (1966 and 1974) were not recommended for "medical curricula" devoted to turning out "practical doctors, trained to go into action," rather than thoughtful physicians.[10] With a more specific focus, *Drugs in Our Society* (1964), based on a conference sponsored by Johns Hopkins University, explored the major problems in making safe and effective drugs.[11] Many issues raised at the conference were still unresolved at the end of the twentieth century, ranging from uncertainties associated with pharmaceutical company-sponsored clinical trials to differences between data from clinical trials and use in everyday practice.

The Patient: A Newfound Voice

By the 1990s, one apparent response of the health care professions to public concerns about medicine (and medicines) was a new emphasis on what was called "patient-centered care." Although this has acquired different shades of meaning, its essence is that diagnosis and treatment must pay attention to *all* the needs and concerns (including concerns about medicines) of a patient; this means exploring the social and emotional context of a disease and the reasons for a visit to a physician. Behind this was a newfound voice by patients and the public in general that readjusted or refocused a long-standing maxim of physicians, namely that *individual* patients are their central concern. Up to the 1960s or so, thoughtful physicians were concerned that insufficient attention was being given to the patient as a person. This was seen as a consequence of the rapid growth of laboratory or "scientific medicine," which overly focused on the disease process. In consequence, the first half of the twentieth century witnessed what historians have called a "patient-as-a-person" movement.[12] One contributor, influential British physician James Mackenzie (1918), asserted that laboratory training—then becoming an increasing part of medical education—*"unfits* a man for his work as a physician" because it accustomed him to mechanistic ways of thinking.[13] Bedside experience was essential.[14] Others took up concerns with reductionism of a patient to a disease entity by developing holistic thinking in various ways. One such school of thought was *constitu-*

tional medicine, which viewed individual responses to disease as related to body type and other characteristics that hinged on heredity.[15]

Although much of the interest in holism had faded by the 1950s, another physician, Michael Balint, influential in Britain well after his death in 1970 if less so in North America, impressed on general practitioners the role that psychotherapy could offer, even in the context of short office visits. As with other physicians, he recognized that "time-famine" (spending too little time with individual patients) was a critical issue in patient care, and he did much to teach how limited time could be used most effectively.[16] As part of a small movement on both sides of the Atlantic, Balint stressed the importance of psychiatry and psychotherapy for general practice.[17] He also raised sensitivities about the "drug doctor," who had a narrow pharmacological focus on dose, timing, toxicity, and so on.[18] In general, Balint's teaching fostered the profession's growing emphasis on personal doctoring and the need to go beyond the diagnosis of disease to the meaning of illness for a particular patient. Some see Balint's originality as merely synthesizing concepts of good medical practice—"everybody knew it all the time, anyway";[19] his work, then, was easy to assimilate and provided fertile ground for allowing the patient's voice into consultations.

Although the views of Mackenzie, Balint, and many others are seen as milestones in the patient-as-a-person movement, the term *movement* becomes much more appropriate from the 1960s onward, when substantial numbers of *nonphysicians*—patients, sociologists, social workers, and others—published or otherwise expressed views that patients' concerns and needs were not being addressed.[20] Moreover, the sentiments of one British physician in 1957 came to the fore: "The basic principle of contemporary clinical medicine [is] the necessity of treating patients as rational beings."[21]

In contrast to well-remembered, earlier times in Newfoundland and elsewhere, when patients asked no questions about diagnosis or therapy during a consultation, the change toward patient-centered care was strikingly rapid as it also gathered support from nurses and, to a lesser extent, pharmacists—in addition to family practitioners, who wanted to make clear that, unlike allegations leveled at medical specialties, their practice was not disease- or physician-centered.[22] Aside from genuine concerns for patients, the new focus helped nursing and pharmacy to increase their professional recognition through new roles. Nursing took new responsibility to "personalize" care in hospitals, palliative care centers, and hospices; pharmacy saw ways to develop potential new clinical roles.

Articulate patients, such as editor and essayist Norman Cousins (1912-1990) with his book *Anatomy of an Illness As Perceived by the Patient: Reflections on Healing and Regeneration,*[23] were particularly influential in adding visibility to a growing movement (including the concept of patients' rights increasingly raised from the 1960s onward) that stressed patients had to be listened to and their autonomy respected. In discussing his decisions to try laughter as a remedy, to stay in a hotel rather than a hospital, and to administer high dosages of vitamin C for his debilitating connective tissue disease, Cousins contributed a reasoned but vibrant tone to discussions on greater patient responsibility. In a foreword to another of Cousins' popular books, physician Bernard Lown wrote that "Cousins's message comes at a critical time, when some physicians are increasingly distancing themselves from the bedside, are abandoning the power of the word as a therapeutic tool, and manifesting indifference to the patient's psychological and spiritual needs." Lown went on to say that the "conventional biomedical model," though giving lip service to the patient, largely ignores psychological factors and subjective concerns as an "irrelevant epiphenomenon."[24]

If Cousins' erudition made him a natural leader, countless contemporaries in local situations were part of a cumulative influence that marshaled people of like mind. This was significant in Newfoundland where the emergence of a body of independent voices depended on growing educational opportunities (especially postsecondary from the 1960s onward) that empowered more and more people to challenge the traditional authority of the priest, the merchant, and the physician. Ambivalence toward, if not mistrust of, doctors (noted in Chapter 4) was still identified in the 1970s.[25] Two items in the *Newfoundland Medical Association Journal* published in 1979 and 1980 are suggestive of people who transformed ambivalence into sharper questioning of physicians. In an open letter to her doctor, a "grateful AL-ANON member" gently chastised her physician for not recognizing that distress and worry, due to her husband's alcoholism, lay behind her complaint of "severe headaches." Although this sounds very much like a physician's failure to appreciate a euphemism for "nerves," the writer admitted she had not been truthful in responding to questions, and that "it was impossible to tell you about [my problems], and so my illness grew worse while I shut myself off from the world." Her recovery was due to her joining an Al-Anon support group, but she asked the doctor "to be patient with people like me."[26] A more challenging message came in a short article titled "Health Care Consumed"; there the writer drew on the wider societal challenges to medicine in stating, "We, the gullible public, decided to accept doctors as heroes, now we, the fickle public, are tired of the god-like image fashioned for us."[27]

Newfoundlanders were soon asking more and more questions of their doctors. As noted later, there seems to have been a clear transition from finding a voice to "the new patient," ready to negotiate many aspects of his or her care.[28] Newfoundland physicians, in looking back on the changing public attitudes that prompted the patient's rights movement and open questioning of doctors, usually suggest such reasons as the impact of Medicare in making many physicians feel like "employees," the strikes by doctors in other parts of Canada, the loss of "traditional" medical values, the "bad" press that arose with lawyers (especially in the United States) encouraging malpractice litigation, and the many new diagnostic tests (e.g., for rheumatoid factor) that came without cures. Only on reflection do physicians recognize the relevance of public concerns over side effects of medicines, of patients not wanting to be blamed for their medical conditions, of barriers created by technology or ineffective communication, and of frustrations over limited time with patients.[29] Little consideration is given to the fact that, by the 1980s to 1990s, public expectations made medicine something of a prisoner of its own success and that for many people problems such as antibiotic resistance were turning earlier successes into hollow conquests.[30]

A number of patients concerned over, for example, rights and adequate informed consent, formed several conspicuous health lobbies within consumer organizations.[31] Those among the latter that focused particularly on medicines include Social Audit (founded in Britain in 1972). Through its publications, which deal with organizations at the center of power in pharmaceutical medicine, Social Audit has international influence in questioning governments and industry. Central to its concerns is the need for patients to know—the need for more public education and knowledge.[32] Another organization, Health

Action International—a global network—has also focused on the pharmaceutical industry and the marketing of medications.[33] Lobby organizations contributed much to what became recognized as "patient power." A noteworthy editorial in the March 2002 issue of the *British Medical Journal* on "The Discomfort of Patient Power" made clear its significance and stated that "medical authorities will have to learn to live with 'irrational' decisions [made] by the public."[34] The term *irrational* is arguable as it tends to overlook the persistently different mind-sets about the safety of medicines noted in Chapter 5 and different worldviews about health and health care.[35]

I close these comments on the patient's voice with a patient's complaint, revealing that communication issues extend beyond misunderstandings over diagnosis and treatment. Although set in the context of Canadian Medicare and physician behavior, rather than medication side effects and errors, it is representative of many patients' "horror" or "scare" stories on both sides of the Atlantic; the overall influence of such negative stories is difficult to determine, but they certainly add to negative media images that are hardly offset by such fictional medical heroes as Dr. Kildare and the doctors of *ER*.[36]

> Some doctors are really wonderful doctors, and there's others. It was only a few years ago I went over to St. Clare's [Hospital] because I was after having attacks of angina. The doctor told me with any pains at all to go over to the hospital because it could be leading to a heart attack. This evening I had pains and I went over and this doctor was on. He examined me and he turns around and he said, "This is what's wrong with the country today," he said, "wasting the tax payers money, people coming in here and nothing wrong with them." It struck me so hard because I had six sons and a husband, working all their lives, half their cheques used to go in taxes. I was so mad, I sat up on the table, I said, "*you* talking about taxes," I said, "if the taxes were added up what my husband and six sons paid in, we'd own this unit." I said to the nurse, "get me my clothes, I'm going home."[37]

The Pharmaceutical Industry and Side Effects of Medications

There seems to be little doubt that book-length critiques by Illich and others[38] from the 1960s to the 1980s helped to make the pharmaceutical industry a lightning rod for criticism about medicines. Added to this was relentless media coverage with exposés and articles (many anecdotal, others culled from authoritative medical journals) written by nonmedical academics, journalists, and social-activist consumer groups from all political angles and ideologies. Some were "straight" media accounts of events, such as the widely reported 1959-1961 U.S. congressional hearings, chaired by Senator Estes Kefauver, on the pharmaceutical industry and the high cost of medicines. Negative stories based on the hearings aroused the public.[39] *Time* magazine, for example, reported that "drugs of high price but low medicinal value are being foisted on doctors"; "a new drug may be marketed, if it cannot be shown that it will probably kill too many people"; and the drug companies treat the nation's physicians as "simpletons."[40]

In general, critics of the industry focused mostly on "greed" through excessively high prices and profits, high-pressure advertising (blamed for much inappropriate physician overprescribing), the constant introduction of "me-too" medicines rather than those offering new advances, the exploitation of developing countries, and inadequate information about safety.[41] That governments could be at the forefront in raising questions, as in Britain following the implementation of the National Health Service, was noted in the Chapter 5's discussion on costs. The phrase "war of attrition with the drug industry," used by the respected British periodical *The Economist* in 1961, foreshadowed a long series of confrontations, if not major battles, over pharmaceuticals.[42]

It is certainly difficult to refute charges—accepted by the courts from time to time—that the industry (at least certain companies) deliberately withheld negative information about the side effects of medicines from doctors and the public. An early notorious case was the 1960s' indictment of the Richardson-Merrell pharmaceutical company for falsifying data, lying to the FDA, and withholding information concerning the hazards of MER/29, an anticholesterol medicine that caused cataracts, among other side effects. Litigation by sufferers continued for many years.[43] The same company, known later as Merrell Dow Pharmaceuticals, faced other litigation from plaintiffs with serious limb defects allegedly due to their mothers taking Bendectin, a product marketed to relieve morning sickness that was voluntarily withdrawn in 1983 but with uncertainty about its safety continuing to reverberate into the 2000s.[44] The 1950s and 1960s also saw the beginnings of a long, drawn-out saga of the dangerous side effects of chloramphenicol—something of a cause célèbre as noted earlier—that also raised questions about manufacturers' truthfulness.[45] Among similar noteworthy episodes to punctuate the second half of the century amid a series of withdrawals of products and changes in recommended dosages are the sagas of Entero-Vioform,[46] Halcion,[47] and Opren;[48] these products contributed to public uncertainty, if only through the public airing of clashes of testimony from experts. These differing viewpoints in the medical community have occurred in other, often extraordinary, controversies, as with the question of whether vitamin C can treat cancer, a theory that began in the 1970s.[49]

Suspicions of the medical industry as a whole were deepened by safety concerns over such nonpharmaceutical products as Dalkon Shield (1970s) and silicon breast implants (1990s), both the subject of thousands of compensation lawsuits for medical complications and ultimate withdrawal from the market.[50] While this was happening, the tobacco industry was increasingly castigated for making misleading statements about the health hazards of smoking.[51] Charges were also made that the pharmaceutical industry used the courts to stifle scientific discussion by obtaining injunctions to prevent the release of reports with negative clinical trial data or to threaten contract university researchers with legal action if they divulged confidential information.[52]

Side Effects

Central to the checkered image of the pharmaceutical industry was the constant thread of public fears over side effects (adverse reactions). Pre-1950 public worries—for example, with calomel and opiate medicines—intensified from the 1950s onward with the increasing use of antibiotics and a host of new synthetic chemicals. Indeed, this became a major issue for health professionals, as witnessed in the spawning of a specialist side-effects literature in the 1950s, when physicians' inexperience in recognizing many symptoms as side effects (e.g., mild to severe allergies) or the interactions between two or more prescribed drugs (e.g., indomethacin and an anticoagulant) prompted much uncertainty.[53]

In 1964 it could be said that the medical profession and the general public were only now becoming fully aware of the magnitude of the hazards accompanying the use of many new and powerful drugs.[54] By the mid-1970s, public worries over the widespread nature of "iatrogenic disease"—as side effects were often called—had become common, especially with published figures that more than thirty million Americans were hospitalized annually for adverse drug reactions, including the interaction between nutrition and medicine, which was then beginning to receive more attention.[55] Perhaps more worrying was a 1974 study indicating that about three million hospital patients suffered an adverse drug reaction *within* the hospital per year.[56]

Up to this time, pharmaceutical industry spokespersons and countless physicians rationalized side effects as an unavoidable evil that accompanies the overwhelming, often triumphal, successes of advances in treatments. For example, Hershel Jick reported in 1974 that, although published evidence can be interpreted as indicating that drugs are very toxic, a re-examination of the data from a "different perspective suggests . . . that drugs are remarkably nontoxic." He suggested that "toxicity is about as low as one could reasonably expect" given the massive exposure to drugs in and out of hospitals.[57]

Although Jick believed drug toxicity to be low, there were still large numbers of cases of significant side effects; this alone produced a climate in which attaching blame for the problem of side effects came easily. For example, the public was blamed on the basis of people's "uncritical belief in the new" and their tendency "to accept advertising and the written word, no matter where and how published, as truth."[58] Physicians, too, have been constantly chastised for inappropriate prescribing. In fact, in 1990 it was said that the medical profession had replaced the pharmaceutical industry as "the target for popular anger."[59] In 2002, comments on a report about withdrawals of prescription products from the market, which received much media attention, seemingly defended physicians and the industry, though that was not the intention. Of 548 new medicines approved between 1975 and 1999 in the United States, just over 10 percent acquired either a "black box warning" in the *Physicians' Desk Reference*—a marker of the most serious adverse reactions—or were removed from the market.[60] Nevertheless, in response to the question whether a physician should be reluctant to prescribe a new drug, editorial comment on the report played down fears so long as the physician considers carefully the reason for the choice, particularly when an equally effective alternative is available. The editorial also said it was incorrect to describe the introduction of unsafe drugs as frequent and added, "if there is sound reason to use a recently approved drug, the physician need not deny the patient this treatment."[61] This might reassure some, but others might continue to have uncertainty.

The issues considered raise something of an apparent paradox. Amidst the many concerns about the safety of medicines, the constant horror stories about them, and doubts about government and pharmaceutical industry truthfulness, there remained at the end of the twentieth century a constant willingness to try new remedies, evidenced by the rising numbers of prescriptions. Some, who view this as continuing public acceptance of physician authority, have questioned whether medicine has lost much of its authority, despite the widespread critiques it has faced; how far it has responded to the concerns and challenges becomes part of the debate.[62] Certainly, pharmaceutical companies in their advertising of medicines continue to extol physician "testimonials." Equally, the impact of negative publicity on the pharmaceutical industry may not be so far-reaching as sometimes supposed, in part because of people's short memories and of the constant dismissal of critics as being one-sided and biased.[63] A 1990 report titled *Critics of the Pharmaceutical Industry* concluded that "the role of outsiders in influencing regulatory policy has been quite limited in the past."[64]

Yet perceptions that physician authority has been less damaged than often stated must not confuse respect and authority with physician power, the latter owing much to expanded gatekeeping roles as discussed in Chapter 5. There is a clear sense that the nature of individual authority has changed. As noted earlier, Newfoundland physicians, in contrast to the priest and merchant, had to earn their authority in the first half of the twentieth century. It would seem that the very status of being a physician often carried much more automatic authority elsewhere. By 2000, physicians everywhere have had to earn their authority on an individual basis in the eyes of Mr. Brown or Ms. Smith; many do, but some fail, with various implications for validating prescription medicines and, as discussed later, compliance with directions about medicines.

Relationships with the Pharmaceutical Industry

Any consideration of public confidence in medicines raises questions about the pharmaceutical industry's interactions with governments, physicians, and pharmacists. Widespread public concern has long been expressed over close industry-government relationships, especially since 1950; charges have been made that this led governments to compromise public safety by favoring the economic well-being of the industry (and its contribution to the export market) through minimizing regulatory hindrances to marketing new medicines. Unfortunately, despite the serious implications of such matters, relatively little detailed historical analysis is available for the second half of the twentieth century on either side of the Atlantic. In one scholarly study, however, sociologist John Abraham argued that similar situations, albeit with significant differences, have existed in both the United States and Britain, where both governments negotiated "with, and between, the interests of the drug trade. Consequently, so far as protection is concerned, legislation has been consistently weak, [and] compromised."[65] Abraham further concluded that "the evidence suggests that corporate bias in the moulding of regulations has been more comprehensive in the U.K. than in the U.S." where "congressional oversight and judicial review are apt to call the [FDA] to account in public for any disengagement from its regulatory responsibilities."[66] In concurring with this, another authoritative observer adds that British "drug regulation is over-secret, cloaked in the veil of secrecy that every government civil servant likes to throw around his or her activities."[67]

Similar issues have been raised about Canada. A 1990 discussion, "Drug Makers and Drug Regulators: Too Close for Comfort," offers the thesis that "while Canadian laws and regulations are some of the strictest in the world," major gaps exist that "ultimately jeopardize the health of the people taking medications."[68] After noting, for example, (1) that various products, e.g., Albamycin T (or Panalba, a combination antibiotic) and Entero-Vioform, were left on the market long after they had been banned elsewhere, and (2) that the FDA had a much stricter auditing system than the Canadian Health Protection Branch, the author stated, "I believe that the underlying factor is the collegial relationship between the Pharmaceutical Manufacturers Association of Canada . . . and the Health Protection Branch." The view is supported by, for example, some crossover of people between government and industry, but more significantly the powerful network associated with industry, informal joint committees (often unrecorded), and the delegation of government authority to companies in such matters as advertising.[69] A more strongly worded statement came in 2001: the Canadian government yields to political pressure both "within and outside the country [and thereby] has let the interests of the pharmaceutical industry prevail over consumer interests when it comes to deciding about drug prices."[70]

A more immediate issue is whether a patient's prescribed medicine was chosen because a physician had developed a close "connection" with a particular company. Since the 1950s, if not earlier, many observers agreed with what was forcibly said in 1984 that, "because of the nature of its dealings with the pharmaceutical industry," the medical profession is in grave danger of "forfeiting public confidence."[71] The concerns arose from wide-ranging pressure promotion aimed at physicians—visits by sales representatives, company gifts, industry-paid continuing medical education (sometimes in exotic places), as well as large financial gifts and research funding to medical institutions and schools—funding that might perpetuate a company name, say, in a building or scholarship. A minority of physicians has always protested publicly about excessive pressure. Although considered less of an issue in Britain (because of its National Health Service) than in the United States, a few British physicians were vigorously complaining in the 1950s and 1960s by recording the number of advertising circulars received in a given number of days (in one practice in 1960, 368 communications in seventy-seven days) or the weight (thirteen pounds received by one physician in February 1960).[72] Despite the constant recognition of conflicts of interest between physicians and the industry, it is hard to discern a collective concern on the part of the medical profession until the 1980s.[73]

Arguably, the biggest influence on physicians has always been sales representatives. Although studies on the impact of representatives offer different assessments, a consensus exists that physician prescribing is commonly affected. One 1988 British investigation found 58 percent of general practitioners stated that their main source of information for a new product was a sales representative, who was also responsible for 39 percent of decisions to prescribe it.[74] Complaints sharpened that representatives presented only selected, usually positive, information about products, perhaps downplaying safety information.[75]

Advertising of medicines has been an equally contentious issue. For example, trends in antihypertensives advertising between 1985 and 1996 seemingly promoted the use of calcium channel blockers over better-substantiated therapies for hypertension.[76] However, such concerns about sales pressures among physicians pale in contrast to a new form of advertising pressure that emerged in the United States during the mid-1980s: the approval of direct-to-consumer advertising of prescription-only medicines, with an additional impetus since 1997, when FDA requirements for television advertising were clarified.[77] Polarized views exist on, for example, whether direct advertising drives up health care costs, its value in educating and empowering patients, and the extent to which it places undue patient pressure on doctors and "upsets" physician-patient relationships. Some believe that "if physicians prescribe [patient-] requested drugs despite personal reservations, sales may increase but appropriateness of prescribing may suffer";[78] others, on the other hand, see a challenge for physicians to develop strategies to help patients evaluate this information and make appropriate informed treatment decisions.[79] In 2003, only New Zealand had joined the United States in allowing direct-to-consumer advertising; strong opposition existed in other countries, though there were signs of it breaking down.[80]

Prescribing Habits and "Inappropriate" Prescribing

> One of the contradictions of pharmacy that I have wrestled with is that some of the stuff I'm putting out there, boy, shouldn't be put out. The patients should be told not to take it. There's a terrible over-use and over-prescribing, over-medicating.
>
> Oral History Collection,
> Newfoundland Pharmaceutical Association,
> Leo Walsh

It is abundantly clear from the account so far that, although simplification, standardization, and legislation "reformed" many preparations or removed them from the market, hosts of new products continued to complicate choices for physicians and patients alike. If nothing else, this exacerbated inappropriate prescribing, which became such a problem for Mr. Brown and Ms. Smith that certain issues need exploring. Inappropriate prescribing most often refers to over- or excessive prescribing (sometimes also referred to as "promiscuous prescribing"), but serious concerns also exist about underprescribing, and the use of inappropriate medications. Errors in prescribing, an aspect of the broad topic of medical errors, has been in the spotlight within the medical profession only since the late 1990s and early 2000s, though the public had long been made aware of it, along with questionable prescribing, through the efforts of consumer watchdog groups.[81]

Although it has a long history, inappropriate prescribing first became an issue in the 1950s, especially in Britain as a result of the National Health Service; it was said that the removal of "patients' inability or unwillingness" to afford medicines led to increased scrutiny of prescribing practices.[82] Costs were a significant matter: at one time "you could dispense things that didn't cost much, but when you're writing out a NHS prescription, it becomes more difficult to prescribe coloured water and therefore you prescribe something that is going to cost more."[83] Tirades became increasingly common about, for instance, the excessive use of sleeping pills, tranquilizers, and antidepressants.[84] A 1976 report, in calling for a systematic review of physician prescribing, revealed striking national differences in the use of, for example, vitamin B_{12}. The report's conclusions noted the need for better training in "pharmacology and medicinal therapy" at undergraduate, postgraduate, and continuing education levels to deal with many "abuses," such as overprescribing to patients (sometimes described as "victims") and pressures on physicians from the pharmaceutical industry and from patients.[86]

Prescribing habits came to be widely studied, often to understand better the failure of physicians to follow guidelines and to control costs. An early British investigation from the University of Edinburgh in 1952, capitalizing on newly available National Health Service prescriptions for study, found that a large number of mixtures were still being prescribed. These included, as was the case in Newfoundland (see Chapter 5), many "elegant and complex recipes [of tonics] which are still manifestly popular, although they must generally be classed as placebos, the justification for which is a matter of considerable current controversy."[87] Another commentator at the time spoke of unnecessary medicines acting as a "mental poultice."[88] The investigation prompted an almost inevitable comment from a general practitioner that a university department of therapeutics knows little of general practice—the type of comment reflecting a general practitioner's view that treatment is determined, in part, by the patient and his or her social circumstances and not by the book.[89]

In fact, the social aspects of prescribing were not ignored in research studies, such that, by the end of the twentieth century, sociologists, anthropologists, physicians, pharmacists, and others had investigated the complexity of factors (from physicians' ages to patients' beliefs) affecting physicians' prescribing decisions. The studies were driven not only by climbing health care costs but also by poor patient compliance in following directions about taking medicines, by growing interest in patient-centered care in the 1990s, and by new professional roles for pharmacists, as well as by the view that "in Canada and other industrialized countries interest in the physician as prescriber has been stimulated by . . . evidence that a substantial proportion of the increasingly large volume of prescriptions written is inappropriate."[90] In general, the studies have revealed more about the diversity of individual prescribing habits than about offering new strategies to improve prescribing skills.[91] However, the studies made clear that quality treatment with effective prescribing—and even the manner in which a prescription is used to close a consultation—can owe much to a physician's understanding of patients' beliefs and attitudes toward medicines.

One consequence of the studies on prescribing practices is that they tend to dispense blame. Physicians constantly blamed patients' demands, especially if they fell into the habit of repeat prescriptions that, particularly in Britain, were often given over long periods of time without seeing the patient.[92] In contrast, studies in the 1990s, mostly from Britain, suggested that less blame should be attached to patients than was generally the case. A 1994 investigation concluded that, on balance, demand from patients for medicines "is probably only one of *many factors* that lead to overprescribing by general practitioners."[93] Patients were often given prescriptions when they didn't expect them, and overprescribing by a general practitioner could be related to how he or she interpreted patients' anxiety and their expectations of management.[94] Another report indicated that, although patients brought expectations to the consultation regarding medication, a doctor's opinion about their expectations was the strongest determinant of prescribing;[95] further, a study on prescribing patterns of proton pump inhibitors for treating gastrointestinal conditions suggested that the use of these medications was initiated primarily by a general practitioner.[96] Such findings are not out of keeping with other investigations that indicated either "little evidence that doctors and patients" shared "information about, and views of, medicines," or that physicians, in failing to follow practice guidelines, used regimens that did not match sources of information that patients might consult.[97]

Blame was, in fact, cast all around among physicians, industry, and patients. At least some observers saw overprescribing as more systemic to particular health care systems as a whole, such as the physician fee for service in Canada. From studies that provided evidence of "a substantial amount of inappropriate prescribing" and a large number of unsuccessful attempts to improve prescribing behavior, one commentator concluded that "alternative forms of physician payment [in Canada] such as capitation or salary are probably necessary to make prescribing more appropriate,"[98] a suggestion obviously irrelevant to Britain.

That widespread, inappropriate prescribing became public knowledge owes much to two classes of medicines: antibiotics and psychoactive medications. In adding here and in the next section comments to discussions on antibiotics and psychoactive medications in Chapter 5, I raise a number of points that may well have puzzled and confused patients, added more uncertainty about medicines, and might even have caused them to go "doctor shopping," perhaps to find a physician with a reputation of prescribing freely.[99]

Antibiotic Resistance and a Time Lag

Patients' demands and liberal prescribing in the early days of penicillin were noted in Chapter 5, and many studies on antibiotic prescribing leave a sense that grossly inappropriate prescribing was common on both sides of the Atlantic.[100] Yet could this have been overstated or misunderstood? Without trying to exonerate bad prescribing practices (e.g., inappropriate prescribing of the relatively toxic chloramphenicol, which could produce aplastic anemia[101]), did critics fail to appreciate the dilemmas facing busy general practitioners in the everyday problem of, say, a sore throat? Do the dilemmas help to explain why forty or so years passed between the discovery of firm evidence of the potential seriousness of antibiotic-resistant bacteria and the real "awakening" of public concern (i.e., the "antibiotic abandon" of the 1950s and the international concerns of the 1990s)?

Penicillin's early, enthusiastic reception was soon tempered by some cautions about safety and potential problems. In part, this arose from experiences with sulfonamides and worries over what might happen if penicillin were abused. Penicillin-resistant strains of staphylococci were described very early in the 1940s and problems were experienced in hospital wards by the 1950s.[102] In fact, the issue of resistance was one factor behind its rapid placement on prescription-only status in Britain, Canada, and the United States. As the British House of Commons was told on June 27, 1946, penicillin was

> one of the most potent cures for certain diseases but was not a universal cure. Its indiscriminate use might be attended by grave consequences. There was a danger of spreading strains of bacteria which were resistant to penicillin if it was improperly used.[103]

Such views contrasted sharply with arguments (e.g., in July 1946) that "there was no excuse whatever for limiting penicillin when anybody could go into a chemist's shop, buy a bottle of aspirins, and kill himself. There [is] a consensus of opinion in the medical profession that penicillin would not do any harm."[104]

In the British parliamentary debates leading to the 1947 Penicillin Act (replacing legislated wartime restrictions introduced because of limited supplies), the government took the prudent approach that "unrestricted access to penicillin would do a grave injury to public health." Aside from repeating that inadequate doses would lead to resistance, concern was expressed specifically over side effects as well as using inadequate dosage to control venereal disease.[105]

Restricting penicillin to prescription-only status hardly prevented public health and other problems from arising. Trotted out was the already noted viewpoint that critics failed to understand the needs and pressures in everyday practice—a failure to recognize, for example, such social factors as patients' education, social class, and even the travel difficulties for patients and physicians' house calls that might call for extra supply.[106] Persistent patients' requests—which were recorded in one physician's practice—were not easy to deal with.[107] A new version of an old skipping song, circulating by 1952, reflected some of this pressure as well as widespread public validation of the new antibiotic.

> Mother, mother, I am ill!
> Call the doctor from over the hill!
> In came the doctor, in came the nurse,
> In came the lady with the alligator purse.
> Penicillin, said the doctor,
> Penicillin, said the nurse,
> Penicillin, said the lady with the alligator purse.[108]

However, it cannot be assumed that all physicians necessarily acceded to demands on grounds other than clinical needs and accepted practices at the time. The high rates of minor infections in Newfoundland—partly because of the fishery—and a spectrum of diagnostic uncertainties have to be considered. Although a superficial glance at some Newfoundland prescriptions at the end of the 1950s suggests that penicillin was overprescribed; many prescriptions were for sore throats and it is salutary that, in 1958, the Newfoundland Medical Association responded to "hundreds—literally hundreds—of streptococcal sore throats in parts of Newfoundland" by encouraging treatment with penicillin:

> Since there are so many different strains of hemolytic streptococci, there is not much point in allowing apparently mild infections to go untreated in hope of producing immunity to one particular strain. Any possible gain is not enough to outweigh the danger of rheumatic fever or nephritis. Any type of hemolytic streptococcus may cause rheumatic fever. . . . Treatment of "strep throats" should aim at eradicating the organisms. It is for this reason that penicillin . . . is preferred to sulphonamides or broad spectrum antibiotics.[109]

The 1950s had witnessed growing public concerns with streptococcal sore throats due to the fear that the offending organism was linked to rheumatic fever (as well as nephritis), a theory that had been growing in acceptance among physicians during the 1940s. In the early 1950s, the American Heart Association encouraged physicians to dispense penicillin even in "suspected" cases.[110] Although the experienced physician might have felt confident in differentiating, on clinical grounds, a streptococcal infection from other causes of sore throat, (even without facilities for throat cultures as usual at the time), it was accepted as good practice to err on the side of caution and to treat.

It must be remembered, too, that around 1960, concerns over resistance were only finally being widely appreciated by the popular media. In the United States, *Time* noted that thanks largely "to overuse and outright abuse of favorite antibiotics—especially penicillin— it has seemed that medical scientists were fighting a losing battle." However, in commenting on some new studies, the magazine hinted that the war could be won by rigorously restricting the use of common antibiotics and imposing strict discipline on doctors and nurses.[111] These views certainly became commonplace, but new semisynthetic penicillins and other antibiotics tended to marginalize the problem. Thus Ernst Chain, a Nobel Prize winner for his contribution to the introduction of penicillin into clinical practice, indicated in 1972 that, because of advances in antibiotics, there were currently no clinical problems, even though one "frequently reads in the daily press, but sometimes also in the medical press, that penicillin therapy is less effective today than . . . when it was introduced into medicine." He added, however, in what almost seems as an afterthought, that there was "no room for complacency and the situation has to be carefully watched."[112] Surprisingly, perhaps, Chain made no reference to the new worry of the 1960s: whether antibiotics in animal and poultry feeds were a health hazard by contributing to the emergence of resistant organisms. It seems that faith in the progress of science, the successes of the pharmaceutical industry, and somewhat muted questioning about overprescribing by the medical and pharmaceutical professions failed to transform fears into general public policies.

This was to change. Precipitating a major challenge was the appearance of methicillin-resistant *Staphylococcus aureus*, which caused increasing problems beginning in the 1980s. Worries were compounded further by the emergence in the 1990s to 2000s of enterococci and *S. aureus* that were resistant to vancomycin, the so-called "last antibiotic" (used as a last resort against bacteria resistant to all other antibiotics). Thus the curtain went up on a new era of doomsday scenarios with new epidemics of infectious disease.[113]

It is not surprising that such trends plus various national and international reports in the 1990s on resistance shifted concerns and control strategies to fire-alarm levels. Members of a 1997 British parliamentary inquiry on antibiotic resistance had "an alarming experience" with their findings, which left them "convinced that resistance to antibiotics and other anti-infective agents constitutes a major threat to public health, and ought to be recognized as such more widely than it is at present."[114] In its response, the British government, in accepting the seriousness of the situation, established a long-term surveillance program of antibiotic use and a multidisplinary advisory committee.[115] New initiatives also came from the United States, Canada, and the World Health Organization.[116]

It became clear that a range of strategies was needed. Increasing efforts to educate the public were under way by 2000, even aside from authoritative, popular books such as *Breaking the Antibiotic Habit: A Parent's Guide to Coughs, Colds, Ear Infections, and Sore Throats* (1999). At the same time, such constructive texts might well have extended Mr. Brown and Ms. Smith's fears over antibiotic resistance and encourage them to try complementary/alternative medicine.[117]

Local investigations can be important in focusing on inappropriate prescribing, if only because the results can be especially meaningful for local medical education. A Newfoundland illustration of potential relevance much further afield was published in 1999.[118] Two physicians, in reporting that rates of antibiotic prescribing in Newfoundland (and Canada as a whole) far exceeded generally accepted rates of bacterial infection, challenged their colleagues to consider a physician's role in excessive prescribing. Specifically, the authors tentatively suggested that fee-for-service payment, rather than salary and the consequent greater volume of patients, contributed to higher antibiotic prescription rates, an explanation noted already for overprescribing in general.

A later Newfoundland study (2001) raised another issue, the influence of physicians' diagnoses on patterns of prescribing.[119] "High prescribers" of antibiotics were, for example, found to diagnose respiratory tract infections (e.g., pharyngitis) significantly more often than "low prescribers," who, in contrast, diagnosed a common cold more frequently. The reasons for the differences in diagnoses are complex, but the activity of high prescribers resonates with the worries in the 1950s (now faded) of sequelae of rheumatic fever and nephritis, as noted earlier.

Psychoactive Medications

Overprescribing psychoactive medications has been as much an issue as antibiotics. Reasons for concern are different—ranging from patients' abuse and dependence to the medicalization of life—but the same question asked of antibiotics has been constant: to what extent is their use justified on strictly medical grounds? Responses to the question are often problematic because of polarized attitudes toward psychiatry. Although the trenchant "antipsychiatry movement" ascendant in the 1960s, particularly associated with psychiatrists R. D. Laing and Thomas Szasz, had faded by 2000, its shadow remains in cynicism and skepticism within and without the discipline of psychiatry.[120]

Questions about overprescribing barbiturates also colored the scene before the "modern" era of tranquilizers and antidepressants began in the 1950s. In 1947, a medical journal editorial stated that practitioners had come to rely on barbiturates

> in the treatment of minor psychiatric disorders and sleeplessness, and for the palliation of many disorders where the diagnosis is uncertain or where no alternative treatment presents itself. These drugs are thus achieving the same status with the doctor that aspirin has long held with the layman.[121]

The editorial also remarked that the extension of uses beyond, say, epilepsy may not be rational, but are "usually defensible"—a reflection of independence of prescribing at the time that could have considerable implications for Mr. Brown or Ms. Smith.

What marked the debates over psychoactive agents during the second half of the twentieth century was the avalanche of conflicting opinions over whether physicians or patients should be blamed for misuse of psychoactive medicines. The U.S. media shifted from generally scathing comments on misuse by patients in the 1960s to mounting censure of physicians in the 1980s for inappropriate prescribing.[122] Such a change seemingly reflected growing concerns and disillusionment with medicine in general; in other words, tranquilizers became something of a lightning rod for criticism. Moreover, a gulf clearly existed between much public and medical opinion, as reflected in two 1980s' publications on the benzodiazepine group of compounds (e.g., Valium). In 1982 the Public Citizen Health Research Group in the United States, along with physician authors, published the book *Stopping Valium.*[123] With such arresting chapter titles as "Drug Companies Push Valium . . ." and "Your Doctor—Who Pushes Them to You?" the book drew public attention to the dangers of taking the benzodiazepines prescribed by doctors, who, it was said, "often dismiss the risks with the assertion that, all in all, these drugs are remarkably safe."[124] Indeed, a medical textbook published shortly afterward told physicians that "the dependence risk factor for the benzodiazepines is low" and that the "dangers to individuals and society are of such a low order that no extension of controls is necessary."[125] This book made no reference to the considerable disagreement among physicians. By 1966, for example, it was reported that "about 80 percent of elderly demented patients" were receiving tranquilizers "unnecessarily."[126]

The 1960s also saw Mr. Brown and Ms. Smith among countless patients whose reasons for taking tranquilizers or antidepressives straddled a blurred line between medical and social reasons. The latter, often characterized by long-term use, focused particular attention on dependence and tranquilizer use as a "social problem," though some users undoubtedly viewed it as an appropriate treatment to regain or maintain emotional health.[127] A 1977 study in Toronto elicited many comments from users about managing stress or lifestyle. One user spoke of taking a tranquilizer after her father died, then tapering it off until she divorced and was "worse than ever." Another used the medication as an "escape":

> Now I am in a situation which I cannot get out of. There is no way I will drop my responsibilities to my husband who is a very fine man, or my children. My husband's and my interests have gone different ways. The communication has diminished, but he's still a very good husband, and he's an excellent father to the children. . . . I can't leave them and because I can't leave them I'm sticking to the Valium. That's my escape.[128]

The widespread social use of psychoactive medications was so embedded in society by the 1970s that changes in advertising them— then directed entirely to physicians—so as to place less emphasis on use of the benzodiazepines for social or living situations, probably had little impact.[129]

It was suggested in Chapter 5 that some inappropriate prescribing in Newfoundland could result from a misunderstanding of the lay meaning of "nerves." However, that could not account for the very high rate of prescribing Valium at the time. In 1979 it was reported in the Newfoundland House of Assembly that perhaps one-third of all prescriptions written in the province were for Valium, or at least it was "by far the most common drug compound used in this Province today."[130] (The issue being raised at the time was possible savings by substituting a generic form of the active substance, diazepam, for the brand Valium.) No information exists as to whether the high usage was clinically justified or reflected indiscriminate physician prescribing; however, studies in Britain at the time suggested that "the treatment of patients with respect to prescriptions for Librium and Valium reflects the doctor's attitudes more than the patient's condition."[131]

By 2000, the number of prescriptions for psychoactive medications was still rising on both sides of the Atlantic; many publications drew attention to this, often to examine consequences ranging from overdoses and suicides to costs.[132] Criticisms of overprescribing remained as acute as ever. These, along with the general critiques of psychiatry, contributed to what the public increasingly saw in the medical profession: a fracturing of medical authority that was evident in the differences of opinion aired in the media and in the growing numbers of malpractice suits.[133] Defensive arguments from physicians rationalized increased prescribing as due to a better understanding of depression. Depression awareness programs mushroomed thanks to support from governments and medical institutions such as the National Institute of Mental Health in the United States (1987) and, in Britain, a Defeat Depression Campaign (1992) by the Royal College of Psychiatrists in association with the Royal College of General Practitioners. Although Mr. Brown and Ms. Smith might be among those accepting messages that came with many programs that proclaimed antidepressant medication is the "treatment of choice," at least for moderate to severe depression, others still had their concerns. Even Prozac, considered to be generally "user-friendly" and a principal reason for the decreasing public stigma toward mental disease, has prompted many concerns about safety.[134] Little doubt can exist that psychoactive agents have produced more uncertainty in the public mind than has any other class of medicines.

Generic Substitution

The last issue to be considered here, in relation to public questioning of prescribing habits and of limiting choices, is the substitution of a less expensive, unbranded (generic) product for a brand-name product. Not only does this illustrate further the impact of rising costs but also the further assault on clinical freedom by third-party insurance schemes (private and public), thus limiting the availability of many medicines for Mr. Brown and Ms. Smith.

Generic substitution (sometimes glossed by insurance companies as "therapeutic interchange programs") has always been contentious. Although long commonplace in hospitals, it became a particular issue in the United States in the 1950s, when many states enacted anti-substitution laws in response to what came to be perceived as a public health problem (one orchestrated by brand-name companies)—namely druggists substituting generic products (cheaper but perhaps inferior) for brand names without consulting the physician.[135] Yet rising costs meant that the generics issue continued to brew. In Britain, in 1963, the authoritative magazine *The Economist* wondered, "Why do doctors continue to prescribe branded drugs" in the face of the Ministry of Health appeals to prescribe generics? "Does 'elegance' have its own therapeutic value or do they recall the prescription for Blogg's Elixir?"[136] Unwittingly, perhaps, this reference to elegance and a preparation well known to a patient touched on factors that could contribute to a placebo effect. The policy of educating physicians to prescribe generic products, unlike mandatory substitution in jurisdictions such as Newfoundland, allowed them to maintain a sense of clinical freedom.[137]

In the United States, economic pressures, including from "social reformers, self-styled economic experts and others," as well as the introduction of Medicare and Medicaid, sparked considerable attention to the issue of generic substitution during the 1960s.[138] In the wake of this, by around 1970 physicians were equally either pro or con to the issue, the latter on the grounds of the uncertain quality of generic products or concerns about further erosion of their clinical freedom. Pharmacists, on the other hand, wanted more responsibility (as drug experts), and in 1970 the American Pharmaceutical Association, albeit to the shock of many pharmacists and others in brand-name companies, reversed previous support of state antisubstitution laws in order to seek their repeal.[139] In fact, the laws were either repealed or amended (the last in 1982), or new laws enacted (as also in Canada) that permitted or mandated generic substitution. Problems of appropriate standards for generic products nevertheless remained. Intense scientific controversies existed especially over equivalence of bioavailability—i.e., whether the same amount of active ingredient is physiologically available in a generic equivalent as in the patented brand.[140] For example, particular worries existed at one time over the availability of the heart drug digoxin, the dose of which always needs precise monitoring.[141] This problem was in large part overcome by the development of a new scientific discipline, biopharmaceutics combined with pharmacokinetics, used to assess such issues as whether two products had the same bioavailability of active constituents.[142]

The Newfoundland contribution to the story of generic substitution not only illustrates certain patterns of control instituted elsewhere but is also a reminder that enigmatic social factors often have relevance to change; in this case, given the economic problems facing the province, the government waited until 1979 to substitute generic drugs for branded prescription drugs, well after most other provinces in Canada. In the House of Assembly debate on the bill ("An Act to Provide for the Provision of Lower Cost Prescription Drugs") it was said to have "taken five or six years to get this bill before the House" and hence it was hardly a "reform."[143] No evidence has been found to suggest that concerns over quality and bioequivalence were any more of an issue in Newfoundland than elsewhere. In fact, substitution had long been happening informally in the province without problems, even outside of hospitals, where it was accepted policy. Publicly, apart from growing costs, it was said that the act was introduced because of concerns that neither the prescriber nor the patient had the assurance that the pharmacist had (1) reviewed appropriate documentation to ensure that the generic brands dispensed were of acceptable quality or (2) selected a lower-cost product than the one prescribed.[144] Nevertheless, there seems to have been an echo at play, albeit faint, of the brown bread saga (see Chapter 3). Perhaps, despite the mind-set of catch-up in the island, there was some wariness about any second-rate products—as some viewed generics—that enhanced feelings of inferiority.[145]

The new act, representative of many acts elsewhere, set out specific standards for generic drugs and the criteria for mandatory substitution for branded versions. It applied to *all* prescriptions, i.e., private and public, unless the prescription "contains a specific written direction to the contrary in the handwriting of the person prescribing the drug." A revised version of the act in 1994 is noteworthy for acknowledging the new societal awareness of patient autonomy and choice such that a person could request that the dispensed prescription "be an equivalent drug listed in the formulary, other than the lowest priced drug listed."[146]

If the latter offered some recognition of patient responsibility, the public felt generally helpless with regard to general controls of costs. In 1987, new Canadian legislation curtailed "compulsory licensing," i.e., allowing generic products to be marketed while the brand name was still under patent protection. In 1993 even this was abolished. The impact on the public, in terms of increased costs, remains a debatable issue.[147] Given such trends, the question remained whether Mr. Brown or Ms. Smith as Canadians and Newfoundlanders were benefiting as much as they might from the generic product regulations. It came as a surprise to many to read in 2001 that Canadians lost out on more than $5.7 million per month in potential savings (by having to buy brand-name products) during 1995 to 1999 because of approval delays for new generic products.[148] Not only were the number of generic prescriptions low (30 percent in 1997), but also the length of registration time for generics varied substantially between provinces. The average number of days for registration ranged from 31.3 (British Columbia) to 384.8 (Prince Edward Island). Newfoundland took 225.7 days. The authors suggested that finding ways to reduce lengthy regulatory approval and delays in provincial reimbursement of generic drugs would bring about substantial savings. Some response to the study dismissed consequent savings as negligible, and stated that a more significant issue is the relative high cost of many generic drugs (they often have no competition) compared with the United States.[149] The same study also served to raise further disquiet about the pharmaceutical industry, which, in North America in general, developed strategies to ensure that brands sustained their share of the market.

Amid an atmosphere of uncertainty and of suspicions of collusion, the question arises, what level of confidence do Mr. Brown and Ms. Smith have in generics? In the United States, where market-driven health care has led to more surveys and analysis than in either Britain or Canada, it seemed that public confidence was relatively high in the 1990s, even after a generic drug "scandal" in the 1980s raised many questions about the quality of products as well as about the integrity of the FDA.[150] A 2000 study, however, showed that respondents who perceived that generic drugs were riskier than brand names varied from around 14 percent to 54 percent, depending on the medical condition being treated.[151] Even so, large financial savings could still sway consumers to set aside concerns.

Self-Care: Over-the-Counter Medicines and the Switch from Prescription Only

In turning now to public questioning of over-the-counter rather than prescription medicines, the story of the inexorable, albeit slow, "reform" during the first half of the twentieth century is continued. A new phase began in the 1960s, most dramatically in the United States. The 1962 Kefauver-Harris Amendments to the 1938 Food, Drug, and Cosmetic Act placed emphasis not only on proof of safety, but also on efficacy of both prescription-only *and* over-the-counter preparations. This included older products marketed since 1938. In consequence, the FDA created seventeen expert panels in 1972, each to review a particular category (e.g., antacids, hemorrhoid treatments, laxatives) of the vast number of over-the-counter products on the market. The protracted review determined those that were "safe and effective" and those that were not—categories I and II respectively; Category III included those on which more data were required. In sending hundreds of products into oblivion, reformulation, and relabeling, choices for the public were obviously reduced "by science," often causing irritations if not frustrations.[152] In the United States, for instance, elderly Mr. Browns or Ms. Smiths might have regretted that, after 1980, they could no longer buy sweet spirits of niter, which they may have used as a home remedy since childhood for fevers and self-diagnosed kidney problems.[153]

Gloomy forecasts at the outset of the FDA review, that the over-the-counter market would decline, did not materialize.[154] Overlooked was the view of many physicians that the public is always ready to self-medicate. Moreover, the consumer movement, the emphasis on taking more responsibility for one's own health, and, as will be seen, government policies of shifting some health care costs to the public, all promoted self-care in general, particularly from the 1970s onward.[155] That physicians often mention self-medication in a deprecating way merely highlights their ambivalence to it—shaped, perhaps, by publications that self-medication abuse was common and constant, and that physicians report only on negative experiences.[156] Although, unlike earlier in the century, references to public gullibility tended to rely more on surveys and reports, the constant use of the term *abuse* registered judgmental attitudes. A 1975 report on abuse of self-medication fueled debate when noting that Americans were more prone to take medicines than Britons; for example, sufficient aspirin was sold in the United States in 1970 to provide every man, woman, and child in the country with 225 tablets each of 320 mg—a clear sign of "a degree of use in excess of any reasonably imaginable need."[157]

Such data flagged cautions in the 1970s and early 1980s about shifting some prescription-only medicines to nonprescription status. ("It is dubious," it was said, that any extension of self-medication by using a limited number of prescription items as over-the-counter products would be "desirable."[158]) This dismissed views expressed in a 1967 article, "Dogma Disputed," in the British journal *The Lancet,* that the public should be allowed to purchase certain existing prescriptions as self-treatment, which would reduce health costs.[159] Oxytetracycline tablets and syrup (a cheap, broad-spectrum antibiotic), for example, should be sold freely with a simple instruction book. Although the article seemingly aroused little interest, the idea of shifting prescription-only to over-the-counter medicines was kept alive by the need to control costs and by such social currents as consumerism becoming more assertive and greater recognition of individual and human rights as applied to health care.[160] Indeed, from the 1970s, the shift slowly escalated. In the United States this was seen as falling "normally and naturally, out of the OTC review," i.e., after the Kefauver-Harris Amendment's efficacy review of over-the-counter preparations, which led to comparisons with prescription medicines.[161] Elsewhere, as in Britain and Canada, the switch was more visibly driven by efforts to reduce national health care costs, although new marketing strategies for companies were also relevant.[162]

Some key national differences emerged that could certainly affect Mr. Brown and Ms. Smith's choices or at least their inclination to purchase. The switch in the United States was to general over-the-counter sales, whereas in Britain and Canada many shifted to pharmacy sales alone, some specifically by the pharmacist ("P-medicines" in Britain are sold only under the supervision of a pharmacist).[163] Business consequences were significant. In 1991, a noteworthy report stated that in Canadian provinces where ibuprofen had been shifted to pharmacist-only sales, it captured only 2.3 percent of the nonprescription analgesic market, whereas in the United States, without pharmacist intervention, it gained 20 percent.[164]

By the mid-1990s, it was said a lack of "consensus in the medical profession" existed, at least in the United States, over greater public access to medication, but that pharmacists were generally supportive.[165] Ambivalence among some physicians and pharmacists drew on the continuing concerns over abuse or misuse of over-the-counter medicines, though definitions of abuse were slippery.[166] Nevertheless, the turn of the century was characterized by a strong sense that the trend to switching would quicken and that self-medication would become an even more conspicuous component in health care.[167] Significantly, some consumers felt that they had sufficient expertise with or validation of the medicines in their own minds to look after their own illnesses without the intervention of the pharmacist.[168]

Natural Health Products: Herbal Medicines

Of all the focal points for the questioning of medicines—indeed, challenges to conventional medicine as a whole—the striking social movement of complementary/alternative medicine has been especially prominent; emerging in the 1960s, it was flourishing by the 1990s. The outline here of key features in the rise of the movement notices both its challenge to conventional medicine and factors that helped to validate it. Moreover, the very availability of herbal medicines (also known as "dietary supplements" or "nutraceuticals"[169])—the focus in this section—and the confidence many people found in their use was only one of myriad practices which constitute the field of complementary/alternative practices, from acupuncture to yoga, that challenged the authority of medicine.

Scholarly interpretations of the late-twentieth-century rise of complementary/alternative medicine vary. Some historians see it as periodic reaction to existing social conditions expressed as clean living movements.[170] Others see it as a specific response to particular issues surrounding, for example, counterculture, high medical costs, and contradictory advice from experts.[171] Yet others see specific responses as renewed interest in a continuum of long-standing ideas that wax and wane over time. Certainly threads of nineteenth-century interest remained evident until the 1960s or so in various places, ranging from "old" herb shops in larger British towns to herbal practitioners in the rural United States.[172] Newfoundlanders, too, who were relying less and less on traditional home medicine by the 1950s, might have tried one of the commercial "natural remedies" available at the time. Sea Tone, for example, a seaweed preparation made from dulce, "makes one of the greatest medicines available for restoring strength, energy and building health."[173]

Signs of a renewal of interest in herbal remedies were numerous in the 1960s.[174] In the United States, the name of Jerome Irving Rodale (1898-1971) was conspicuous. His initial promotion of organically grown food led to a flagship publication, *Prevention,* with the general philosophy that "nature" or a natural approach to health is always superior.[175] Many of the growing number of popular books in the 1970s on nutrition (often with herbal content) were, in some ways, an expansion of Rodale's messages. Joining the most popular author of all, Adelle Davis (1904-1974),[176] were, for example, Ruth Adams (e.g., with Frank Murray, 1973, *Megavitamin Therapy*),[177] W. Pritzker (1971), *Natural Foods, Eat Better, Live Longer, Improve Your Sex Life,*[178] and R. J. Williams (1971), *Nutrition Against Disease: Environmental Prevention.*[179] Other books focused on diet for preventing or treating specific conditions, with cancer high on many lists. Laetrile, commonly promoted as a vitamin (B_{17}), acquired much support (as it still has) despite vigorous condemnation as a quack medicine by health care professionals and medicines regulators.[180] Of particular interest in linking to the food-for-nerves theme considered in Chapter 3 is H. L. Newhold's (1975) *Mega-Nutrients for Your Nerves.*[181] Newhold, an advocate of "nutritional psychiatry," promoted concepts from earlier decades. For example, the lack of such vitamins as B_1, described as "the granddaddy" of the nerve vitamins, could result in "almost any nervous manifestation you can name: depression, difficulty in concentration, fatigue, tension, hyperactivity, confusion, disorientation, hallucinations, numbness in the arms or legs, and many more."[182] Implicit and explicit in all such books were critiques of conventional medicines and sometimes the failure of medical education to teach nutrition.

The welter of such books, coupled with influential discussions by journalists and academics from the late 1950s and an emphasis on deep historical roots, gave, by 1980 or so, an increasing number of people a sense of a pedigree to alternative medicine.[183] For many, the new movement fulfilled a diversity of needs and concerns, e.g., finding a complementary/alternative medicine practitioner who devoted more time to listen than did most conventional practitioners; new ways of discovering meanings to an illness; finding a new level of support for more personal control in health and illness, whether it be for chronic problems or life-threatening situations; and catering to beliefs that it is prudent to try out new health ideas, even when scientists disagree about effectiveness.

Conceptually, complementary/alternative medicine did reinvigorate many long-standing beliefs about health and disease, a reinvigoration that was spread widely through testimonials (from relatives, friends, and others), advertising, conventional physicians who embraced complementary/alternative medicine, and other ways. Unlike the weakness story (Chapter 3), no one overriding concept underpins the use of a wide range of herbal medicines. However, long-standing notions of revitalizing and of purifying the body became particularly evident in the last decades of the 1900s. The concept could be found in academic as well as popular health books. *Complementary Therapies for Pregnancy and Childbirth,* for example, a textbook for nurses published in 2000, supported the use of herbs with reference to, for example, the properties of spring tonics. Such tonics are said to "stimulate the liver, invigorate the digestion and thereby increase the body's vitality by promoting more effective assimilation and elimination."[184] Often implicit in such accounts is the importance of maintaining balance (including balancing energy) for good health. In validating this, Mr. Brown or Ms. Smith might draw on traditional Chinese medicine, anthroposophical medicine, and even concepts heard within conventional medicine such as "balancing brain chemicals" with psychoactive drugs. Relevant, too, were growing concerns over the difficulty of maintaining a "balanced diet" because of decreased nutritional values due to late twentieth-century food processing.

Another concept discussed in Chapter 3, *autointoxication*, was also very much in evidence in the popular literature of the 1980s and 1990s on herbs/dietary supplements. For many people, the concept seemed to be intuitively correct; it was even reinforced by e-mail spam that referred to malnutrition and autointoxication as being due to plaques of mucoid in the gastrointestinal canal.[185] This prompted recommendations to use blood purifiers and laxatives, sometimes promoted on the basis of their historical "pedigree" (perhaps now known as "immunomodulators") to "build up" or strengthen the immune system.[186]

Helping to meld the diversity of complementary/alternative medicine into a movement was the notion of *holistic care* (alternatively, "wholistic"), a term that began to be widely used from the late 1970s onward.[187] Unfortunately, it has meant different things to different people. At one level, it is usually used within complementary/alternative medicine as an approach to a person that takes into account the interrelationships of body, mind, and spirit.[188] An important practical consequence of this is that time must be given to listening empathically to a patient's entire story, their worries and conflicts. On another level, holism tends to be equated with taking responsibility for prevention and wellness.

Discussions on holism have often been set in the context of "there's trouble in health care"; indeed, this became a constant refrain.[189] Specifically, "reductionism" in medicine was often critiqued, i.e., perceptions—sometimes real, sometimes not—that licensed physicians consider the disease only, and only in terms of physiological or biochemical changes. In 1978 an American university professor of health services, in critiquing conventional medicine after pointing out that there "has been a gradual transformation of health care in the United States that has been *initiated by the patients*," stated:

> What a wonderful natural concept it is, this idea that has been dubbed holistic healing. *Holism* refers to the principle in which the living organism is seen as a whole that is more than the mere sum of its interacting parts.[190]

Medical opposition to complementary/alternative medicine has been vigorous, generally with no appreciation that different cultures and worldviews often exist between physician and patient. Health beliefs such as those just mentioned have often been castigated as nonrational, noncritical thinking on the part of the public resulting from poor scientific literacy, anti-intellectualism, antiscientific attitudes, piggybacking on New Age mysticism, and susceptibility to vigorous marketing. If any success is made above and beyond the natural healing process, critics dismissed it as due to placebo action.[191]

In commenting further on the widespread public validation of herbal medicines amid such hostility, I look at insights offered by the Newfoundland scene.

The Newfoundland Contribution

The growth of complementary/alternative medicine saw many parallels on both sides of the Atlantic, with much influence from specific authors and from centers often associated with New Age thinking. The relative isolation of Newfoundland, well away from such centers, meant that around the mid-1980s, Newfoundland's Mr. Brown and Ms. Smith were unlikely to have much appreciation of the new movement. That this had changed quite dramatically by 1990 illustrates further the consolidation and deepening of the movement.

The first "infiltration" or "awakening"—words used by more than one Newfoundland observer looking back to the 1980s—was the opening around 1986 of Mary Jane's, a baker/grocery/herb store in downtown St. John's. Established by an American (a "come-from-away," as foreigners are still known in Newfoundland), the store sold a wide variety of herbs, both loose and in capsulated form. It became a port of call for many who had already recognized the social trend of changing lifestyles and healthy foodways; some even saw the store as a Newfoundland shadow—admittedly a very pale one—of the "New Age," indeed a catch-up.

A second "awakening" was the opening of the Wellness Centre in 1991 by a licensed physician. It flourished immediately by offering both complementary and conventional therapy, especially the former. Other practitioners (e.g., of acupuncture and naturopathy) were added. A leading businessman in St. John's and a strong supporter of the center frequently argued that it was time for society to shift paradigms:

> Those in the medical profession build strong boxes around themselves; they are boxed in by the education they have received and by the validation from drug companies. . . . Most doctors do not have the time or the interest to go beyond the paradigm box, to get out and check other cultures.[192]

By 2000, the Wellness Centre faced competition from many practitioners of complementary/alternative medicine, but continued to be viewed as a seminal force, in large part because of the role of its licensed physician.

Apart from continuing education courses at Memorial University in the early 1990s, which helped to raise awareness of the new movement, in the wake of a growing number of complementary/alternative practitioners much consolidation of the movement came from the Cancer Coalition for Alternative Medicines, founded in 1996 under the dynamic enthusiasm of Jeff Blackwood. With experience working in the media and supporting his wife through breast cancer with alternative therapy, Blackwood brought together and helped to sustain a flourishing support group through monthly meetings, a locally published free magazine titled *Hope: The Alternative Medicine Magazine for Cancer Patients and Care Givers,* the sponsorship of an annual "Natural Health Fair" (commenced in 1997), and the publication of a directory of complementary/alternative services in Newfoundland.[193] The upsurge of self-help or support groups—sometimes interpreted as part of a general protest against dominant values and institutions of society—was significant.[194] The "energy" of the movement alone widened interest, and for some it was a validation, as it encouraged many people to try herbs/nutraceuticals, to make lifestyle changes, to take "charge" of one's health, and to get second opinions from physicians.

One hope of many members of the Cancer Coalition—many of whom had paid no attention to complementary/alternative medicine prior to their illness—has been for more understanding of complementary/alternative treatments by physicians, in fact some level of integration of care with conventional medicine. Concerns over possible incompatabilities of herbal remedies with prescription medicines have increased since around 2000, as have demands for "scientific" evidence of efficacy, even among some complementary/alternative practitioners with much skepticism about the value of randomized, double-blind clinical trials for assessing their practices. In fact, scientific support was emerging; one example was St. John's wort, which attracted as much interest in Newfoundland as elsewhere in self-treatment of depression—in part through efforts to gather the herb from the wild.[195]

The story of St. John's wort and acceptance by many of its scientific validation—i.e., identification of constituents with pharmacological evidence as well as clinical data from acceptable clinical trials—contrasts (even if it is contestable) with countless other herbs and dietary supplements having much less supporting evidence.[196] As mentioned, there is no overriding concept such as weakness that rationalizes a wide variety of products. Public acceptance and validation is commonly drawn from countless factors that include the long-standing pedigrees of historical usage and perhaps commercial products, compatibility with long-standing health beliefs, and testimonial support from within the complementary/alternative movement (users and popular texts). In addition, suggestions that scientific "validation" may be around the corner are increasingly common (e.g., presence of antioxidant activity), all of which suggests to many that it is prudent or "common sense" to try it. Any sense of "feeling better" after a course of a herbal product may contribute to validation.

A significant aspect of validation is the belief that side effects are not a problem as with prescription products. In fact, when the subject of side effects is raised by health agencies, users often consider that some form of collusion exists between the pharmaceutical industry and government. This happened with the emergence of controls such as the placing of St. John's wort on prescription-only status in Ireland in 2000, purportedly because of "the inherent toxicity of the herbal substance itself and its interactions with orthodox medicines [cyclosporin, the Pill, warfarin, theophylline]."[197]

THEME 4: CHANGING RELATIONSHIPS— FROM COMPLIANCE TO CONCORDANCE

In the area where I work, most of the patients I deal with are non-compliant with treatment and do not wish to take prescribed medicines. In order to cope with this problem, medicines must be offered as part of a package of care, some of which is seen as desirable by patients. A more multidisciplinary approach is called for ... to get patients to buy the idea that medicines are helpful.

Philip Harrison-Reed,
British physician[198]

Paralleling the increased questioning of the safety and, sometimes, effectiveness of medicines—often inseparable from criticism of physicians and the pharmaceutical industry—much debate existed on changes in physician-patient relationships, of which the emphasis on patient-centered care, mentioned earlier in this chapter, is one manifestation. The changes have been driven not only by the patient's new voice, but also by the concerns of health care practitioners. One particular issue, becoming conspicuous in the 1970s, is why do many patients fail to take their medicines "three times a day"? Why do they disregard, ignore, or forget directions given to them by physicians and pharmacists, or on labels and information sheets? As a response to such questions and to provide context I comment on the terms *physician-patient relationships* and *therapeutic relationships* (as used from the 1970s onward), on the changing roles of pharmacists, on lay attitudes toward medicines, and on compliance.

Relationships and the "New" Patient

Although both physician-patient and therapeutic relationships are often viewed as synonymous, discussions on the former have focused more on "models" of relationships, such as the "priestly," the "engineering," the "friendly," the "fiduciary," and the "contract," but with the recognition that relationships can shift during the course of an illness.[199] Specifically, with regard to physicians' prescribing patterns, such characteristics have been translated into (1) a dominant-doctor model (the physician controls the encounter); (2) a consumer-patient model (the consumer-patient leads and the physician aims to please and retain the patient); and (3) a cooperation model (the physician and patient cooperate to define the patient's problem and decide how to solve it).[200]

The latter model is nearest to what would be described as a therapeutic relationship, which is often viewed more in the language of subjective outcomes, especially from a patient's perspective.[201] Thus, it might mean no more than feeling better, even though objective signs (e.g., laboratory test results) may not have improved. The concept of the therapeutic relationship is long-standing, though until recent times it rested on the authority of the physician and the establishment of patient confidence as discussed in Chapter 4. The concept was clearly articulated in the early twentieth century through the work and influence of Sigmund Freud. By the 1960s to 1970s, however, it was increasingly discussed in such other areas of health care as nursing and "office" psychotherapy with the goal of helping the patient feel better. Since the 1990s it has been promoted as a matter for all practitioners, especially in complementary/alternative medicine. Some saw effective therapeutic relationships resulting from *holistic* approaches, a term that, as already discussed, became popular in health care from the late 1970s onward. Indeed, in some people's minds therapeutic relationships and holism were synonymous in contributing to *quality of life,* an idea becoming increasingly popular from the late 1970s which, in turn, often brought out the sentiment that "the cure is worse than the disease."[202]

The 1970s crystallized trends that had a major bearing on changing physician-patient relationships and a divorce from the "bad" paternalism of physicians—or what was so interpreted—in past physician-patient relationships (see Chapter 4). Patients were urged to question, rather than be passive with, physicians and to take more responsibility for their care. The dubbing of the United States in the 1970s as shifting "from unhappy patient to angry litigant" reflects some of the change that was under way.[203] However, as forcibly argued by consumer organizations that have focused on medicines (e.g., Social Audit and Health Action mentioned earlier), obtaining appropriate information for the public to make responsible decisions has commonly met resistance from the medical and pharmaceutical professions, the pharmaceutical industry, and governments.

An early illustration of this relates to resistance in the 1950s and 1960s to dispensing prescriptions that were labeled with the name of the medicine and other information. In 1957 the Association of Teaching Hospital Pharmacists in Britain accepted the value of labels "in some instances" but pointed out disadvantages and risks with indiscriminate use. For instance, they could encourage indulgence in self-medication; a patient might recommend his or her prescription to others with "'similar' symptoms"; demands on physicians could be increased; and leftover tablets might be used on a later occasion. The association concluded that, unless instructed otherwise, "the pharmacist will continue to maintain the secrecy which we believe he has always done in the past."[204] Apart from the need to respect the autonomy of patients, practical issues (e.g., rapid identification in poisoning cases) won the day for labeling, though few went so far as one labeling advocate, who wrote to the *New England Journal of Medicine* in 1969, suggested: "many 'hippies' are pilfering medication from their parents." If "the number of capsules are on the bottle, a suspecting parent can count the number of pills and check pilferage readily."[205]

Similar, if not more intense, resistance and accompanying debates occurred over educational patient package inserts (PPIs). As noted in the discussion on hormones in women's health (Chapter 5), PPIs were introduced in the United States in the early 1970s. A markedly different approach was taken by Britain and Canada, which was oriented more toward changing physician prescribing habits. The PPI in the United States, where it received more attention than elsewhere in the 1970s and early 1980s, subsequently had a checkered career, running into much opposition when the FDA wanted to extend the concept to other products.[206] In addition to opposition on the basis of costs and logistics from the pharmaceutical industry and the hands-off policies of Ronald Reagan's presidency, many physicians strongly opposed it. The latter used the same arguments as they had with oral contraceptives, in addition to suggesting that providing patient information would encourage both self-diagnosis as well as patients passing on their medications to others.

Much of the medical opposition seemingly reflected the "old" paternalism. Perhaps it was a persistence of attitudes expressed in a 1960 book, *The Management of the Doctor-Patient Relationship*, namely that doctors had to learn to "change the attitudes of patients so that, within the physician-patient relationship, patients will behave more maturely and will be more appreciative and cooperative."[207] Even those who felt there was some value in inserts argued that information had to be limited to, for example, side effects and such "don'ts" as what foods to avoid with the medication.

By around 1990, PPIs were coming into general use, often on a voluntary basis by companies. By that time, however, they joined what can be described as the full flood of a populist search for health information that called upon an unending variety of sources, from the *Physicians' Desk Reference* to the Internet. This new attitude of entitlement owed much to consumer groups that had been lobbying for years for more, as well as accurate, patient information.[208] Yet the new movement brought many tensions, such that the comfort level of Mr. Brown and Ms. Smith with the information they had about the medicines they were taking could depend a great deal on the practitioners they were consulting. A not uncommon attitude was that the public could not possibly understand modern medicine and hence should have limited responsibility with medications. As was said in 1988, a depressingly huge literature existed on the problem of "functional incompetence" of consumers. British examples included: "Four out of ten people cannot read railway timetables, and one in four adults cannot work out the change they should receive from a £5 note after purchasing a single article."[209] This same author, however, made clear that part of the medicines problem was that the consumer was continuing to be left in the dark, and that more patient education was required. It is noteworthy that, although health literacy has long been recognized as a significant problem, the matter has received relatively little attention in the literature generally read by physicians, despite the increasing importance attached to informed consent from the 1970s onward.[210]

Notwithstanding tensions about information—accentuated by the American direct-to-consumer advertising of prescription medications—it was evident that, by 2000, "new" patients were impacting on health care, patients who were not just voices asking for clarification about medications but who wished to discuss their newfound knowledge on the latest medicines, patients interested in negotiating their treatment. That is not to say that, despite all the questioning of the authority of physicians, trust in a practitioner did not remain in the 2000s as the generally accepted cardinal feature of the physician-patient relationship. However, as noted earlier, more than ever confidence and trust has to be earned by a practitioner on an individual basis. Moreover, in the new world of practitioner-patient negotiation, trust can be a less important issue. Interesting perspectives arise from a study of patients visiting either general or complementary/alternative practitioners in Toronto from 1994 to 1995:

> While there are overarching differences in the nature of the therapeutic relationship that exist in medicine and in alternative care, both kinds of relationships are nevertheless positive and valuable, and not mutually exclusive. The physician relationship is based primarily on trust in expertise, while the complementary/alternative medical relationship is based principally on partnership in healing.[211]

Changing Roles for Pharmacists: Toward Patient-Centered Care

As relationships between physicians and Mr. Brown or Ms. Smith had been under revaluation in the last decades of the twentieth century, so had relationships with pharmacists in Britain and North America. The authority druggists gave to physicians in matters of medicines—certainly up the 1970s—has been made clear. However, amid some slow but quite dramatic changes in the drugstore or pharmacy, which raised questions about whether medicines, especially over-the-counter ones, were viewed as medicines or commodities, pharmacists began to take on a new role as the experts on medicines.

Clear changes within pharmacies began in the 1950s with the rapid rise in numbers of prescriptions, most conspicuous in Britain following the 1948 introduction of the National Health Service with free prescriptions for all. One historian has suggested that, from 1948 to 1982, this led to the "disappearing" pharmacist, who, in order to cope with the new workload, disappeared into the dispensary at the back of the shop and became less available to customers.[212] Equally significant were the general changes that were occurring in community pharmacies, albeit more slowly in places such as Newfoundland. In the 1950s Newfoundland customers appreciated that druggists, now tending to be called pharmacists, continued to face such quality-control frustrations as medicinal preparations freezing during cold winter nights.[213] Slowly and inexorably, however, the commercial momentum was impinging on the character of pharmacies as had already happened in cities elsewhere. One pharmacist in a small Newfoundland community remembers increasing sales pressure from pharmaceutical companies, a measure of the industry's efforts to permeate all corners and opportunities. "Even though I was down out of the way in Bonavista, I'd hate to see the representatives coming through the door from big drug companies—Ayerst Laboratories, Parke, Davis, Burroughs Wellcome. Everybody wanted their share of my business."[214]

Such company sales pressures, along with the retirement of elder physicians, helped to complete the transition from the dispensing of extemporaneously prepared medicines to the counting of manufactured tablets. Even so, rather than leading to the "disappearing pharmacist," as noted for Britain from the 1950s, the shift away from compounding complex prescriptions in places such as Newfoundland, where post-1950 pharmacists were not overwhelmed by large numbers of prescriptions, allowed more time for customers.[215] By this time, too, pharmacists had generally ceased to make their own over-the-counter medicines[216] and no longer counter prescribed or provided first aid, such as "cleaning up cuts, split lips, falls on milk bottles with some peroxide and alcohol—you became afraid of being sued."[217]

One small detail, the growing use of paper bags, underscores as much as any other activity the sense of a loss of traditional practices and values often felt by pharmacists as well as changing relationships with medicines: "Previously some felt it was a disgrace to the profession to use a bag or sack for a dispensed medicine rather than wrapping it by hand. 'Sir, where do you think you are? In a grocery store? Or, in a drugstore?'"[218] As mentioned in the discussion on the bottle of medicine in Chapter 4, the amount of care that seemingly went into a bottle of medicine could well have contributed to a placebo response. Certainly Mr. Brown or Ms. Smith had difficulty in seeing that same level of care in a dispensed bottle of tablets made by a "big" company.

The somewhat aristocratic place of medicines within pharmacies was also challenged by increasing business pressures in the 1960s, albeit again more gradual in Newfoundland than elsewhere.[219] Small but significant steps in the 1960s registered change with, for example, the introduction of cigarettes and newspapers, which fell in line with a local newspaper report in 1959 that druggists in Canada were facing serious problems "as a result of revolutionary changes in merchandising including the sale of the traditional drugstore lines by food stores, and by increases in door-to-door selling."[220] Pharmacy's dilemma was spelled out in the article, namely that "carrying lines too far from those generally recognized" would detract from "professional prestige." Some resistance existed to new trends. Hogan's Drug Store in St. John's, for example, "wouldn't carry nylons that were becoming available after the War; he had an old-fashioned store."[221] However, small-scale professional "protests" were no match for the growth of supermarket or discount pharmacies, where pharmacies essentially became a dispensing "counter" in one section of a store.[222]

Broad social movements also drove change. Pharmacists, for example, had a place in the shift to more open attitudes toward sexuality. The silence over sexual matters between generations in the early decades of the century was as pronounced in Newfoundland—if not more so—than elsewhere in North America and Britain. The contraceptive Pill, introduced as a prescription-only drug in 1960 (see Chapter 5), was just one factor that affected the "atmosphere" of the drugstore, just as the distinctive odor from herbs, liquid medicines, and compounded preparations was generally fading. In 1960s Newfoundland, no longer were boxes of sanitary napkins (Kotex and Modess) individually wrapped in brown or green paper, tied with red string, and placed in a special place in the store. Female customers, who knew where they were, would take them to the counter—to "one of the *girls*" (not the male pharmacist) and "nothing was said."[223]

The new visibility and availability of condoms also highlighted a new era. In previous years, teenage boys would get a laugh by getting one of their peers to go to a Catholic druggist for condoms and "get chewed out." One drugstore—that of celebrated Newfoundlander Thomas Ricketts, a Victoria Cross hero of World War I—was well known for selling condoms. One recollection likened a scene in the movie *Summer of '42* (1971), in which two teenagers were plucking up courage to buy a condom and dealing with Ricketts because his was

> the only place in town where you could buy a condom. You know, you were 16 or 17, you were dying to get one, even just to look at. But we were afraid to go in there. Even if you were 19.[224]

New Challenges

The loss of so many traditional roles—minor medicine, dispensing of multi-ingredient prescriptions, "control" over contraception—along with the growth of consumerism, the patient's newfound voice, and ultimately the new patient contributed to an unsettled time for community pharmacy in Britain and North America during the last decades of the twentieth century. The new circumstances did not lend themselves to the paterfamilias role that community pharmacists readily assumed in earlier years. In fact, the "professional" (some might say "respectable") areas within pharmacy in the late 1950s and 1960s were hospital pharmacy and the pharmaceutical industry (research, formulating medicines, and analytical control), not community pharmacy. The latter began to search for new directions.

In Britain and North America new programs and philosophies emerged from the 1960s and 1970s that, in their different ways, not only challenged the physician as the authority on medicines but were also forerunners to patient-centered care approaches. It is beyond the present discussion to consider the extent to which this drew on (1) the development of the concept of patient-centered care within the medical and nursing professions, (2) the concerns of patients about medicines (as well as new emphases on patients' rights), and (3) the policies of the profession to expand the educational and professional boundaries of pharmacy. However, little doubt exists that all made some contribution to changing mind-sets that had focused largely on the quality and guardianship of medicines. The first step was a clinical pharmacy movement that promoted the pharmacist as the drug expert, capitalizing on the new medicines, their actions, side effects, and incompatibilities.[225] One outcome is that, by around 1970, patients' medication profiles were being kept in more and more pharmacies, primarily to spot incompatibilities between the medicines they were taking.[226]

However, clinical pharmacy only really found a home in hospital pharmacy, rather than community pharmacy. Nevertheless, clinical pharmacy set the stage for pharmacy to focus not so much on the pharmacist as an "expert" compared with the physician but as a *counselor* for patients and their needs (not dissimilar to the role many community pharmacists had had in the past). This new phase, from 1990 onward, came to be known as "pharmaceutical care." Many different shades of meaning have been attached to the term around the world, but one definition, published under the auspices of an American Pharmaceutical Association publication, captures many aspects. The definition states that for every dilemma or difficulty faced by a patient (e.g., in managing multiple medicines or the inability to afford a necessary medication), pharmacists should

> find out what was really going on with the patient, pinpoint unidentified problems that may exist, and work with the patient and his or her physician to make sure the appropriate care is rendered and that the patient achieves the desired effect from treatment.[227]

Pharmaceutical care and therapeutic relationships embrace the same concerns of improving therapeutic outcomes, but a sharp difference exists in that pharmaceutical care, as practiced, generally focuses on medications alone rather than the much broader approach of care for patient well-being as discussed in Chapter 7. Moreover, the extent that pharmaceutical care is implemented depends on individual pharmacists, their environment, and economic situations. Many found it impossible to implement; others say that, because modern dispensing takes much less time than it did decades ago, more counseling is possible—even to the point of helping "out with domestic disputes and so on."[228] "We do a lot more now in pharmaceutical care. We're doing a lot of patient counselling. And you'd be surprised how many people phone you and ask your advice about medications, which they never did in the old days."[229]

Patients' Attitudes

A clear purpose of pharmaceutical care is to help patients carry out directions in taking a medicine. But the pharmacy is the setting for other considerations. For instance, were a person's attitudes toward medicines shaped by changes in the atmosphere of pharmacies to a more commercial environment? By 2000, the Newfoundland scene, no longer different from elsewhere, was felt by some to have reached a new level of impersonal service ("they don't seem to have the time for their customers like a small pharmacy").[230] "The chain stores are forced into keeping up with the competition and down-sizing and offering the dispensary only in the back of a grocery store and charging a dollar ninety-nine for this or that." Loss leaders were a particular problem, as were rising costs.

The problem goes right back to my day that we did not educate the consumer what a fee was. When I graduated there was a markup system and no one knew what fees were. All of a sudden we decided to be "professional" and we wanted a dispensing fee. The public still don't understand what a fee for service is. They think you're making money on your drugs anyway and this fee is a little extra, you know.[231]

There are no general answers to questions about how patients' attitudes toward medicines affect whether they follow directions because of the unending number of variables that shape individual behavior. In addition to long-standing beliefs about blood purification, side effects of medicines, with their huge impact on the public as already made clear, are related to opinions that medications will become less effective if taken continuously, that they can be minimized by taking a "rest" from the medication, or that all medicines are toxic.[232] Such concerns are expressed in different ways, e.g., that "all medicines to an extent are carcinogenic" if taken over a long period of time, or that antibiotics stop the immune system from "performing."[233] Widely held views such as medicines being a "quick fix" are also a consideration. In many ways, the latter is hardly new, but what senior citizens see as different is much less stoicism toward illness than in the past, despite the growth of interest in self-care and preventive medicine in the last decades of the twentieth century.[234] Observations on declining stoicism hint at the growth of public preoccupation with the emotional health, most conspicuous from the 1970s onward. In the United States, attitudes of "let it all hang out" to express one's feelings encouraged more attention to adjusting lifestyles by medications, as well as relying more on both self-care and health care practitioners.[235]

Another matter relevant to attitudes is whether a medicine, particularly an over-the-counter medicine, was increasingly seen as an everyday commodity far removed from the mystique of the prescription bottle of medicine. The term *commodity,* which perhaps implies a "limited warranty," came with the terminology of business and economics that has increasingly engulfed all aspects of health care since the 1980s.[236] Commodity mind-sets are hardly discouraged by pharmacies with such names as Supreme Drug *Mart* and Shoppers Drug *Mart,* and the pleasurable images of rows of products that make you "glamorous, heal you, or give you sexual power."[237]

Professionals, certainly pharmacists, object strenuously to views that medicines are not "special"—i.e., different from commodities—on the basis that viewing them as general merchandise encourages indiscriminate use, such as happened with nutrition supplements.[238] Unfortunately, patients can sometimes feel that the special nature of medicines is treated cavalierly by health professionals—more so with over-the-counter medicines. This is suggested when limited opportunity exists to ask pharmacists questions, perhaps about the "warranty" of safety. As one Briton reported:

If you mean do I stand out in the corridor and "chin-wag" with the [pharmacist]. No, it's just a case of handing in the script and out again. They [pharmacists] don't have much to say at all. As I say, it's a silent world. They are frightened to say in case you come back on them and sue them or something you know.[239]

Many physicians, too, have not helped patients to understand issues surrounding their medicines or inquired into patients' thinking about medicines. Issues of withholding information about medicines persist: Doctors "withhold this information [on side effects] because they don't feel it's good for us. It's like treating us like children, and we should have all the information so we can determine whether or not we want the drug."[240]

From Compliance to Concordance

The various issues raised so far are just some of the variables that surround what is recognized as a frustrating phenomenon of noncompliance with directions and advice in taking medicines or changing diet and lifestyles (see Figure 6.1). Depending on the attitudes of Mr. Brown or Ms. Smith, even though relationships with their physicians might include a strong element of trust, their compliance with directions in taking a medicine could be undermined by consuming worries over potential toxic effects.

Concerns with patients' poor compliance became increasingly evident in the late 1960s and mushroomed in the 1970s with an appreciation that, for example, a large number of patients were not taking the prescribed regimens for the care of their hypertension.[241] One researcher at the time said that it finally "dawned on him that his hypertensive patients' unpredictable and often disappointing responses to

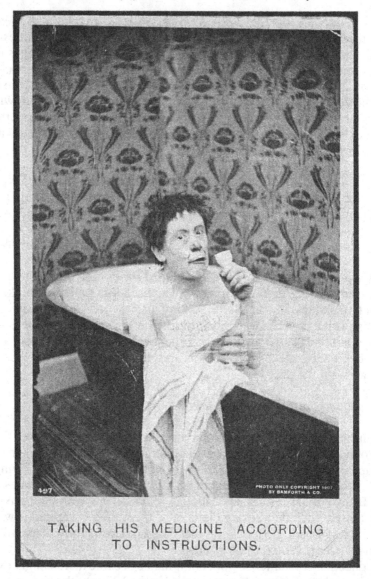

TAKING HIS MEDICINE ACCORDING
TO INSTRUCTIONS.

FIGURE 6.1. Of the countless factors affecting compliance in following directions on taking medicines, effective communication is especially important. Cartoonists commonly poked fun at misunderstandings, as in this comic postcard (c. 1907) in which the medicine label says "Take in Cold Water." (*Source:* Author's collection.)

therapy were the result of neither 'resistant' disease nor inadequate drugs, but were due to low compliance."[242] In the 1980s the literature on the issue of compliance continued to mushroom; in 1986 it was said

> hundreds of articles and dozens of books have been written about patients' compliance. . . . Yet the need for more information and for better understanding is great because the management of this problem is still poor, and 50 percent of patients are still noncompliers.[243]

Studies on the low compliance rates from the 1970s onward pointed to countless factors—more than 200 culled from the literature—and suggested innumerable strategies to overcome the phenomenon.[244] Aside from counseling patients about their negative views and educating them about medicines, attention has been given to the difficulties patients had with complex regimens of multiple medicines.[245] However, what psychologists judgmentally call the "flaws of the human condition" continue to frustrate practitioners, who often fall back and blame patients.[246] The issue of blame is implicit, if not explicit, in much of the literature, which tends to overlook the very real and complex regimens that many patients face, but few record.[247]

A common assumption—one that persists—is that "rational" behavior will result from appropriate education. The history of health education, however, questions time and again the wisdom of this view. Whether this will change with the new emphasis on patient responsibility, new sources of readily accessible information (e.g., both scientifically valid and invalid), and the erosion of the medical monopoly on medical knowledge remains to be seen.

Concordance and Validation

In the 1970s concerns existed that the term *compliance* was coercive and inappropriate to the calls to change physician-patient relationships. Moreover, the term *noncompliance* was viewed as being judgmental of patients and casting all blame on them.[248] However, in the 1990s, in keeping with the recognition of the patient's new voice, emphasis on patient-centered care, and so on, a new term emerged with the hope that it would replace *compliance*. *Concordance* was to be the goal whereby physicians, pharmacists, and patients negotiate agreements that take into account a patient's beliefs, preferences, and concerns about medicines.[249] The basic push behind this change was the continuing need to control costs by reducing wastage of expensive medicines. However, if the concept flourishes, it will take into account the new relationships, the attitudes of new patients, and a better understanding of patients' attitudes, and much more.

The concordance mandate clearly has a potentially important role in addressing the extent to which a patient has accepted and validated a medicine. Though many patients, as I have made clear, still have unquestioned trust in the authority of doctors and pharmacists, others are less certain. For those patients, partnership and negotiation can do much to ensure an understanding of the latest review information, the concept of evidence-based treatments, and risk-benefit data. What has been said about doctors—"if physicians are truly to connect with patients as partners in care, they must change their mindset and develop skills to involve patients in meaningful ways"[250]—now applies to all health professionals.

Hope Amid Uncertainty

Readers may wonder what happened to the theme of hope included in the chapter title. After all, much has been said to challenge the confidence of Mr. Brown or Ms. Smith in prescribed medicines. On the other hand, the continuing rise in the twenty-first century in numbers of prescriptions on both sides of the Atlantic shows that patients visit their doctors in droves and are dependent on them, even if ultimately their compliance with taking medicines is uncertain.

Hope has always been a singularly strong driving force in health care, and most people look for it wherever it might be found. Physicians themselves commonly talk about their *hope* that this or that treatment will help. The quote that opened this chapter echoes long-standing physicians' views.[251] Although there is no reason to think that hope is any less a therapeutic tool in 2003 than it was in 1973, a new emphasis on respecting patients' autonomy and ensuring fully informed consent has led to patients being told "everything" in any situation. The extent to which this can extinguish hope, perhaps demoralize a patient when told about a life-threatening disease, is a dilemma that doctors, in following the lead of society, have perhaps unwittingly been asked to bear. In fact, hope receives relatively little attention, at least in the medical literature compared with the nursing literature.[252] Patients, especially those with chronic or life-threatening illness, who fail to find hope in conventional treatment, often look to complementary and alternative medicine. In concluding his book *Doctors on Trial,* physician John Bradshaw (1978) offered thoughts that were to be pursued by many, namely that "Western doctors are certainly more productive, directly or indirectly, of ill-health, in every sense, than of health." He adds,

> We must look for hope, not to doctors, but to those, whether or not they are medically qualified, who see the need to create a new society, of which health will be an integral part as ill-health is of ours.[253]

This may not be in tune with the thinking of all "new" patients, but widespread hope of some fundamental changes in health care certainly exists, perhaps in line with a suggestion discussed in the epilogue that follows.

Epilogue

Do We Need a "New" Therapeutics?

New medicines, and new methods of cure, always work miracles for a while.

William Heberden, 1802

Among the greatest discoveries of medicines are the generally belated ones that some treatments are utterly useless.

Richard Gordon, 1993

Treatment is far more than handing out pills. It's the way the doctor hands you those pills.

Misel Joe, 2000[1]

The quotes that head this epilogue (the first two from physicians)—more or less two hundred years apart—reflect two threads running throughout this book: uncertainty, sometimes cynicism, about medicines, and feeling that there is more to treatment than just handing out a medication. In Chapter 6, the suggestion was made that the concept of concordance could make a useful contribution to helping those people—at least those who are looking for a partnership in decision making—who have difficulty with validating prescription medicines. Since part of the intention of this book is to help bring into focus questions about people's relationships with medicines, I close by going one step further than concordance to suggest that the concept of a new therapeutics is wanted by many people.

A long-standing dichotomy of views between patient and physician is captured in the opening quote, "Treatment is far more than handing out pills." There have been subtle shifts over long periods of time toward physicians focusing on medicines alone. As early as 1850, Robley Dunglison stated that:

> Therapeutics is a branch of Medical Science which comprises the doctrine of the management of disease. Generally, however, the term is restricted to a description of the *modus operandi* of medicines and the department is commonly associated in our Institutions with Materia Medica.[2]

Dunglison had concerns that the "therapeutist" did not have a broad understanding of disease, its natural history, and various, intangible factors affecting its course. In fact, emphasis on the modus operandi of medicines gathered momentum, beginning in the second half of the nineteenth century, with, for instance, the rise of pharmacology as an experimental science and of rational therapeutics, along with growing emphasis on the goal of finding medicines with specificity of action and of reforming the "old" medicines. Significantly, the modus operandi became central in twentieth-century medical and pharmaceutical education on medicines and fostered scientific methodology, rather than so-called anecdotal experience of individual practitioners, as the gold standard for validating medicines.[3]

Today, in an analogous way to Dunglison's views, countless patients seem to want and often ask for a return to the "management" or care of their illness that embraces a broad understanding of the many factors—e.g., body, mind, and spirit—that affect its course and treatment. Although other patients still prefer to accept the authoritative statements of physicians and/or wish to retain as much of their privacy as possible, calls for broader holistic approaches to many conditions are widespread, at the very least, that practitioners spend sufficient time with a patient to listen to their concerns and needs. In many respects, this may be little more than what was behind various trends and issues throughout the 1900s: the patient-as-a-person movement up to the 1950s or so; the chastisement by general practitioners of academic/scientific colleagues for failing to understand everyday practice and the value of clinical experience;[4] the patient-centered-care philosophy from the 1970s onward; the discussions on therapeutic relationships; and the recent arguments for a new philosophy of concordance.

In essence, I suggest that what many people want is a more catholic approach to therapy, what is increasingly spoken of today as integrative medicine or integrative care. This is integration both within conventional medicine—e.g., dealing with the splintering of care by specialists—and without it by incorporating aspects of complementary/alternative medicine, ranging from herbal treatments to breathing exercises or yoga.

To cover such public wants, I suggest that the term *therapeutics* be resurrected as the *"new" therapeutics*. It would contrast sharply with the term *therapy*, which is reserved for specific treatments such as prescription medicines or a recommended over-the-counter herbal medicine. It would be reflective of Dunglison's view of a broad approach to management, an approach that would embrace what many physicians see as the art of medicine—one that calls into play a broad knowledge of health experience and clinical judgment, or, to meet today's demands, humane clinical judgment; the latter expression underscores that judgments are always being made in complex social environments for which an understanding of the human condition, as offered by the humanities and the social sciences, can be invaluable.[5]

Earlier in this book it was stated that no one—within governments, health care professions, and the public—was ready for the rapid rise in costs that came with the new medicines and insurance schemes of the 1950s and 1960s. Fifty years later, although the continuing rise in costs is at least anticipated, finding a solution remains a conundrum. The chances are high that trends and approaches already in train will persist, such as further limiting physicians' clinical judgment in prescribing, hence restricting the availability of certain medicines to Mr. Brown or Ms. Smith; changes in professional authority with new professional roles for nurses and pharmacists; and giving patients more responsibilities by downgrading prescription medicines to over-the-counter status.[6] However, such trends could well consolidate an emphasis on therapies rather than the public request for therapeutics, unless commitments are made to the latter.

A positive mind-set toward a new therapeutics would alert all practitioners within both conventional and complementary/alternative medicine to keep constantly in mind that treatment may need to go beyond their special knowledge of drugs, acupuncture, homeopathic medicines, and so on. "To be taken three times a day" would remain a common, but less directive than agreed-upon strategy that allows Mr. Brown and Ms. Smith to have not only a sense of responsibility for their own health but also their own identified role in validation.

Notes

Chapter 1

1. Quoted in M. Bliss, *William Osler, A Life in Medicine*, Toronto: University of Toronto Press, 1999, p. 189, from Osler's "Recent Advances in Medicine," *Science*, 27 March, 1891, pp. 170-171. This oft-quoted remark reflected Osler's belief that physicians be as conservative as possible in using medicines, perhaps to consider "a little more exercise, a little less food, and a little less tobacco and alcohol."

2. Although in 1979 it was said by Charles Rosenberg that historians find therapeutics an awkward piece of business and respond by ignoring it, many books and articles have since appeared that highlight milestone events and/or provide a sense of sociocultural factors impacting on therapy and, more often, drug discovery. Recent books that focus on the general story or aspects of medicines in the twentieth century by looking at a broad category of remedies include L. R. Basara and M. Montagne, *Searching for Magic Bullets: Orphan Drugs, Consumer Activism, and Pharmaceutical Development*, Binghamton, NY: Pharmaceutical Products Press, 1994; O. Faure (ed.), *Les Thérapeutiques Savoirs et Usages* (Therapeutics: Theory and Practice), Lyons: Marcel Merieux, 1997; J. Goodman and V. Walsh, *The Story of Taxol: Nature and Politics in the Pursuit of an Anticancer Drug*, Cambridge, UK: Cambridge University Press, 2001; D. Healy, *The Antidepressant Era*, Cambridge, MA: Harvard University Press, 1997; G. J. Higby and E. C. Stroud (eds.), *The Inside Story of Medicines*, Madison, WI: American Institute of the History of Pharmacy, 1997; R. Landau, B. Achilladelis, and A. Scriabine (eds.), *Pharmaceutical Innovation: Revolutionizing Human Health*, Philadelphia: Chemical Heritage Press, 1999; J. Mann, *Murder, Magic, and Medicine*, Oxford: Oxford University Press, 2000 (a popular work useful for all readers); H. M. Marks, *The Progress of Experiment: Science and Therapeutic Reform in the United States, 1900-1990*, Cambridge, UK: Cambridge University Press, 1997; W.-D. Müller-Jahncke and C. Friedrich, *Geschichte der Arzneimitteltherapie* (History of Medicines and Treatment), Stuttgart: Deutsche Apotheker, 1996; R. Porter and M. Teich (eds.), *Drugs and Narcotics in History*, Cambridge, UK: Cambridge University Press, 1995; M. C. Smith, *A Social History of the Minor Tranquilizers: The Quest for Small Comfort in the Age of Anxiety*, Binghamton, NY: Pharmaceutical Products Press, 1991; W. Sneader, *Drug Discovery: The Evolution of Modern Medicines*, Chichester, UK: Wiley and Sons, 1985; J. P. Swann, *Academic Scientists and the Pharmaceutical Industry*, Baltimore: Johns Hopkins University Press, 1988; M. J. Vogel and C. E. Rosenberg, *The Therapeutic Revolution, Essays in the Social History of American Medicine*, Philadelphia: University of Pennsylvania Press, 1979; J. H. Warner, *The Therapeutic Perspective: Medical Practice, Knowledge, and Identity in America, 1820-1885*, Cam-

248 A Social History of Medicines in the Twentieth Century

bridge, MA: Harvard University Press, 1986; M. Weatherall, *In Search of a Cure: A History of Pharmaceutical Discovery*, Oxford: Oxford University Press, 1990.

There are, too, a growing number of works on single drugs, as well as journal articles, many of which are utilized in this book. Examples of a wide range of general works also called upon include A. Digby, *The Evolution of British General Practice 1850-1948*, Oxford: Oxford University Press, 1999; J. Le Fanu, *The Rise and Fall of Modern Medicine*, New York: Carroll and Graf, 1999; R. Cooter and J. Pickstone (eds.), *Medicine in the Twentieth Century*, Amsterdam, Netherlands: Harwood, 2000.

3. Smith, *A Social History of the Minor Tranquilizers*, pp. 2-3. Smith is primarily interested in the life cycle of psychoactive drugs, but the notion has been applied to others. For example, see E. Jawetz, "Infectious Diseases: Problems of Antimicrobial Therapy," *Annual Review of Medicine*, 5(1954), 2-26.

4. Healy, *The Antidepressant Era*.

5. For medicines as cultural events, see D. Healy, *The Psychopharmacologists II*, London: Altman, 1998, p. xi.

6. C. Hoyle and J. W. Linnell, "The Misuse of Some Common Remedies," *The Practitioner*, 136(1936), 94.

7. Quoted in G. B. Risse, "The Road to Twentieth-Century Therapeutics: Shifting Perspectives and Approaches," in Higby and Stroud, *The Inside Story of Medicines*, p. 51. Recently published histories of medicine carry the same message, although perhaps not quite so emotively; for example, see R. Porter, *The Greatest Benefit to Mankind: A Medical History of Humanity*, New York: Norton, 1999, pp. 674-676.

8. J. W. McGrath, "Casual Memories from Half a Century of Medical Practice in Newfoundland," *Newsletter Newfoundland Medical Association*, 16(4)(1974), 9-11. We might add that pharmacists have also been equally ready to chastise medicines of the past. In 1992, a retired Newfoundland pharmacist subjectively felt that many doctors' prescriptions, even in the 1960s and 1970s, were of little value (Oral History Collection, Medical Communication Group, English Department, Memorial University of Newfoundland, file 007, p. 10).

9. P. Beeson, "Changes in Medical Therapy During the Past Half Century," *Medicine*, 59(1980), 81.

10. Cf. C. E. Rosenberg, "The Therapeutic Revolution: Medicine, Meaning, and Social Change in Nineteenth-Century America," *Perspectives in Biology and Medicine*, 20(1977), 485-506.

11. Social studies on science and medicine that emphasize the way social factors shape science and its interpretation have mushroomed in recent years. The sentiment used here is from L. Bryder, "'We Shall Not Find Salvation in Inoculation': BCG Vaccination in Scandinavia, Britain, and the USA, 1921-1960," *Social Science and Medicine*, 49(1999), 1157-1167.

12. For discussion on the council and rational therapeutics, see Marks, *The Progress of Experiment*.

13. For example, see A. Dally, *Fantasy Surgery, 1880-1930: With Special Reference to Sir William Arbuthnot Lane*, Amsterdam, Netherlands: Rodopi, 1996; J. D. Pressman, *Last Resort: Psychosurgery and the Limits of Medicine*, Cambridge, UK: Cambridge University Press, 1998.

14. It is always important to appreciate that diagnostic labels, meanings, and etiologies of disease can often be in a state of flux; see R. A. Aronowitz, *Making Sense of Illness, Science, Society, and Disease*, Cambridge, UK: Cambridge University

Press, 1998. For views on the concept of nondisease, see R. Smith, "In Search of Non-Disease," *British Medical Journal,* 324(2002), 883-885; see also letters to the editor, Ibid., 912-913.

15. Points listed here are also identified in surveys from the 1970s onward about patients' beliefs and their attitudes toward medicines (see Chapter 6).

16. L. Payer, *Medicine and Culture: Varieties of Treatment in the United States, England, West Germany, and France,* New York: Holt, 1988.

17. Ibid., p. 24. For a more recent discussion on the differences between Japan and Western countries in the use of antidepressives and anxiolytics, see D. Healy, *The Psychopharmacologists III,* London: Arnold, 2000, pp. 286-288 (interview, "Psychopharmaceuticals in Japan," with Toshi-Hiro Kobayakawa).

18. J. P. Griffin, "Therapeutic Conservatism or Therapeutic Fossilisation," *International Pharmacy Journal,* 9(1)(1995), 23.

19. Discussed in C. G. Helman, *Culture Health and Illness,* Oxford: Butterworth-Heinemann, 2000. This raises questions about different cultural values in validation, cf., H. Fabrega Jr., "Medical Validity in Eastern and Western Traditions," *Perspectives in Biology and Medicine,* 45(2002), 395-415.

20. Cf. T. L. Savitt and J. H. Young (eds.), *Disease and Distinctiveness in the American South,* Knoxville: University of Tennessee Press, 1988.

21. V. Berridge, "Fenland Opium Eating in the Nineteenth Century," *British Journal of Addiction,* 72(1977), 275-284.

22. See J. K. Crellin, *Patent Medicines in North Carolina,* Revised Edition, Bailey, NC: Country Doctor Museum, 1993. I am grateful to Mrs. Elsie Booker for highlighting this topic.

23. See R. Hoffenberg, *Clinical Freedom,* London: The Nuffield Provincial Hospitals Trust, 1987, p. 19.

24. The province is actually Newfoundland *and* Labrador. The latter, part of the mainland, became part of Newfoundland in 1927. With a population of around 28,000 (in 2000), it is sparsely populated and I intentionally omit its particular medical story.

25. "Business News," *The Pharmaceutical Journal,* 75(series 4)(1905), 446.

26. For references and further comment, see discussion on syphilis in Chapter 5.

27. R. Rompkey (ed.), *The Labrador Memoir of Dr. Henry Paddon (1912-1938),* Montreal: McGill-Queen's University Press, 2003, p. xxx. See also M. Macleod, *Peace of the Continent,* St. John's: Harry Cuff, 1986, pp. 31-48. For a general account of Grenfell, see R. Rompkey, *Grenfell of Labrador: A Biography,* Toronto: University of Toronto Press, 1991. I am grateful to Dr. Rompkey for the prepublication review of the Paddon transcript.

28. The majority of the volunteers were associated with the Grenfell Mission and served the Northern Peninsula of Newfoundland and Labrador; see Rompkey, *Grenfell of Labrador,* pp. 242-245.

29. For the remarkable career of Olds see G. L. Saunders, *Doctor Olds of Twillingate. Portrait of an American Surgeon in Newfoundland,* St. John's: Breakwater, 1994.

30. Recent relevant discussions on the illicit drug scene in the United States and Britain include P. Jenkins, *Synthetic Panics: The Symbolic Politics of Designer Drugs,* New York: New York University Press, 1999; and A Working Party of the Royal College of Psychiatrists and the Royal College of Physicians, *Drugs: Di-*

lemmas and Choices, London: Gaskell, 2000. Both raise questions about existing policies.

31. P. Starr, *The Social Transformation of American Medicine,* New York: Basic Books, 1982.

32. For an overview of the situation in the United States, see N. Tomes, "Merchants of Health: Medicine and Consumer Culture in the United States," *Journal of American History,* 88(2001), 519-546.

33. J. Parascandola, "The Drug Habit: The Association of the Word 'Drug' with Abuse in American History," in R. Porter and M. Teich (eds.), *Drugs and Narcotics in History,* Cambridge, UK: Cambridge University Press, 1995, pp. 156-167.

34. St. John's, the capital city of Newfoundland, is only relatively urban. The population in 1951 was about 51,000; in 2001, about 99,000. However, if only as a port, it faced social issues beyond its size.

35. A. Hardy, *Health and Medicine in Britain Since 1860,* Basingstoke, UK: Palgrave, 2001, p. 103.

36. *First Interim Report of the Royal Commission on Health and Public Charities, June 1930,* St. John's: King's Printer, 1930, p. 18.

37. Quoted in R. S. Morton, *A Woman Surgeon. The Life and Work of Rosalie Slaughter Morton,* New York: Grosset and Dunlop, 1937, p. 199.

38. For an introduction to macho medicine, see A. Dally, "Women and Macho Medicine," in L. Conrad and A. Hardy (eds.), *Women and Modern Medicine,* Amsterdam, Netherlands: Rodopi, 2001, pp. 9-21.

39. *The Dewar Report. The Highlands and Islands Medical Service Committee Report,* 1912, available online at <www.rarari.org.UK/documents/Dewar_Report. doc>, accessed August 2003. For this information, I am indebted to Megan J. Davies for access to her manuscript, "Rural Medicine in the Scottish Highlands and Islands before 1939," read to the Canadian Society of the History of Medicine Annual Meeting, May 2002. The manuscript centers on the Dewar Report.

40. For more on Appalachia, see S. L. Barney, *Authorized to Heal. Gender, Class, and the Transformation of Medicine in Appalachia 1880-1930,* Chapel Hill: University of North Carolina Press, 2000, p. 27. It is safe to generalize on the universality of rural use of over-the-counter medicines, cf. L. Finch, "Soothing Syrups and Teething Powders: Regulating Proprietary Drugs in Australia, 1860-1910," *Medical History,* 43(1999), 74-94.

41. In Newfoundland, homemade remedies persisted much longer in rural areas than in towns such as St. John's; see J. K. Crellin, *Home Medicine. The Newfoundland Experience,* Montreal: McGill-Queen's University Press, 1994; for the United States in the twentieth century, see J. K. Crellin and J. Philpott, *Trying to Give Ease, Tommie Bass and the Story of Herbal Medicine,* Durham, NC: Duke University Press, 1997, pp. 66-82. Accounts of twentieth-century home medicine (as distinct from earlier periods) have been looked at more from the discipline of folklore than history; for a recent bibliography see E. Brady (ed.), *Healing Logics: Culture and Medicine in Modern Health Belief Systems,* Logan: Utah State University Press, 2001, pp. 211-277 and various sections. For a different approach to commercial medicines, see J. H. Young, *The Medical Messiahs: A Social History of Health Quackery in Twentieth-Century America,* Princeton, NJ: Princeton University Press, 1992.

42. A. E. Hertzler, *The Horse and Buggy Doctor,* New York: Harper and Bros., 1938, p. 34.

43. J. T. Hart, "Going to the Doctor," in Cooter and Pickstone (eds.), *Medicine in the Twentieth Century,* pp. 543-557.

44. It seems evident from surviving copies and recollections back to the 1950s that journals, such as the British *Practitioner* with its short, up-to-date reviews, were widely appreciated in Newfoundland. For a textbook reading, see J. K. Crellin, "Medical Books: For Information or Learning? Reflections on the Books of Three Newfoundland Physicians, c. 1860 to c. 1970," *Canadian Bulletin of Medical History,* 12(1995), 339-350.

45. See P. I. Crellin and J. K. Crellin, *By the Patient and Not by the Book: Constancy and Change in Small Town Doctoring,* Durham, NC: Acorn Press, 1988, pp. 36-42.

46. Hertzler's book focuses on Kansas.

47. Grenfell's own account, reprinted a number of times, originally appeared in W. T. Grenfell, *Adrift on an Ice Pan,* Boston: Houghton Mifflin, 1909.

48. Cf. Rompkey, *Grenfell of Labrador,* pp. 141-149.

49. Recounts of various instances of difficult, often unnecessary house calls appear in R. S. Ecke, *Snowshoe and Lancet: Memoirs of a Frontier Newfoundland Doctor 1937-1948,* Portsmouth, NH: Randall, 2000.

50. J. W. Heath, "Presidential Address," *Newsletter Newfoundland Medical Association,* 2(6)(1960), 2-3. Another rather condescending remark made in 1930 by a British-trained physician merits noting. In seeing "little improvement in sanitation" in Newfoundland outports over forty-two years, he cited Ferryland, where night soil was deposited as manure heaps by about 90 percent of the population and then spread on fields and gardens in the spring. This, along with rotting cods-heads—also spread as fertilizer in the same gardens and fields—was said to be the reason why "outports are pestered" with a public health menace of "myriads of flies." (R. J. Freebairn, presidential address to Newfoundland Medical Association. Unpublished typescript, September 1930, kindly brought to my attention by Dr. M. Braden.)

51. Davies, "Rural Medicine in the Scottish Highlands and Islands before 1939."

52. J. R. Martin, *Leonard Albert Miller, Public Servant,* Toronto: Associated Medical Services and Fitzhenry and Whiteside, 1998, p. 122. Besides being used by individual physicians, institutions such as the Grenfell Mission and the hospital at Twillingate relied on the book system even before the approach became part of the government-operated cottage hospital scheme in rural Newfoundland.

53. For some discussion in Britain see: A. Digby, *Making a Medical Living: Doctors and Patients in the English Market for Medicine, 1720-1911,* Cambridge, UK: Cambridge University Press, 1994, pp. 224-253, and A. Digby, *The Evolution of British General Practice 1850-1948,* Oxford: Oxford University Press, 1999, discussion on costs, pp. 241-246.

54. Lutterloh "charity" prescriptions (1934), Sanford, N.C. Author's collection.

55. See R. E. Durden, *Lasting Legacy to the Carolinas: The Duke Endowment 1924-1994,* Durham, NC: Duke University Press, 1998, pp. 29-88.

56. I am particularly indebted to Dr. Paddy Warwick for discussions on this point.

57. H. T. Englehardt, "The Doctor's Role in the Evolution of Human Society," in S. G. Wolf and B. B. Berle (eds.), *Limits of Medicine: The Doctor's Job in the Coming Era,* New York: Plenum Press, 1978, pp. 1-10.

58. D. Porter, "The Healthy Body," in Cooter and Pickstone (eds.), *Medicine in the Twentieth Century,* pp. 201-216. Despite much agreement among historians on issues contributing to the development of public health at particular time periods, some differences of opinion exist. This partly reflects that certain themes (e.g., control of infectious disease) are continuous, whereas interest in the general environment and health has waxed and waned; further, it is relevant that the public health movement in the United States has been much less tied to the medical profession than in Britain. Cf. various discussions in E. Fee and R. M. Acheson (eds.), *A History of Education in Public Health: Health That Mocks the Doctors' Rules,* Oxford: Oxford University Press, 1991.

59. J. H. Cassedy, *Medicine in America: A Short History,* Baltimore: Johns Hopkins University Press, 1991, p. 121.

60. This Newfoundland story has yet to be written, but it seems unlikely that the role of women matched the situation in Appalachia, which faced similar socioeconomic problems in the first few decades of the 1900s. See Barney, *Authorized to Heal: Gender, Class, and the Transformation of Medicine in Appalachia, 1880-1930.* For an example of active individuals in Newfoundland concerned with broad public health issues, see H. MacDermott, *MacDermott of Fortune Bay Told by Himself,* London: Hodder and Stoughton, 1938, especially pp. 120-142. In Newfoundland, NONIA (Newfoundland Outport Nursing Industrial Association) was important.

61. The term *social medicine,* in currency by the 1940s, reflected the view that medicine was a social science involved in political reform to improve society. See D. Porter, "Introduction," in D. Porter (ed.), *Social Medicine and Medical Sociology in the Twentieth Century,* Amsterdam, Netherlands: Rodopi, 1997, pp. 1-31. It is arguable whether Grenfell's work is to be seen as social medicine or as social reform, especially as his work was set in a Christian rather than political setting. However, Grenfell recognized that social change was necessary for improved health and that government involvement was needed (compare with R. Rompkey, *Grenfell of Labrador*). For government activities, see J. Lewis and M. Shrimpton, "Notes Toward an Assessment of Health Policy Under Commission Government," unpublished manuscript, Founders' Archive, Faculty of Medicine, Memorial University of Newfoundland, file no. 003/5.09.002. It should be noted that the Commission Government did build on the Newfoundland Health and Welfare Act of 1932. For typical problems with respect to inadequacy of public health diagnostic services, see the Josephson manuscript, History of Medicine Collection, Faculty of Medicine, Memorial University of Newfoundland.

62. It would seem that Newfoundlanders became just as concerned with the germ-carrying potential of flies. Cf. N. Rogers, "Germs with Legs: Flies, Disease, and the New Public Health," *Bulletin of the History of Medicine,* 63(1989), 599-617.

63. Labeling is significant; *public health*—or *social medicine*—became redefined as *community medicine* with the emphasis on epidemiology and population health with implications for preventive medicine and medications.

64. In the English-speaking world, Selye's 1956 book, *The Stress of Life,* New York: McGraw-Hill, was significant, following his earlier work published in Ger-

man in the 1930s. In Canada, a 1974 government document, *A New Perspective on the Health of Canadians,* Ottawa: Information Canada (also known as the Marc LaLonde report), had far-reaching influence in accelerating interest in prevention. It encouraged a shift away from treatment facilities and toward prevention and the reduction of illness associated with lifestyle and environmental factors. For context see J. Cassel, "Public Health in Canada," in D. Porter, *The History of Public Health and the Modern State,* pp. 276-312.

65. The concept of *healthy communities* has deep roots, but the term only became popular in the medical literature in the 1980s. Texts such as P. A. Keller and J. D. Murray, *Handbook of Rural Community Mental Health,* New York: Human Sciences Press, 1982, document interest in community psychiatry in the 1970s. For a Newfoundland contribution see B. Neis and B. Grzetic, "Restructuring and Women's Health: The Fisheries Crisis in Newfoundland," available online at <www.cewh-cesf.ca/bulletin/v2n2/page6.html>, accessed August 2003. Community and individual social stress was conspicuous in the 1990s relating to the unparalleled decline in northern cod stocks, which led the federal government to impose a moratorium on the cod fishery; this continued (aside from minor relaxations) into 2002 with no sign of being lifted.

66. Beginning around the turn of the twentieth century, the events that lay behind these upheavals were the establishment of rail transport, forest industries and pulpwood production, and mining that began to break the "truck" system, in which merchants supplied fishing families with provisions and gear on credit and were to be repaid by the season's catch. From the late 1940s onward, industrialization further impacted Newfoundland's fishing industry with the increase in capital ownership of fleets of large mechanized groundfish trawlers and fish processing plants. These became the economic backbone of major "fish plant towns" or, as politicians called them, "growth centers," many of which failed to flourish.

67. A. Best, "Voices from the Outports," *Maclean's,* 114 (August 13, 2001), 26. This quote reflects the feelings of many Newfoundlanders who contributed reminiscences for this book, even though many now realize that it was a good move for their children.

68. For recent discussions, see S. Marks, "What Is Colonial About Colonial Medicine? And What Has Happened to Imperialism and Health?" *Social History of Medicine,* 10(1997), 205-219, and M. Worboys, "Colonial Medicine," in Cooter and Pickstone (eds.), *Medicine in the Twentieth Century,* pp. 67-80.

69. Quoted in P. Neary (ed.), *White Tie and Decorations: Sir John and Lady Hope Simpson in Newfoundland 1934-1936,* Toronto: University of Toronto Press, 1996, p. 67.

70. Taken from Frederick Treves' preface to W. T. Grenfell, *Vikings of To-day,* London: Marshall Brothers, 1895. See also Rompkey, *Grenfell of Labrador,* p. 84.

71. Although the celebrated work of Wilfred Grenfell and the Grenfell Mission was associated with Labrador, which became part of Newfoundland in 1927, its influence had already impacted Newfoundland even beyond the Grenfell headquarters at St. Anthony on the Northern Peninsula of the island. Cf. Rompkey, *Grenfell of Labrador.*

72. Stafford Allen and Sons, *The Romance of Empire Drugs,* London: Stafford Allen and Sons, n.d. (c. 1932), p. 64. Stafford Allen was a British company that produced chemicals and essential oils.

73. Oral History Collection, Newfoundland Pharmaceutical Association, Bill O'Mara.

74. "Trade Notes," *The Pharmaceutical Journal,* 75(series 4) (1905), 446.

75. As one pharmacist remembered of the 1940s, "We carried wets and dries and we labelled those in our own dispensary." Some were made (e.g., camphorated oil) and others just bottled in small containers (Oral History Collection, Newfoundland Pharmaceutical Association, John Stowe).

76. Two other establishments identified in part by their wholesale/manufacturing and brand-name preparations were McMurdo's (for "ACME" products) and Connors (for "EXCEL"). The Imperial Manufacturing Company (without a retail outlet) also produced a line of essences and other products (Collections, O'Mara Pharmacy Museum, Newfoundland Pharmaceutical Association).

77. For a sense of long-standing debates on local versus exotic remedies, see A. Wear, "Making Sense of the Health and the Environment in Early Modern England," in A. Wear (ed.), *Medicine in Society: Historical Essays,* Cambridge, UK: Cambridge University Press, 1992, pp. 119-147.

78. For some introduction to this see P. Palladino, "Medicine Yesterday, Today, and Tomorrow," *Social History of Medicine,* 14(2001), 539-551.

79. For a good example, see D. Geier and M. Geier, "The True Story of Pertussis Vaccination: A Sordid Legacy," *Journal of the History of Medicine and Allied Sciences,* 57(2002), 249-284.

80. See A. I. Marcus, *Cancer from Beef: DES, Federal Food Regulation, and Consumer Confidence,* Baltimore: Johns Hopkins University Press, 1994.

81. For a recent example, see R. Mahomed, C. Paton, and E. Lee, "Prescribing Hypnotics in a Mental Health Trust: What Consultant Psychiatrists Say and What They Do," *The Pharmaceutical Journal,* 268(2002), 657-659.

82. For useful comments on problems of access to records in the United States, see J. P. Swann, "In Search of the Historical Record," *Pharmacy in History,* 41(1999), 131-136.

83. It is difficult to decide which terms—*druggist* or *pharmacist* (or *drugstore* or *pharmacy*)—to use consistently throughout the book. I have elected to use *druggist* and *drugstore,* the terms that are appropriate to North America, except in Chapter 6. However, in Newfoundland the British terms *chemist* and *druggist* and *pharmacy* were also evident in the nineteenth century, continuing into the twentieth. In Newfoundland (and elsewhere in North America) *pharmacists* and *pharmacy* (as well as *pharmaceutical chemist,* which appeared on the Newfoundland registration certificate after 1954) have come to be terms for the "new" or modern practitioner, hence our use in Chapter 6. *Drugstore,* rather than *pharmacy,* however, remains commonplace.

84. See A. Helmstädter and C. Staiger, "Cain and Abel or Siamese Twins?: Defining Essential Considerations for a Successful Cooperation of Physicians and Pharmacists in the 21st Century—an Historical Review," *Pharmaceutical Historian,* 32(2002), 33-40.

85. Oral History Collection, Medical Communication Group, file 010.

86. Observations on tensions over commercialism are widespread in discussions on the profession, for example, see L. J. Muzzin, G. P. Brown, and R. W. Hornosty, "Professional Ideology in Canadian Pharmacy," *Health and Canadian Society,* 1(1993), 319-345.

87. Advertisement of G. J. Brockelhurst, Carbonear, in *McAlpine's Newfoundland Directory, 1894-1897*, Halifax, Nova Scotia: McAlpine, 1894, p. 492.

88. For this aspect of the Newfoundland story see Crellin, *Home Medicine: The Newfoundland Experience*.

89. For a discussion on values among Newfoundlanders, see R. Andersen, J. K. Crellin, and B. O'Dwyer, *Healthways: Newfoundland Elders, Their Lifestyles and Values*, St. John's: Creative Publishers, 1998.

90. Quoted in J. O. Breeden, "Disease As a Factor in Southern Distinctiveness," in Savitt and Young (eds.), *Disease and Distinctiveness in the American South*, p. 1.

91. See J. Bornat, R. Perks, P. Thompson, and J. Walmsley (eds.), *Oral History, Health, and Welfare*, London: Routledge, 2000.

92. In many ways popular writings reinforced other "exposés," such as the Kefauver Senate Hearings (1960-1962) on the pharmaceutical industry. Muckraking—reminiscent of the critiques of over-the-counter medicines of the late nineteenth and early twentieth centuries—is overly strong for many of the writings, but compare M. A. Bealle's *The Drug Story*, Washington, DC: Columbia Publishing, 1949, a forerunner of countless others that attacked the pharmaceutical industry, the FDA, etc.

93. See J. Gabe, "Benzodiazepines As a Social Problem: The Case of Halcion," *Substance Use and Misuse*, 36(2001), 1233-1259.

94. Many writings, e.g., Young, *The Medical Messiahs*, avoid a sense of snobbery, but nevertheless provide an establishment, rather than populist, view.

95. The A.W. Chase Company was marketing from the United States and Canada. For different labels in Canada and the United States, see A. J. Cramp, *Nostrums and Quackery: Articles on the Nostrum Evil, Quackery, and Allied Matters Affecting the Public Health. Reprinted with or Without Modifications from the Journal of the American Medical Association*, Chicago: AMA, 1912, Volume 1, pp. 494-496. That is not to say that advertising copy was not changed when companies exported their products to places with more stringent regulations, as between Britain and the United States in 1906. See Young, *The Medical Messiahs*, illustration 1.

One example where Newfoundlanders saw new labeling because of legislative changes elsewhere was on a favorite medicine in Newfoundland, Dodd's Kidney Pills, produced in Canada. The recommendation for treating diabetes was only dropped around September 1935, many years after the introduction of insulin—obviously due to new Canadian controls on advertising. Cf. advertisements in *The Twillingate Sun*, August 31, 1935, p. 2, and September 14, 1935, p. 2. In 1934, a list of disorders that could not be mentioned in advertisements to the public (including insulin) was added to Schedule A of the Canadian Food and Drugs Act of 1920. See G. L. Kalbfleisch, "Pharmaceutical Legislation 1907-1957," *Canadian Pharmaceutical Journal*, 90(1957), 726, 728.

96. This subject has been much discussed, but for a useful introduction see T. J. J. Lears, "American Advertising and the Reconstruction of the Body, 1880-1930" in K. Grover (ed.), *Fitness in American Culture: Images of Health, Sport, and the Body 1830-1940*, Amherst: University of Massachussetts Press, 1989, pp. 48-66.

97. For a full account of vitamins and advertising in the United States, see R. D. Apple, *Vitamania: Vitamins in American Culture*, New Brunswick, NJ: Rutgers University Press, 1996.

98. *The Evening Telegram*, July 23, 1937, p. 7.

99. In Newfoundland, two St. John's newspapers (*The Evening Telegram* and *The Daily News*) were of particular influence, though papers published for the outports were also important (many, however, were short-lived, with exceptions such as *The Twillingate Sun*). They all carried identical advertising to the St. John's papers.

100. A fascinating photograph of a derelict building with peeled wallpaper to reveal newspaper insulation with adverts such as for Gin Pills (c. 1930) appears in a photographic exhibition, "Unsettled," by Scott Walden. For title (no picture), see the exhibition catalog published by Art Gallery of Newfoundland and Labrador, 2001, item 43. Obviously this is not to say such use was a constant reminder of the medicine, if only because newspaper insulation was generally covered by regular wallpaper.

101. See Crellin, *Home Medicine. The Newfoundland Experience.*

102. *The Daily News,* July 18, 1900, p. 2. For further information on Pierce's volume and general background see N. Gevitz, "Domestic Medical Guides and the Drug Trade in Nineteenth-Century America," *Pharmacy in History,* 32(1990), 51-56.

103. *Dodd's Almanac 1960,* n.p., n.d., p. 2.

104. For more on Doyle and his other activities, see Crellin, *Home Medicine. The Newfoundland Experience,* especially pp. 18-21.

Chapter 2

1. *Public Ledger,* August 31, 1830, p. 3. This advertisement described Henry Bisset of the London Medical Establishment as "bred in the Apothecary and Druggist line."

2. For a review and summary of earlier literature, see R. L. Numbers (ed.), *Medicine in the New World: New Spain, New France, and New England,* Knoxville: University of Tennessee Press, 1987, pp. 1-11. The book emphasises that "medical practice changed remarkably little in transit from the established societies in the Old World to the new settlements in the Americas" (p. 157).

3. It is appropriate to notice that the story of colonial North America has generally focused on French, Spanish, and English settlements from New England southward. The richness of the archaeology of the two stone-built English settlements in Newfoundland has only been recognized in recent years; along with the substantial written record, they can add much to the story of health in British colonial North America.

An essential source for relevant early documents is G. Cell (ed.), *Newfoundland Discovered: English Attempts at Colonization 1610-1630,* London: Hakluyt Society, 1982. This work retains seventeenth-century spelling and punctuation. In contrast, P. Pope, "Six Letters from the Early Colony of Avalon," *Avalon Chronicles,* 1(1996), 1-20, has published a small proportion of the same material transcribed into modern English.

4. See D. L. Cowen, "The Impact of the Materia Medica of the North American Indian on Professional Practice," *Veröffentlichungen der Internationalen Gesellschaft für Geschichte der Pharmazie* (Proceedings of the International Society for the History of Pharmacy), 53(1984), 51-63.

Contacts between the Beothuk people and settlers at Cupids and Ferryland were minimal. (See I. Marshall, *A History and Ethnography of the Beothuk,* Montreal:

McGill-Queen's University Press, 1996, pp. 23-41, Chapter 2, "The Seventeenth Century Colonization, Trade and Encroachment.") Of course, a possibility exists of information reaching the settlers from local knowledge acquired over decades by migratory fishermen, who, in turn, may well have interacted with native people. On the other hand, given the migratory habits of both fishermen and Beothuks (and the latter's apparent reluctance to develop trading relationships with Europeans), it seems unlikely that local medical knowledge was incorporated into the common stock of knowledge available to settlers. By the same token, given the Newfoundland setting, it is not altogether surprising that any new observations did not enter into the mainstream or the maze of suggestions for scurvy.

5. For a useful review, see J. W. Estes, "The European Reception of the First Drugs from the New World," *Pharmacy in History,* 37(1995), 3-23.

6. See D. L. Cowen, "The History of Pharmacy and the History of the South," *Report of RhoChi,* 3(1967), 18-25.

7. D. L. Cowen, "The British North American Colonies As a Source of Drugs," *Veröffentlichungen der Internationalen Gesellschaft für Geschichte der Pharmazie,* 28(1966), 47-59.

8. Letter, Henry Crout to Percival Willoughby, Willoughby Papers, 1610-1613. Mix file no. 1/13 B43 (Microfilm copy, Memorial University of Newfoundland, Marine Archives).

9. W. Vaughan, *Directions for Health: Naturall and Artificiall,* London: Roger Jackson, 1617, p. 1. For additional information on Vaughan, see the *Dictionary of Canadian Biography,* Toronto: University of Toronto Press, 1966, Volume 1, pp. 654-657.

10. It is appropriate to mention here a discussion on "the dietary basis for the origin of human medicines" in T. Johns, *With Bitter Herbs They Shall Eat It: Chemical Ecology and the Origins of Human Diet and Medicine,* Tucson: University of Arizona Press, 1990, pp. 251-291.

11. J. Mason, *A Briefe Discourse of the New-Found-Land,* Edinburgh: Andro Hort, 1620, p. 7. For more on the cultivation of medicinal plants in the Virginia settlements, see Cowen, "The History of Pharmacy and the History of the South."

12. Letter, Edward Wynne to George Calvert, August 17, 1622, reprinted in Pope, "Six Letters from Avalon," p. 14.

13. For another version of the scurvy story, see J. K. Crellin, "Early Settlements in Newfoundland and the Scourge of Scurvy," *Canadian Bulletin of Medical History,* 17(2000), 127-136.

14. R. Hayman, *Quodlibets, Lately Come Over from New Britaniola, Old Newfoundland,* London: All-de, 1628, p. 33, No. 88.

15. Letter, Captain Edward Winne to Sir George Calvert, August 20, 1621, in Cell, *Newfoundland Discovered,* p. 257.

16. Cf. K. J. Carpenter, *The History of Scurvy and Vitamin C,* Cambridge, UK: Cambridge University Press, 1986, pp. 239-246.

17. See ibid., pp. 200-204, for a discussion on low vitamin reserves. William Vaughan (*The Newlander Cure,* London: Constable, 1630, pp. 71-72) offered detailed advice on early treatment to the person "that scares or suspects himselfe tainted": (1) "change or ayre his apparrell, putting on clean shifts and linnen"; (2) "sleepe in boorded Roomes," and have the "Chamber Wainscotted, or well dryed of those dampish fauours, which stone or earthen walls are want to euaporate and

breath out"; (3) "beate and burne one Acre of Land rounde about [the] dwelling"; and (4) eat an appropriate diet.

18. Letter, John Guy to Percival Willoughby, October 6, 1610, in Cell, *Newfoundland Discovered*, p. 62.

19. *Cochlearia officinalis* is no longer found around Cupids (P. Scott, personal communication). Although reported for the Avalon Peninsula, it is usually restricted to coastal habitats influenced by salt water, such as salt marshes, brackish water, and sea beaches. It is not improbable that it was once much more common in the area. For more on habitat, see S. J. Meades, S. G. Hay, and L. Brouillet, *Annotated Checklist of the Vascular Plants of Newfoundland and Labrador*, 2000, available online at <www. nfmuseum.com/meades.htm>, accessed August 2003, p. 55.

20. John Guy's "Journal of a Voyage to Trinity Bay," in Cell, *Newfoundland Discovered*, p. 70.

21. Journal of Henry Crout, *The Willoughby Papers*. Middleton manuscripts, University of Nottingham, p. 27.

22. Brooklime has not been reported for the island. *Nasturtium officinale* is an introduced species. See Meades, Hay, and Brouillot, *Annotated Checklist of the Vascular Plants of Newfoundland and Labrador*, p. 59.

23. Mason, *A Brief Discourse of the New-Found-Land*, p. 7.

24. R. Whitbourne, *A Discourse and Discovery of New-Found-Land*, London: Kingston, 1620, p. 7. The reference to juicing the plants is tantalizing. R. E. Hughes, "The Rise and Fall of the 'Antiscorbutics': Some Notes on the Traditional Cures for 'Land Scurvy,'" *Medical History*, 34(1990), 52-64, indicates that expressed juices of antiscorbutic plants "lose almost all their vitamin C within a matter of minutes of preparation" (p. 61).

25. Letter, N. H. to W. P., August 18, 1622, in Pope, "Six Letters from the Early Colony of Avalon," p. 19.

26. See J. K. Crellin and J. Philpott, *Trying to Give Ease: Tommie Bass and the Story of Herbal Medicine*, Durham, NC: Duke University Press, 1997, pp. 18-22.

27. See Hughes, "The Rise and Fall of the 'Antiscorbutics,'" p. 53.

28. See Vaughan, *The Newlander Cure*, p. 73; J. Woodall, *The Surgions Mate*, London: Laurence Lisle, 1617, p. 186, notes wormwood's use for symptom management.

29. The view that the origin of plant medicines is derived largely from diet has been forcibly put forward by Johns, *With Bitter Herbs They Shall Eat It*. It is noteworthy that the rutabaga, popularly called "turnip" or "winter turnip" by Newfoundlanders, contains vitamin C; however, its introduction to Newfoundland probably occurred in the early 1900s.

30. For more on the effectiveness of turnip juice, see Carpenter, *The History of Scurvy and Vitamin C*, p. 184; Carpenter also notes John Wesley's eighteenth-century treatment recommendation "to live on turnips for a month" and suggests that this may be linked to John Guy's experience around 1610 (p. 45). This is always a possibility but is more likely to be independent knowledge. The effects of different growing conditions on vitamin C are not known.

31. J. W. Estes, "The Therapeutic Crisis of the Eighteenth Century," in G. J. Higby and E. C. Stroud (eds.), *The Inside Story of Medicines. A Symposium*, Madison, WI: American Institute History of Pharmacy, 1997, p. 40.

32. For more on Yonge see F. N. L. Poynter (ed.), *The Journal of James Yonge 1647-1721, Plymouth Surgeon,* London: Longmans, 1963, p. 59. It seems that other plants were also included: "tops of spruce, wild vetches, and agrimony, a sort of wild succory (called here scurvy leaves) steept in beer, and bathing them in decoctions of the same" (p. 59). Yonge also stated that scurvy, at least acute scurvy, is a "disease not curable by all the medicines which can be carrried there, but easily by a few vegitives of the country" (p. 59).

33. J. Josselyn, *New-England's Rarities Discovered,* London: Widdowes, 1672, p. 64. Carpenter, *The History of Scurvy and Vitamin C,* p. 229, says that spruce beer was used during the sixteenth century as a beverage by sailors in the Baltic Sea.

34. J. Quincy, *Compleat English Dispensatory,* London: Bell, 1719, p. 502. For seventeenth-century reference to scorbutic beers, see Hughes, "The Rise and Fall of the 'Antiscorbutics.'"

35. For Cook, see B. J. S. Harley, *The Legacy of James Cook,* Corner Brook, Canada: Harkin, 1998, pp. 25-28. For Banks see A. M. Lysaght, *Joseph Banks in Newfoundland and Labrador, 1766: His Diary, Manuscripts, and Collections,* Berkeley: University of California Press, 1971, pp. 139-140.

36. A. Thomas, *The Newfoundland Journal of Aaron Thomas, Able Seaman in H.M.S. Boston: A Journal written during a Voyage from England to Newfoundland and from Newfoundland to England in the years 1794 and 1795, addressed to a friend,* J. M. Murray (ed.), London: Longmans, 1968, pp. 59-60. Added interest comes from Peter Kalm's earlier observation, recorded in Montreal during 1749, that spruce beer was sometimes drunk but seldom "by people of quality" (P. Kalm, *Travels into North America by Peter Kalm,* J. R. Forster [trans. and ed.], Barre, MA: Imprint Society, 1972, p. 504.) Kalm, in fact, notes the use of white spruce. See also references in C. Erichsen-Brown, *Use of Plants for the Past 500 Years,* Aurora, Canada: Breezy Creeks Press, 1979, pp. 7-14.

37. J. Lind, *A Treatise on Scurvy,* London: Crowder, 1772, p. 146.

38. Ibid., pp. 201-202.

39. Lysaght, *Joseph Banks in Newfoundland and Labrador,* p. 140.

40. William Buchan, *Domestic Medicine,* London: Johnson, 1810, p. 279.

41. G. H. Napheys, *The Prevention and Cure of Disease,* Springfield, MA: Holland and Co., 1875, p. 804.

42. For Franklin, see Carpenter, *The History of Scurvy and Vitamin C,* p. 230. A home medicine book (c. 1890) suggested that merchant seamen be given spruce beer instead of rum, but with the pragmatic comment: "we are afraid the men would fail to appreciate the change" (Anonymous, *The Family Physician: A Manual of Domestic Medicine,* London: Cassell, n.d., p. 361).

43. See R. E. Griffith, *A Universal Formulary,* Philadelphia: Lea, 1866, p. 490.

44. W. T. Fernie, *Meals Medicinal with "Herbal Simples,"* Bristol: Wright, 1905, p. 93.

45. R. E. Hughes, "James Lind and the Cure of Scurvy: An Experimental Approach," *Medical History,* 19(1975), 342-351. See also Carpenter, *The History of Scurvy and Vitamin C,* p. 226, for a discussion on vitamin C concentrations.

46. C. J. Lawrence, "William Buchan: Medicine Laid Open," *Medical History,* 19(1975), 20-35.

47. B. Ellis, *The Medical Formulary,* Philadelphia: Lea and Blanchard, 1849, p. 229.

48. See J. Duffin, *Langstaff: A Nineteenth-Century Medical Life,* Toronto: University of Toronto Press, 1993, p. 81.

49. In "'Pray Let the Medicines Be Good': The New England Apothecary in the Seventeenth and Early Eighteenth Centuries," *Pharmacy in History,* 41(1999), 87-101. N. Gevitz notes that occupational boundaries in early New England were nebulous.

50. Although a British colony, the French influence in Newfoundland, most marked up to the Treaty of Utrecht in 1713—not discussed in this book—has been considerable. See J. R. Smallwood (ed.), *Encyclopedia of Newfoundland and Labrador,* St. John's: Harry Cuff, 1993, Volume 4, pp. 317, 407-415; and Volume 2, pp. 407-415.

51. Advertisement of a Mr. Dobie, *Newfoundland Mercantile Journal,* January 5, 1826, p. 3.

52. See N. Rusted (compiler), *Medicine in Newfoundland c. 1497 to the Early 20th Century. The Physicians and Surgeons, Biographical Gleanings,* St. John's: Faculty of Medicine, Memorial University of Newfoundland, 1994, p. xiv, for numbers registered under the "Act to Regulate the Practice of Medicine and Surgery in the Colony."

53. The issue of ethics in selling products was raised from time to time on both sides of the Atlantic. For some context in Britain, see J. K. Crellin, "Revisiting Counter Practice Amid Pharmacy and Medical Reform in 19th-Century Britain," *Pharmaceutical Historian,* 30(2000), 44-49.

54. For reference to the London Medical Establishment, see *The Newfoundlander,* July 3, 1838, p. 3, and *Public Ledger,* August 31, 1830, p. 3, which specifically notes dispensing by a "young gentleman thoroughly bred in the Apothecary and Druggist line in one of the first Apothecary Halls in Scotland." For Wilson, established 1828, see *The Newfoundlander,* July 3, 1828, p. 3. McMurdo's store always claimed to be established in 1826.

55. *The Newfoundland Patriot,* July 18, 1840, p. 3. It seems very unlikely that the term *apothecary* here meant *general medical practitioner.*

56. *The Newfoundland Patriot,* August 20, 1833, p. 22.

57. The diverse activities of drugstores have been noted many times; for an interesting perspective, one that discusses the appearance of many drugstores in the United States, see W. H. Helfand, "The Design of American Pharmacies, 1865-1885," *Pharmacy in History,* 36(1994), 26-37. For other North American examples, see J. Collin, "Entre Discours et Pratiques Les Médecins Montréalais Face à la Thérapeutique, 1869-1890" (Between Discourse and Practice: Montreal Physicians and Therapeutics, 1869-1890) *Revue d'Histoire de l'Amerique Francaise* (Review of the History of French America), 53(1999), 61-92. Cf., Box 2.1.

58. McMurdo advertisment, *Hutchinson's Newfoundland Directory for 1864-65,* St. John's: McConnan, 1864, p. 154.

59. Cf. J. K. Crellin, "Domestic Medicine Chests: Microcosms of 18th and 19th Century Medical Practice," *Pharmacy in History,* 21(1979), 122-131.

60. *The Daily News,* December 29, 1915, p. 1. See also J. J. Keilley advertisement, "Ships' Medicine Chests supplied and refilled at Shortest Notice," *Newfoundland Directory, 1928,* St. John's: The Newfoundland Directories, 1928, p. 278.

61. See Duffin, *Langstaff: A Nineteenth-Century Medical Life,* especially Chapter four, "Medical 'Knowledge' in Therapy: Old Stand-bys, Innovations and Intangibles."

62. The story of aspirin and the context of other synthetic chemicals has been told a number of times; see C. C. Mann and M. L. Plummer, *The Aspirin Wars: Money, Medicine, and 100 Years of Rampant Competition,* New York: Knopf, 1991. For interesting discussions, illustrating anecdotes, and controversies that often surround discoveries see T. J. Rinsema, "One Hundred Years of Aspirin," *Medical History,* 43(1999), 502-507; and W. Sneader, "The Discovery of Aspirin: A Reappraisal," *British Medical Journal,* 321(2000), 1591-1594.

63. For more on research see J. P. Swann, *Academic Scientists and the Pharmaceutical Industry: Cooperative Research in Twentieth-Century America,* Baltimore: Johns Hopkins University Press, 1988.

64. J. Savory, *A Compendium of Domestic Medicine,* London: Churchill, 1952, p. 339. Savory gives interesting historical background to the situation in the 1840s. The quotation has, probably by coincidence, echoes of the Doctrine of Signatories, as Newfoundland's fishing grounds, like the island, had a reputation of damp and cold. For a general review see R. A. Guy, "The History of Cod Liver Oil As a Remedy," *American Journal of Diseases of Children,* 26(1923), 112-116.

65. For more on the use of cod-liver oil in the Massachusetts General Hospital see H. H. Warner, *The Therapeutic Perspective: Medical Practice, Knowledge and Identity in America, 1820-1855,* Cambridge: Harvard University Press, 1986, pp. 117, 145. Studies on usage in hospitals have not been undertaken, but if the large quantities employed in St. George's Hospital, London, during the final decades of the nineteenth century is also representative, then hospitals did much to promote the product. See J. K. Crellin, "Glimpses of Hospital Pharmacy Economics in the Nineteenth Century," *M and B Pharmaceutical Bulletin,* 10(1961), 75-76.

66. E. Souther, *A Treatise on the Use of Cod-Liver Oil,* Boston: Mead's Press, 1848, p. 8.

67. For reference to dark oil, see W. B. Willmott, *Glycerin and Cod Liver Oil,* London: Ballière, 1860, p. 97. Many other references have been made to the onetime popularity of the dark oil; e.g., J. Rayner, *Cod-Liver Oil: Its Uses, Mode of Administration,* New York: Rushton, Clark and Co., 1849.

68. See *Hutchinson's Newfoundland Directory for 1864-65,* pp. 99 and 369 for three drugstores, W. H. Thompson, Thomas McMurdo and Co., Alfred Dearin and J. J. Dearin. In 1860, Willmott (*Glycerin and Cod Liver Oil,* p. 32) said that while many preferred homemade British oil, the Newfoundland oil (presumably raw) "assimilates in physical character to the [British] home-made, and is considered by many to be superior in beneficial effect" (p. 32).

69. See J. Carson, *Synopsis of the Course of Lectures on Materia Medica and Pharmacy Delivered in the University of Pennsylvania,* Philadelphia: Blanchard and Lea, 1851, p. 81. Carson classifies the oil as a tonic and notes positive effects on nutrition.

Immunity was replacing *resistance* around the 1950s, as in an advertisement for Brick's Tasteless Cod Liver Oil under the heading, "How Nearly Immune Are You?" The copy went, "Seldom does anyone feel safely immune against those infections, that are so generally known as 'common colds and coughs.' Yet it is the neglected cold or cough that can and often does become a serious menace to health...."

Thousands owe their present vigour and good health, their ability to resist the common infection to Brick's Tasteless." *Western Star,* December 5, 1957, p. 8.

70. Oral History Collection, Medical Communication Group, English Department, Memorial University Newfoundland, 1992, file 010.

71. R. R. Andersen, J. K. Crellin, and B. O'Dwyer, *Healthways, Newfoundland Elders: Their Lifestyles and Values,* St. John's: Creative Press, 1998, p. 66.

72. Oral History Collection, Medical Communication Group, file 014.

73. G. F. Butler, *A Text-Book of Materia Medica, Therapeutics, and Pharmacology,* Philadelphia: Saunders, 1900, p. 138.

74. *The Evening Telegram,* December 19, 1902, p. 2.

75. For reference to disputed constituents, see A. A. Stevens, *Modern Materia Medica and Therapeutics,* Philadelphia: Saunders and Co., 1904, p. 297. Nowadays, the term *alterative* is commonly defined as an agent that increases resistance to physical, chemical and biological stress, and builds up general vitality, including the physical and mental capacity for work.

76. H. C. Thomson, "Cod-Liver Oil. Notes on a Visit to Newfoundland," *Chemist and Druggist,* 66(1905), 255-256.

77. See "Trade Notes," *Chemist and Druggist,* 63(1903), 786; Ibid. 66(1905), 834.

78. *Twillingate Sun,* January 31, 1942. For background with particular reference to cod-liver oil, see A. B. Davis, "The Rise of the Vitamin-Mineral Illustrated by Vitamin D," *Pharmacy in History,* 24(1982), 59-72; see also R. D. Apple, *Vitamania: Vitamins in American Culture,* New Brunswick, NJ: Rutgers University Press, 1996.

79. *The Evening Telegram,* July 2, 1947, p. 10.

80. See R. D. Apple, *Vitamania,* especially pp. 54-74.

81. R. S. Ecke, *Snowshoe and Lancet Memoirs of a Frontier Newfoundland Doctor,* Portsmouth: Randall, 2000, p. 93.

82. For recent commentary, see P. R. Fortin, R. A. Lew, M. H. Liong, M. H. Wright, L. A. Beckett, T. C. Chalmers, and R. I. Sperling, "Validation of a Meta-Analysis: The Effects of Fish Oil in Rheumatoid Arthritis," *Journal of Clinical Epidemiology,* 48(1995), 1379-1390.

Chapter 3

1. This reference, occurring at intervals in various chapters, refers to phrases heard in the Outpatient Department at the hospital in Twillingate. American-trained physician John Olds (in Newfoundland from 1932 until 1985) recorded remarks by his Newfoundland patients over many years. They commonly reflect the feelings and worries of patients everywhere, and highlight potential communication problems. The quotes are generally taken from a transcript of a selection in the History of Medicine Collection, Faculty of Medicine, Memorial University of Newfoundland. A somewhat different selection can be found in G. L. Saunders, *Doctor, When You're Sick You're Not Well: Forty Years of Outpatient Humour from Twillingate Hospital,* St. John's: Breakwater, 1988, which provides further information on the background of OPDisms.

2. Anon., *The Modern Materia Medica,* New York: The Druggists Circular, 1906.

3. For a discussion on "spot of land" in Southern Appalachia, see J. K. Crellin and J. Philpott, *Herbal Medicine Past and Present,* Volume 1: *Trying to Give Ease,* Durham, NC: Duke University Press, 1990, p. 58.

4. Oral History Collection, Medical Communication Group, English Department, Memorial University of Newfoundland, file 010.

5. In times of severe economic hardship, as in the 1930s, residents in the city of St. John's often felt that people in the outports were better off than themselves; this reflected a tradition of self-help amid a long history of rural poverty and dependence on the state; see P. Neary, *Newfoundland in the North Atlantic World, 1929-1949,* Montreal: McGill-Queen's University Press, 1988, p. 10.

6. The diagnosis of subclinical vitamin conditions became part of the Newfoundland scene as illustrated by physician R. F. Dove in his 1943 discussion "The Diagnosis and Treatment of the Subclinical Dietary Deficiency Disease," *Northern Medical Review,* 1(1)(1943), 7-9. After noting that "70 percent of the population exhibited signs and symptoms referable to deficiencies of the B complex and 70 percent of the population had normal ranges of blood vitamin C for only 2 months of the year," Dove reviewed for readers early symptoms of various vitamin deficiency disorders.

7. R. R. Andersen, J. K. Crellin, and B. O'Dwyer, *Healthways, Newfoundland Elders: Their Lifestyles and Values,* St. John's: Creative Publishers, 1998, p. 33.

8. J. K. Crellin, "A Candid View of Newfoundland Patients," *MunMed* (Memorial University of Newfoundland) 13(1)(2001), 3.

9. See K. J. Carpenter, *Beriberi, White Rice, and Vitamin B: A Disease, a Cause, and a Cure,* Berkeley: University of California Press, 2000, pp. 177-178.

10. G. Jones, *'Captain of All these Men of Death': The History of Tuberculosis in Nineteenth and Twentieth Century Ireland,* Amsterdam: Rodopi, 2001, p. 2, outlines the recent controversies and literature on the history of tuberculosis.

11. E. House, *Light at Last: Triumph over Tuberculosis in Newfoundland and Labrador,* St. John's: Jesperson Press, 1981, p. 7.

12. Andersen, Crellin, and O'Dwyer, *Healthways,* p. 54.

13. *The Evening Telegram,* February 26, 1936. Quoted in J. K. Crellin (compiler), *The White Plague in Newfoundland Medical and Social Responses 1900-1970 and Beyond,* St. John's: Faculty of Medicine, Memorial University of Newfoundland, 1990, p. 45.

14. For A. E. Rutherford, "Tuberculosis," *Rutherford Manuscript,* p. 24. History of Medicine Collection, Faculty of Medicine. For other medical comment—e.g., about "confusion worse confounded" with respect to tuberculosis and its treatment—see M. Paterson, "Pulmonary Tuberculosis: The Present Position of Treatment," *The Practitioner,* 87(1911), 758-763; and L. R. Williams and A. M. Hill, "The Use of 'Patent Remedies' by Tuberculosis Patients," *Journal of the American Medical Association,* 94(1930), 1292-1294. For some historical appraisals and patent medicines see, B. Bates, *Bargaining for Life: A Social History of Tuberculosis, 1876-1938,* Philadelphia: University of Pennsylvania Press, 1992, pp. 35-36, and pp. 252-254. For a discussion of remedies under attack see F. B. Smith, *The Retreat of Tuberculosis 1850-1950,* London: Croom Helm, 1988, pp. 150-162.

15. A. M. Tizzard, *On Sloping Ground. Reminiscences of Outport Life in Notre Dame Bay,* edited with an introduction by J. D. A. Widdowson, St. John's: Breakwater, 1984, p. 81.

16. G. B. Risse, "Brunonian Therapeutics: New Wine in Old Bottles," *Medical History Supplement,* (8)1988, pp. 46-62.

17. See W. B. Campbell, *Hand-Book of Modern Treatment and Medical Formulary,* Philadelphia: Davis, 1919, p. 41.

18. For more on asthenic or senile pneumonia see W. Osler and T. McCrae (eds.), *Modern Medicine: Its Theory and Practice,* Volume 2, Philadelphia: Lea Brothers, 1907, p. 583.

19. For context see J. C. Whorton, *Crusaders for Fitness: The History of American Health Reformers,* Princeton, NJ: Princeton University Press, 1982.

20. A. E. Rutherford, "Health and Hygiene," *Rutherford Manuscript,* p. 10, History of Medicine Collection, Faculty of Medicine. The remarks on getting fresh air in the lungs between the dinner table and the desk hardly applied to most Newfoundlanders.

21. For general discussion see D. Porter, "The Healthy Body" in R. Cooter and J. Pickstone (eds.), *Medicine in the Twentieth Century,* New York: Harwood Academic, 2000, pp. 201-216. For emphasis on roles in promoting popular health see E. Toon and J. Golden, "'Live Clean, Think Clean, and Don't Go to Burlesque Shows': Charles Atlas As Health Advisor," *Journal of the History of Medicine and Allied Sciences,* 57(2002), 39-60. For background, including a discussion of Macfadden, see Whorton, *Crusaders for Fitness,* pp. 298-304.

22. Cf. Whorton, *Crusaders for Fitness,* pp. 201-238. For detail on the issue of sexual drive see S. Nissenbaum, *Sex, Diet, and Debility in Jacksonian America: Sylvester Graham and Health Reform,* Westport, CT: Greenwood Press, 1980.

23. For context see H. Kamminga and A. Cunningham, "Introduction: The Science and Culture of Nutrition, 1840-1940," in H. Kamminga and A. Cunningham (eds.), *The Science and Culture of Nutrition, 1840-1940,* Amsterdam, Netherlands: Rodopi, 1995, pp. 1-14.

24. See L. M. Barnett, "'Every Man His Own Physician': Dietetic Fads, 1890-1914," in H. Kamminga and A. Cunningham (eds.), *The Science and Culture of Nutrition,* Amsterdam: Rodopi, 1995, pp. 155-178.

25. C.A. Sharpe, "'The Race of Honour': An Analysis of Enlistments and Casualties in the Armed Forces of Newfoundland 1914-1918," *Newfoundland Studies,* 4(1)(1988), 27-55.

26. For comment on shock among the American people see J. J. Walsh and J. A. Foote, *Safeguarding Children's Nerves: A Handbook of Mental Hygiene,* Philadelphia: Lippincott, 1924, p. vii.

27. Oral History Collection, Medical Communication Group, file 001.

28. Cf., C. Putney, *Muscular Christianity, Manhood and Sport in Protestant America, 1880-1920,* Cambridge: Harvard University Press, 2001; and G. L. Mosse, *The Image of Man, The Creation of Modern Masculinity,* Oxford: Oxford University Press, 1996.

29. R. Rompkey, *Grenfell of Labrador: A Biography,* Toronto: University of Toronto Press, 1991.

30. For background see L. S. Goodwin, *The Pure Food, Drink, and Drug Crusaders, 1879-1914,* Jefferson: McFarland, 1999; and C. A. Cappin and J. High, *The Politics of Purity: Harvey Washington Wiley and the Origins of Federal Food Policy,* Ann Arbor: University of Michigan Press, 1999.

31. Advertisement of Tessier and Co., *The Evening Telegram,* July 12, 1907, p. 1.

32. For an overview of the situation in early twentieth-century America see J. C. Whorton, "Popular Concepts of Diet, Strength and Energy in the Early Twentieth Century," in K. Grover (ed.), *Fitness in American Culture: Images of Health, Sport, and the Body, 1830-40,* Amherst: University of Massachussetts Press, 1989, pp. 86-122.

33. For a discussion of health foods at the beginning of the 1900s, cf., W. T. Fernie, *Meals Medicinal with "Herbal Simples" or Edible Parts,* Bristol: Wright, 1905.

34. For breakfast cereals in the context of a food fad, see Barnett, "'Every Man His Own Physician.'"

35. *The Evening Telegram,* December 6, 1907, p. 6.

36. *The Evening Telegram,* July 17, 1902, p. 5.

37. *The Evening Telegram,* July 7, 1930, p. 2.

38. Andersen, Crellin, and O'Dwyer, *Healthways,* p. 54.

39. J. Friedenwald and J. Ruhräh, *Diet in Health and Disease,* Philadelphia: W. B. Saunders, 1909, p. 107.

40. *Journal of the American Medical Association,* 58(1912), 2029-2030.

41. Ibid., p. 2038. See also Carpenter, *Beriberi, White Rice, and Vitamin B,* p. 140.

42. For more on Graham see S. Nissenbaum, *Sex, Diet and Debility in Jacksonian America.* See also Whorton, Crusades for Fitness, pp. 46-49.

43. Some commercial promotion of brown flour occurred in 1907. Newfoundlanders were told that Beaver Flour ("a blend of the choice Manitoba Spring Wheat [and] Ontario Fall Wheat") contained "all the nutrient—all the blood, brain and muscle-building properties—of the wheat kernel" (*The Evening Telegram,* December 3, 1907, p. 5). For the British story see M. Weatherall, "Bread and Newspapers: The Making of 'A Revolution in the Science of Food,'" in H. Kamming and A. Cunningham (eds.), *The Science and Culture of Nutrition, 1840-1940,* Amsterdam, Netherlands: Rodopi, 1995, pp. 179-212.

44. In 1914 Little's work was extended, at his suggestion, to interesting experiments on diets given to chickens. These experiments supported views that a diet consisting largely of white bread was a large factor, if not the single factor, in the cause of beriberi in Newfoundland's Northern Peninsula and in Labrador; see W. R. Ohler, "Experimental Polyneuritis: Effects of Exclusive Diet of Wheat Flour, in the Form of Ordinary Bread, on Fowls," *Journal of Medical Research,* 31(1914), 239-246.

45. See Rompkey, *Grenfell of Labrador,* p. 242; and J. Overton, "Brown Flour and Beriberi: The Politics of Dietary and Health Reform in Newfoundland in the First Half of the Twentieth Century," *Newfoundland Studies,* 14(1)(1998), 1-27.

46. Weatherall, "Bread and Newspapers."

47. *The Evening Telegram,* July 20, 1937, p. 7. In 1932, under the heading "No More Indigestion," Newfoundlanders were told that barrels and bags of flour could be purchased "for your health" by eating and enjoying "delicious Brown Bread made from Quaker 100 p.c. Whole Wheat Flour" (*The Evening Telegram,* July 21, 1932, p. 18).

48. Oral History Collection, Medical Communication Group, file 011.

49. Although details of the introduction of brown flour cannot be given, brief comment is useful to notice the role of science. On February 16, 1934, in order to

avoid bankruptcy, Newfoundland self-government was suspended and replaced by a Commission Government appointed in Britain. The new commissioners recognized that social reform had to happen if the island was ever to become self-supporting again. One immediate issue was the need to improve on existing food relief—white flour, tea, molasses, pork and beef, salt, and yeast—for the high number of dole recipients (see Neary, *Newfoundland in the North Atlantic World, 1929-1949*, p. 54). Although plans to introduce brown flour were in the pipeline before the new government was established, reformers such as Charles Parsons (medical director of the Notre Dame Memorial Hospital) felt it necessary to lobby the commission by eliciting testimonies of international scientific authorities, such as Gowland Hopkins in England, E. V. McCollum in the United States, and Frederick Tisball in Canada, to vouch for brown flour as a preventative against beriberi (correspondence, History of Medicine Collection, Faculty of Medicine).

50. Letter, History of Medicine Collection, Faculty of Medicine.

51. R. S. Ecke, *Snowshoe and Lancet: Memoirs of a Frontier Newfoundland Doctor 1937-1948*, Portsmouth, NH: Randall, 2000, p. 213.

52. L. G. Graves, *Foods in Health and Disease*, New York: Macmillan, 1932, p. v. Home economics teaching, mostly by women, was an important means for the spread of nutrition advice.

53. For the science and commerce of babies' milk and infant foods, see R. D. Apple, *Mothers and Medicine: A Social History of Infant Feeding 1890-1950*, Madison: The University of Wisconsin Press, 1987. For colonial issues, such as milk to "defend" the empire, see S. Marks, "What Is Colonial About Colonial Medicine," *Social History of Medicine*, 10(1997), 205-219; and M. Lewis, "The 'Health of the Race' and Infant Health in New South Wales: Perspectives on Medicine and Empire," in R. MacLeod and M. Lewis (eds.), *Disease, Medicine and Empire: Perspectives on Western Medicine and the Experience of European Expansion*, London: Routledge, 1988, pp. 301-315.

54. *The Practitioner*, 83 (October 1909), lvi.

55. See R. Hutchison, *Food and the Principles of Dietetics*, New York: William Wood, 1917, table facing p. 468.

56. *The Daily News*, December 29, 1915, p. 2.

57. *The Evening Telegram*, July 6, 1932, p. 2.

58. In contrast to a similar product, Fry's Malted Milk Cocoa with Eggs. *The Evening Telegram*, July 22, 1932, p. 11.

59. *The Evening Telegram*, July 9, 1937, p. 5. For reference to vitamins and Cocomalt see *The Evening Telegram*, July 13, 1937, p. 10. Recollections of Newfoundland school experiences with Cocomalt testify to its extraordinary impact; for instance, teachers of the combined school/chapel in Trout River School "would send one of the bigger boys out to the brook for water [for the cocomalt]. The kettle was put on early on the potbelly stove because it would take hours for the water to boil" (*History of Trout River*, available online at <http://www.k12.nf.ca/jakeman/united.htm>, accessed August 2003).

60. For tests for malt see P. W. Squire, *Squire's Companion to the British Pharmacopoeia*, London: Churchill, 1916, pp. 327-328.

61. Kepler's extraction, typical of many efforts to standardize extracts at the time, secured "the fullest possible percentage of those constituents of Barley Malt, to which authorities attribute chiefly the nutritive influence." Aside from diastase,

these included "soluble albuminoids and soluble phosphates; and carbo-hydrates (a group of dextrins associated with maltose)." The dextrins were said to increase the secretion of the enzyme pepsin, "thus adding materially to the digestive powers of the gastric process," an important aspect of "the constitutional treatment of disease" by food digestants. (Such claims were made many times, but see trade catalog, *Burroughs Wellcome and Co., Manufacturing Chemists*, London, 1896 (February), p. 10.

62. *The Evening Telegram*, December 16, 1902, p. 3.

63. For constituents of Bovril see S. O. L. Potter, *Therapeutics, Materia Medica, and Pharmacy*, Philadelphia: Blakiston's Son, 1913, p. 94.

64. *The Evening Telegram*, July 5, 1902, p. 3.

65. *The Evening Telegram*, July 13, 1937, p. 9.

66. Advertisements in *The Practitioner*, 1907-1910.

67. *The Newfoundland Quarterly*, 11(4)(1912), 27.

68. *The Evening Telegram*, December 2, 1927, p. 9.

69. See W. H. Martindale and W. W. Westcott (eds.), *The Extra Pharmacopoeia of Martindale and Westcott*, London: Lewis, 1906, p. 794.

70. J. V. Shoemacker, *A Practical Treatise on Materia Medica and Therapeutics*, Philadelphia: Davis, 1896, p. 71.

71. J. K. Crellin, *Home Medicine. The Newfoundland Experience*, Montreal: McGill-Queen's University Press, 1994, p. 228.

72. Olds OPDism, History of Medicine Collection, Faculty of Medicine, Memorial University of Newfoundland.

73. Oral History Collection, Medical Communication Group, file 002.

74. Oral History Collection, Medical Communication Group, file 005.

75. For discussions on these plants, see J. K. Crellin, *Home Medicine. The Newfoundland Experience*.

76. *The Evening Telegram*, March 6, 1925. Quoted in Crellin, *Home Medicine. The Newfoundland Experience*, p. 227.

77. See *The Evening Telegram*, December 1, 1917, p. 8. For context see B. C. Torbenson, J. Erlen, and M. S. Torbenson, "Lash's Bitters: From the Bathroom to the Barroom," *Pharmacy in History*, 43(2001), 14-22.

78. Bottle label, James O'Mara Museum, Newfoundland Pharmaceutical Association.

79. Bottle label, James O'Mara Museum, Newfoundland Pharmaceutical Association.

80. Anderson, Crellin, and O'Dwyer, *Healthways*, p. 98. (Newfoundland informant, b. 1921.)

81. *Canadian Medical Association Journal*, 1935, p. ix.

82. For the phrase "germ panic," see N. Tomes, "The Making of a Germ Panic, Then and Now," *American Journal of Public Health*, 90(2000), 191-198. G. Feldberg, in *Disease and Class. Tuberculosis and the Shaping of Modern North American Society*, New Brunswick: Rutgers University Press, 1995, indicates that the notion of building up resistance, both physiological and sociological, was gaining popularity.

83. Oral History Collection, Medical Communications Group, file 001. It is of interest that one of the first companies to promote a range of disinfectants in Newfoundland was Calvert and Co., of Manchester, England, a pioneer in the use of phe-

nol as a disinfectant (J. K. Crellin, "Disinfectant Studies by F. Crace Calvert and the Introduction of Phenol as a Germicide," *Veröffentlichungen der Internationalen Gesellschaft für Geschichte der Pharmazie* [Proceedings of the International Society for the History of Pharmacy], 28[1966], 61-67). Numerous advertisements promoted the concept of germs around 1900 onward, especially in treating colds and bad chests—for example, Catarrhozone, Minard's Liniment (an "enemy to Germs" [*The Evening Telegram,* December 18, 1922, p. 14]), Buckley's Mixture (dealing with "Cold Germs [that] revel in an Acid Poisoned System" [*The Evening Telegram,* December 5, 1932, p. 3]), Stuart's Catarrh tablets, which "destroy the catarrhal germs wherever found" (*The Daily News,* December 8, 1900, p. 2), and Cresolene Antiseptic Tablets ("a simple and effective remedy for sore throats and coughs. They combine the germicidal value of Cresolene with the soothing properties of slippery elm and licorice" [Bottle label, Museum of the Newfoundland Pharmaceutical Association]). On the other hand, long-standing treatments—e.g., applying to the chest anything from goose grease to Vicks VapoRub—remained standard, as did cough mixtures for relief and expectorant action (e.g., the popular Dr. Chase's Syrup of Linseed and Turpentine) or laxatives (e.g., Laxative Bromo-Quinine). Quarantine more forcibly raised the specter of germs. Yellow quarantine signs outside homes with diphtheria and scarlet fever were commonplace. For example, these quotes refer to living under quarantine: "We used to live on a road, and it was all barred off from horses, nothing could come around" (Andersen, Crellin, and O'Dwyer, *Healthways,* p. 106); "And there would be no passing of money" (Oral History Collection, Medical Communication Group, file 109).

84. *The Daily News,* December 10, 1910, p. 6, and December 14, 1910, p. 3. Tonics contrast with a few products such as Catarrhozone promoted to attack the offending germs: "Catarrhozone cures more quickly than ordinary remedies because it is the only antiseptic yet discovered that is volatile enough to reach the root of the trouble in remote parts of the lungs and bronchial tubes, and impregnate every particle of the air breathed with its healing, germ-killing vapor" (*The Evening Telegram,* July 14, 1902, p. 3).

85. *The Evening Telegram,* December 7, 1912, p. 2.

86. See Anonymous, *The Modern Materia Medica,* New York: The Druggists Circular, 1912, p. 114.

87. *The Daily News,* December 4, 1905, p. 5.

88. Rutherford, "Tuberculosis," *Rutherford Manuscript,* p. 24, History of Medicine Collection.

89. For more on Ayer's Cherry Pectoral and consumption see *The Daily News,* December 3, 1900, p. 3. For quote see advertisement for "Nox a Cold Specific 108," *The Evening Telegram,* December 5, 1912, p. 3.

90. *The Evening Telegram,* December 15, 1902, p. 2.

91. *The Evening Telegram,* December 8, 1902, p. 3.

92. *The Evening Telegram,* December 4, 1907, p. 2.

93. *The Daily News,* December 11, 1905, p. 3.

94. Andersen, Crellin, and O'Dwyer, *Healthways,* p. 44. Although recorded in 1992, the practice extends back to the early 1900s and earlier.

95. For an article interesting for its title, see W. M. Fowler, "Chlorosis—an Obituary," *Annals of Medical History,* 8(1936) 161-177.

96. See K. Wailoo, *Drawing Blood: Technology and Disease Identity in Twenti-eth-Century America,* Baltimore: Johns Hopkins University Press, 1997, 17-45.

97. See W. Osler, *Principles and Practice of Medicine,* New York: Appleton, 1892, p. 686.

98. See K. Wailoo, *Drawing Blood,* pp. 21-26.

99. A. A. Stevens, *Modern Materia Medica and Therapeutics,* Philadelphia: Saunders, 1904, p. 537.

100. For more on autointoxication see E. Lloyd Jones, *Chlorosis: The Special Anaemia of Young Women, Its Causes, Pathology, and Treatment: Being a Report to the Scientific Grant's Committee of the British Medical Association,* London: Baillière, Tindall, and Cox, 1897, p. 156.

101. *The Evening Telegram,* July 23, 1912, p. 5. For background on the vast range of over-the-counter preparations, their wide usage, and notions of iron and strength see M. R. Harris, "Iron Therapy and Tonics," in K. Grover, *Fitness in American Culture: Images of Health, Sport, and the Body, 1830-1940,* Amherst: University of Massachussetts Press, 1989, pp. 67-85.

102. See *The Evening Telegram,* July 18, 1912, p. 6.

103. See *The Daily News,* July 17, 1915, p. 7.

104. *The Daily News,* July 13, 1905, p. 3.

105. Some companies (e.g., Crookes Laboratories), however, still used the term *chlorosis* in the 1920s. The company promoted Collosol Ferro Malt in the treatment of anaemia, chlorosis, convalescence, and all conditions of asthenia (Leaflet of the Crookes Laboratories, London, 1925, Museum of the Newfoundland Pharmaceutical Association).

106. Oral History Collection, Medical Communications Group, file 006.

107. *The Daily News,* December 21, 1910, p. 2.

108. The surviving 1920s and 1930s prescriptions of physicians I. H. Lutterloh and Hayden Lutterloh in North Carolina were, in contrast to those from Newfoundland doctors, for more men than women. A favored one was elixir of iron, quinine, and strychnine. The directions given suggested this prescription was often given as an appetite stimulant.

109. Cf., G. B. Wood, *A Treatise on Therapeutics and Pharmacology or Materia Medica,* Philadelphia: Lippincott, 1868, Volume 1, pp. 426-427.

110. Osler, for one, noted that he had had the "greatest success" with the preparation. *The Principles and Practice of Medicine,* 1892, p. 695.

111. Prescriptions, Newfoundland Pharmaceutical Association and History of Medicine Collection, Faculty of Medicine, Memorial University of Newfoundland.

112. Prescriptions of Drs. Cluny Macpherson and A. C. Tait, History of Medicine Collection, Faculty of Medicine, Memorial University of Newfoundland.

113. One of the three Newfoundland brands, Excel, offered only dose information ("for Adults, one teaspoonful in a little water three times a day, for children of 10 years, half a teaspoonful, one year, ten drops"). In contrast, Parrish's Chemical Food, Dr. F. Stafford and Son, Chemists and Druggists, had a "Shake Before Using" reminder on the bottle and promotional information on constituents and uses: "A solution of the soluble phosphates of potash, lime, soda and iron in combination with phosphoric acid. This preparation will strengthen and restore the blood, impart vitality to wasting tissue, invigorate the brain and spinal column, increase bone structures in growing children and build up weakened constitutions." Precise dos-

ages were also stated: "Under 10 years, 1/4 to 1/2 teaspoonful; between 10 and 15 years, 1/2 to 1 teaspoonful; from 15 years upwards, 1 to 2 teaspoonfuls. Always give with plenty of water and after each meal"(Bottles in the Collections of the Museum of the Newfoundland Pharmaceutical Association). The third brand, McMurdo's Syrup of the Phosphates of Lime, Iron, Potash and Soda, stated it was "an acknowledged improvement on the original formula devised by Mr. Parrish." Recommended doses—"for adults, one teaspoonful in a table-spoonful of water twice a day"—did not specify dosages for children as the other two did.

114. Oral History Collection, Medical Communications Group, file 106.

115. Osler, *The Principles and Practice of Medicine,* 1907, p. 1086.

116. See T. Lutz, "Varieties of Medical Experience: Doctors and Patients, Psyche and Soma in America," in M. Gijswijt-Hofstra and R. Porter (eds.), *Cultures of Neurasthenia: From Beard to the First World War,* Amsterdam, Netherlands: Rodopi, 2000, pp. 51-76.

117. For discussions on neurasthenia and national characteristics in Britain, Germany, and the Netherlands see M. Gijswijt-Hofstra and R. Porter (eds.), *Cultures of Neurasthenia: From Beard to the First World War.*

118. Osler, *The Principles and Practice of Medicine,* 1892, p. 980.

119. Osler's observation on men did not appear in the 1907 edition of his book, *Principles and Practice of Medicine.* For some discussion on neurasthenia in Britain see M. Thomson, "Neurasthenia in Britain," in Gijswitjt-Hofstra and Porter (eds.), *Cultures of Neurasthenia: From Beard to the First World War,* pp. 77-95.

120. For a sense of influence see Osler, *Principles and Practice of Medicine,* 1907, p. 1095. B. Sicherman, "The Uses of a Diagnosis: Doctors, Patients, and Neurasthenia," *Journal of the History of Medicine and Allied Sciences* (1977) 33-54, notes that "several physicians—mistakenly—considered neurasthenia a male disease at a time when the profession rarely lost an opportunity to decry the ill-health of American women" (p. 42). It is not clear that "mistaken" is entirely appropriate, at least in the 1890s as noted above.

121. A. A. Stevens, *Modern Materia Medica and Therapeutics,* Philadelphia: Saunders, 1904, p. 630. See also M. Neve, "Public Views of Neurasthenia: Britain, 1880-1930," in Gijswijt-Hofstra and Porter (eds.), *Cultures of Neurasthenia: From Beard to the First World War,* pp. 141-159.

122. For an extended discussion on the critiquing of medicines and interest in mental therapeutics see F. G. Gosling, *Before Freud: Neurasthenia and the American Medical Community,* Urbana: University of Illinois Press, 1987, pp. 108-142. See also Neve, "Public Views of Neurasthenia: Britain, 1880-1930." For specific interest in psychotherapy at the time see J. J. Walsh, *Psychotherapy,* New York: Appleton, 1912, pp. 555-561.

123. For context see F. G. Gosling, *Before Freud: Neurasthenia and the American Medical Community 1870-1910,* p. 109. Neve, "Public Views of Neurasthenia: Britain 1830-1930," p. 145, notes that "Scottish accounts of avoiding neurasthenia put great weight on the need for vigorous exercise throughout life, careful diet and varieties of muscular Christianity." See R. Rompkey, *Grenfell of Labrador: A Biography,* Toronto: University of Toronto Press, 1991, for a discussion of Grenfell and muscular Christianity. It is worth pointing out that sleep, like rest, was viewed as enabling the patient to build up and store nerve force, hence the use of sleep aids such as sedatives (See Gosling, *Before Freud,* p. 116).

124. See T. Lutz, "Varieties of Medical Experience: Doctors and Patients, Psyche and Soma in America."

125. J. J. Walsh and J. A. Foote, *Safeguarding Childhood Nerves: A Handbook of Mental Hygiene,* Philadelphia: Lippincott, 1924, p. 15.

126. For example, in a series of papers in *The Practitioner,* 86(1909), 1-192, no reference was made to phosphorus medicines.

127. A. A. Stevens, *Modern Materia Medica and Therapeutics,* p. 294.

128. See T. Lauder Brunton, *A Text-Book of Pharmacology, Therapeutics and Materia Medica,* Philadelphia: Lea Brothers, 1888, p. 627. In 1924 W. Hale-White stated that "in some cases they appear to have done good [but] there is no satisfactory evidence of their value" (W. Hale-White, *Materia Medica Pharmacy, Pharmacology and Therapeutics,* Toronto: Macmillan, 1924, p. 244).

129. *The Evening Telegram,* July 17, 1902, p. 5.

130. Oral History Collection, Medical Communications Group, file 109.

131. A.W. McCann, *Starving America,* New York: Doran, 1912, p. 70.

132. Advertisements in *The Practitioner,* 1907-1912.

133. The suggestion that Newfoundland physicians prescribed phosphates more than many other physicians is a supposition that needs further exploration. Certainly the Lutterlohs in North Carolina prescribed very few (Lutterloh prescriptions, author's collection).

134. Prescriptions of Drs. Skully, MacPherson, Mitchell, and others, History of Medicine collection, Faculty of Medicine.

135. *The Evening Telegram,* July 29 and December 9, 1922, pp. 2 and 4 respectively. Italics added. Both commercial prescriptions and prescriptions containing lecithin generally contained other phosphates, notably glycerophosphates. Another widely advertised product for nerves or neurasthenia in the St. John's papers was "The New French Remedy, Therapion No. 3" (for neurasthenia, nervous exhaustion, chronic weaknesses). Well known on both sides of the Atlantic, it was said to contain calcium glycerophosphate. An analysis published by the British Medical Association in *Secret Remedies: What They Cost and What They Contain,* London: British Medical Association, 1909, pp. 172-174, indicated the presence of calcium glycerophosphate (plus gentian and damiana). Therapion No. 3, widely promoted in 1900 (e.g., *The Daily News,* December 1, 1900, p. 2), was still being promoted as "the new French remedy" in the late 1930s for neurasthenia and chronic weaknesses (*The Evening Telegram,* July 30, 1937, p. 2).

136. Oral History Collection, Medical Communication Group, file 002. Another remark: "Her nerves would get bad and she couldn't eat or couldn't sleep, so she'd take Dr. Chase's Nerve Food and *build herself up* and she'd be all right again." If a local supply was not available, outporters often ordered it from St. John's (Ibid., italics added).

137. In commenting on neurasthenia remedies in Germany, H-P. Schmiedebach, "The Public's View of Neurasthenia in Germany: Looking for a New Rhythm of Life," in Gijswijt-Hofstra and Porter (eds.), *Cultures of Neurasthenia: From Beard to the First World War,* pp. 219-231, divides the over-the-counter medicines as those acting on the basis of (1) the anatomical-mechanistic approach and (2) the more energetic approach that lay behind electrotherapies. The nutrition approach fits with (1), but with overlap to (2).

138. See Carpenter, *Beriberi, White Rice and Vitamin B,* p. 60.

139. In Canada Dr. Chase's Ointment was promoted as a "food" for the skin.

140. *The Evening Telegram,* July 18, 1922, p. 11.

141. Ibid. Another example of Chase's advertising, "The Pallor of Anaemia Calls for Reconstructive Treatment," *The Evening Telegram,* December 5, 1917, p. 3.

142. *The Evening Telegram,* December 9, 1932, p. 15.

143. *The Evening Telegram,* July 8, 1922, p. 5. For context with respect to body weight see A. Offer, "Body Weight and Self-Control in the United States and Britain Since the 1950s," *Social History of Medicine,* 14(2001), 79-106.

144. *The Evening Telegram,* July 1, 1907.

145. *The Daily News,* December 2, 1910.

146. From bottle label, c. 1910. Sample in Patterson's Country Mill Museum, Chapel Hill, North Carolina.

147. *The Evening Telegram,* July 27, 1912, p. 5.

148. *The Daily News,* December 2, 1910, p. 2. "Female" remedies have often been chastised as euphemisms for abortifacients. Many could have been effective at times as drastic purgatives or through having a direct action on the uterus. Communities in general had a stock of social knowledge about abortifacients. For Newfoundland, cf., Crellin, *Home Medicine,* pp. 57-62. Among the commercial remedies promoted, Newfoundlanders were mostly assailed by Dr. de Van's Female Pills, "a reliable French regulator; never fails. These pills are exceedingly powerful in regulating the generative portion of the female system" (*The Evening Telegram,* 3 December, 1912, p. 9). Later, major pharmaceutical companies sold "utero-ovarian sedatives and tonics," sometimes containing the same herbs as in the Lydia Pinkham and Pierce treatments.

149. *The Evening Telegram,* July 1, 1907, p. 3.

150. The 1917 edition was unchanged from nineteenth-century editions (e.g., 1895). The promotion included posters, notebooks, and much more.

151. *The Evening Telegram,* July 23, 1907, p. 3.

152. Bottle label, James O'Mara Museum, Newfoundland Pharmaceutical Association. For general background see S. Stage, *Female Complaints: Lydia Pinkham and the Business of Women's Medicine,* New York: Norton, 1979.

153. Cf., J. H. Young, "Sex Fraud," *Pharmacy in History,* 35(1993), 65-69.

154. *The Evening Telegram,* July 22, 1912, p. 3.

155. Oral History Collection, Medical Communications Group, file 116. Newfoundland informant (b. 1927).

156. G. H. Brieger, "Dyspepsia: The American Disease? Needs and Opportunities for Research," in C. E. Rosenberg (ed.), *Healing and History: Essays for George Rosen,* New York: Science History Publications, 1979, p. 182.

157. See D. Steven and G. Wald, "Vitamin A Deficiency: A Field Study in Newfoundland," *Journal of Nutrition,* 21(1941), 526-531.

158. Oral History Collection, Medical Communications Group, file 012. Squashberry's scientific name is *Viburnum edule.*

159. Osler, *The Principles and Practice of Medicine,* p. 421.

160. W. Alvarez, *Nervousness, Indigestion, and Pain,* New York: Hoeber, 1943, p. 177. Alvarez's issue with autointoxication had been long-standing. See also J. C. Whorton, *Inner Hygiene Constipation and the Pursuit of Health in Modern Society,* New York: Oxford University Press, 2000, pp. 81-84.

161. Alvarez, *Nervousness, Indigestion, and Pain,* p. 266.

162. Ibid., p. 310.

163. For context and general interest in autointoxication and focal infection among many physicians and surgeons see A. Dally, *Fantasy Surgery, 1880-1930: With Special Reference of Sir William Arbuthnot Lane,* Amsterdam, Netherlands: Rodopi, 1996, pp. 66-83.

164. F. Christopher, *Minor Surgery,* Philadelphia: W. B. Saunders, 1936, p. 311.

165. The one Newfoundland physician who strongly supported focal infection in the 1930s and 1940s often viewed the cervix as the offending site (recollection from Dr. Nigel Rusted). For reference to this in England c. 1940, see W. L. Rees (in conversation with David Healy), "The Place of Clinical Trials in the Development of Psychopharmacology," *History of Psychiatry,* 8(1997), 1-20.

166. See Whorton, *Inner Hygiene, Constipation, and the Pursuit of Health in Modern Society,* p. 213, for more information on food faddists.

167. For example, Buckley's Mixture for colds and sore throats proclaimed in 1932: "Cold Germs Revel in the Acid Poisoned System. Buckley's is highly alkaline and neutralizes the excess acids that cause colds" (*The Evening Telegram,* December 5, 1932, p. 3). Newfoundlanders, as elsewhere, in the "Beauty Chats" columns of Edna Kent Forbes in local newspapers were warned in the early 1930s about particular foods (e.g., tomato juice) that had a special tendency toward acidity (e.g., *The Evening Telegram,* July 13, 1932, p. 8).

168. Alvarez, *Nervousness, Indigestion, and Pain,* p. 178.

169. *The Evening Telegram,* July 8, 1912, p. 3. The tonic was manufactured at the Stafford drugstore by the early 1900s and was still popular in the 1930s.

170. *The Evening Telegram,* July 17, 1922, p. 7. A typical testimonial added that "three bottles of Tanlac rid me of indigestion, the nervousness and dizziness" (*The Evening Telegram,* July 7, 1922, p. 3).

171. For a discussion on artificially digested foods see H. C. Wood and H. C. Wood Jr., *Therapeutics: Its Principles and Practices,* Philadelphia: Lippincott, 1907, pp. 13-14.

172. *The Evening Telegram,* December 2, 1912, p. 2.

173. *Daily News,* December 4, 1905, p. 2.

174. *The Evening Telegram,* December 14, 1922, p. 2.

175. *The Evening Telegram,* July 7, 1922, p. 12. In the late 1950s, the "vegetable" laxative Carter's Little Liver Pills also linked inadequate flow of bile to feeling "sluggish, headachy, [and] nervous," although at the time the concept was fading (*The Evening Telegram,* December 2, 1959, p. 16).

176. *The Daily News,* December 23, 1905, p. 7; for other aspects of Cascarets advertising see J. C. Whorton, *Inner Hygiene, Constipation, and the Pursuit of Health in Modern Society,* Oxford, 2000, pp. 88-89.

177. *The Evening Telegram,* December 14, 1912, p. 2.

178. Cf. J. S. Haller Jr., "Samson of the Materia Medica: Medical Theory and the Use and Abuse of Calomel in Nineteenth Century America," *Pharmacy in History,* 13(1971), 27-34, 67-76.

179. Mercurous chloride, a medicine with a long and fascinating history, is often considered to have disappeared from therapy following nineteenth-century concerns about its side effects of mercury poisoning when large doses were taken. However, many doctors continued to prescribe it as a laxative until well into the 1930s

and beyond. This was despite numerous advertisements for over-the-counter medicines proclaiming the dangers of calomel. A favored prescription was calomel with sodium bicarbonate, a combination that encouraged alkalinity in the intestine to ensure the release of mercury, which was thought to stimulate peristalsis. It is of interest to speculate here whether "pink disease"—a condition of babies and toddlers with pink-colored, often peeling skin—was prevalent in Newfoundland. The condition became generally recognized in the 1920s. The cause baffled physicians and was variously attributed to germs and nutrition deficiencies until the 1940s, when mercury was identified as the causative agent. The principal culprits were considered to be teething powders containing calomel and/or diaper rinses. When mercury was withdrawn from most teething powders after 1954, the condition almost disappeared. However, depending on the doctor, children could be subjected to prescribed calomel or encounter it in other preparations used in Newfoundland (A. Dally, "The Rise and Fall of Pink Disease," *Social History of Medicine,* 10[1997], 291-304).

180. E.g., see advertisement Diotox, *The Evening Telegram,* December 8 and 12, 1932, pp. 15 and 8, respectively.

181. The *Evening Telegram,* July 22 and 29, 1937, pp. 15 and 15, respectively.

182. Many references to its expense appeared in the 1930s. For example, V. J. Woolley, "Favourite Prescriptions. No. X—The Pharmacopoeia of St. Thomas's Hospital," *The Practitioner,* 135(1935), 393-602. For Newfoundland prescribers of bismuth preparations, see the prescription book of Drs. Cron and Strap, Historical Collections, Newfoundland Pharmaceutical Association.

183. *The Evening Telegram,* July 22, 1937, p. 11.

184. *The Evening Telegram,* July 29, 1912, p. 4.

185. *The Evening Telegram,* July 26, 1937, p. 8.

186. *The Evening Telegram,* December 6, 1932, p. 10.

187. *The Evening Telegram,* July 26, 1937, p. 8, and July 25, 1932, p. 7.

188. *The Evening Telegram,* December 6, 1937, p. 13 and July 29, 1937, p. 13.

189. For discussion on Haig and the intriguing influences of his uric acid promotion, see J. C. Whorton, *Crusaders for Fitness: The History of American Health Reformers,* Princeton, NJ: Princeton University Press, 1982, pp. 239-269.

190. *The Daily News,* December 15, 1905, p. 3.

191. *The Daily News,* July 28, 1900, p. 2. That "people could go to town on them" is a recollection of many Newfoundland elders. See, for example, Oral History Collection, Medical Communication Group, file 010.

192. See *The Daily News,* July 18, 1900, p. 2.

193. *Twillingate Sun,* April 4, 1942, p. 2. Among other products claiming to deal with uric acid was Cystex. "Get rid of Uric Acid and Rheumatism" (*The Evening Telegram,* December 1, 1932, p. 16). Also, a "Remarkable Remedy for Rheumatism, Neuritis and 'acid' complaints. Not a drug nor medicinal compound but a tropical plant called HERVEA." The 1937 advertisement for this went on to invite all sufferers from rheumatism and acid complaints in Newfoundland to write to an accredited agent, "namely Mr. Cornelius McIsaac, South Branch, Newfoundland" (*The Evening Telegram,* July 22, 1937, p. 3).

An added comment on Dodd's Pills is appropriate since they were one of the most popular over-the-counter preparations on the island. Like the equally well-known Gin Pills and Chase's Kidney and Liver Pills, they were commonly used for backache, bladder troubles, "stopped water," headaches, and much more. In New-foundland they pushed aside traditional remedies, such as a tea made from juniper for "stopped water," honey and vinegar for bladder infections, and rubs for back-ache: "I heard them talk about kidneys. They used to say it was from getting cold, a bad cold used to cause their kidney problem. I don't know if it was. Had a problem with their water sometimes. You'd rub their back with things a lot of the time. Lini-ment or Minard's liniment, on their back" (Oral History Collection, Medical Com-munications Group, file 005).

194. See British Medical Association, *Secret Remedies,* pp. 69-71; A. J. Cramp, *Nostrums and Quackery: Articles on the Nostrum Evil, Quackery, and Allied Mat-ters Affecting the Public Health. Reprinted, With or Without Modification from the Journal of the American Medical Association,* Volume 2, Chicago: AMA, 1921, p. 215. Gin pills, particularly popular in Newfoundland, also contained methylene blue used by physicians for infections. Newfoundland seniors commonly remember that the pills turned the urine green. Dodd's Pills also contained potassium nitrate, powdered fenugreek, pine resin, and oil of juniper, all of which were accepted kid-ney medications in medical textbooks (e.g., see R. A. Hare, *A Textbook of Practical Therapeutics,* Philadelphia: Lea and Febiger, 1916).

195. A. J. Cramp, *Nostrums and Quackery and Pseudo-Medicine,* Volume 3, 1936, p. 69. Conspicuous in the 1910s and 1920s among Newfoundland physicians was Urotropine (a brand of hexamethyleneamine). In fact it was a fairly standard preparation in Britain and the United States. One Newfoundland physician learned of it from his Canadian medical school (Nigel Rusted, student notebook, 1933, still in his possession): "In pyelitis due to B. coli, sod. benz (5-10 grs) with hexamine is good." Hexamine was also recommended for cystitis compounded with infusion of buchu and tincture of belladonna.

196. Cf., W. B. Campbell, *Handbook of Modern Treatment and Medical Formu-lary,* Philadelphia: Davis, 1920.

197. See V. E. Tyler, "Was Lydia E. Pinkham's Vegetable Compound an Effec-tive Remedy?" *Pharmacy in History,* 37(1995), 24-28. Tyler lists the constituents of the Vegetable Compound as unicorn root, life root, black cohosh, pleurisy root, fenugreek seed, and alcohol (18 percent). Pierce made no secret of his formula, stated to be, "Golden Seal root, Lady's Slipper root, Black Cohosh root, Unicorn root, and Blue Cohosh root." See, for example, R. V. Pierce, *The People's Common Sense Medical Adviser,* Bridgeburg and Buffalo: World's Dispensary Medical Asso-ciation, 1914, p. 351. See also, *The Evening Telegram,* July 23, 1907, p. 3.

198. *The Evening Telegram,* December 7, 1912, p. 3.

199. *The Evening Telegram,* December 9, 1912, p. 2.

200. W. Grenfell, *Yourself and Your Body,* New York: Scribner's Sons, [1924] 1946, pp. viii, 1-2.

201. E. F. Bowers, *Side-Stepping Ill Health,* Boston: Little, Brown, 1916, p. 2.

202. G. B. Risse, "The Road to Twentieth-Century Therapeutics: Shifting Per-sepctives and Approaches," in G. J. Higby and E. C. Stroud (eds.), *The Inside Story of Medicines: A Symposium,* Madison: American Institute of the History of Phar-macy, 1997, p. 69.

Chapter 4

1. R. S. Ecke, *Snowshoe and Lancet: Memoirs of a Frontier Newfoundland Doctor 1937-1948.* Portsmouth: Randell, 2000, p. 130.

2. In fact, some do not limit the rising authority to 1900 onward but suggest c. 1880 to c. 1970. See R. Cooter and J. Pickstone (eds.), *Medicine in the Twentieth Century,* New York: Harwood, 2000, p. xvii. An issue, however, was the need for visibility, much of which came later.

3. For some lead references see M. C. Smith, *Pharmacy and Medicine on the Air,* Metuchen: Scarecrow Press, 1989, pp. 101-109. See also J. Turow, *Television, Storytelling, and Medical Power,* New York: Oxford University Press, 1989. For a general overview, see S. E. Lederer and N. Rogers, "Media," in Cooter and Pickstone (eds.), *Medicine in the Twentieth Century,* pp. 487-502.

4. Questions about placebo responses in clinical trials and with inert substances have been questioned. See G. S. Kienle and H. Kiene, "A Critical Reanalysis of the Concept, Magnitude, and Existence of Placebo Effects," in D. Peters, *Undestanding the Placebo Effect in Complementary Medicine,* Edinburgh: Churchill Livingstone, 2001, pp. 31-50; See also A. Hróbjartsson and P. C. Gøtzsche, "Is the Placebo Powerless? An Analysis of Clinical Trials Comparing Placebo with No Treatment," *New England Journal of Medicine,* 344(2001), 1594-1602, which found little evidence of clinical placebo effects under the conditions of clinical trials. Note also editorial comments by J. C. Baillar III, "The Powerful Placebo and the Wizard of Oz," *New England Journal of Medicine,* 344(2001), 1630-1632.

5. For an earlier history, especially as a "control" in the assessment of therapies, see T. J. Kaptchuk, "Intentional Ignorance: A History of Blind Assessment and Placebo Controls in Medicine," *Bulletin of the History of Medicine,* 72(1998), 389-433; see also T. J. Kaptchuk, "Powerful Placebo: The Dark Side of the Randomised Controlled Trials," *Lancet,* 351(1998), 1722-1725.

6. W. Osler, *The Principles and Practice of Medicine,* New York: Appleton, 1907, p. 1095. Relevant also is Osler's essay, "The Faith That Heals," *British Medical Journal,* 2(1910), 1470-1472.

7. T. J. Kaptchuk, "Powerful Placebo," p. 1722.

8. *The Daily News,* July 15, 1905, p. 2.

9. Osler, *Principles and Practice of Medicine,* p. 1094.

10. A. E. Hertzler, *The Horse and Buggy Doctor,* New York and London, 1938, p. 97.

11. D. Gilfond, *I Go Horizontal,* New York: Vanguard Press, 1940, p. 11.

12. This has been discussed exhaustively for the United States, but it was a factor elsewhere. See J. H. Warner, *The Therapeutic Perspective: Medical Practice, Knowledge, and Identity in America, 1820-1885,* Cambridge, MA: Harvard University Press, 1986.

13. The emphasis on empirical tradition in English medicine has often been noted. See C. Lawrence, "Edward Jenner's Jockey Boots and the Great Tradition in English Medicine," in C. Lawrence and A.-K. Mayer (eds.), *Regenerating England: Science, Medicine and Culture in Inter-War Britain,* Amsterdam, Netherlands: Rodopi, 2000, pp. 45-66. From 1935 to 1936 *The Practitioner* ran a series of articles of "Favourite Prescriptions" from various hospital formularies, revealing many in-

sights into constancy and change. The first was "The Pharmacopoeia of St. Bartholomew's Hospital," *The Practitioner,* 134(1935), 96-108.

14. W. M. Mendel, "Authority: Its Nature and Use in the Therapeutic Relationship," *Hospital and Community Psychiatry,* 21(1970), 367-370. Perhaps this shift was less evident in Britain. Views about general practitioners expressed in 1950 still carried and reflected a view of therapeutic authority. "In a world of ever-increasing management, the power of senior managers are petty compared with the powers of the doctor to influence the physical, psychological and the economic destiny of other people" (M. Bevan, "Career Choice and the Life Histories of General Practitioners," in J. Bornat, R. Perks, P. Thompson, and J. Walmsley (eds.), *Oral History, Health and Welfare,* London: Routledge, 2000, pp. 21-47).

15. For some background on the role of ethicists, see A. R. Jonsen, *The Birth of Bioethics,* New York: Oxford University Press, 1998, pp. 336-337.

16. J. T. Hart, "Going to the Doctor," in Cooter and Pickstone (eds.), *Medicine in the Twentieth Century,* p. 548. The comment was made with respect to Britain in the 1950s, but it applies wherever general practice and house calls flourished in earlier years.

17. M. Gothill and D. Armstrong, "Dr. No-body: The Construction of the Doctor As an Embodied Subject in British General Practice 1955-97," *Sociology of Health and Illness,* 21(1999), 6. By the 1930s tests were already a dominant aspect of diagnosis, at least in hospitals; for an interesting patient account of this, see Gilfond, *I Go Horizontal.*

18. Elder Newfoundlanders commonly recall the difficulties many physicians faced, including traveling to various communities for clinics: "Dr. Whelan, he had half the Southern Shore to look after." (Oral History Collection, Medical Communication Group, English Department, Memorial University of Newfoundland, file 012; of course, finances were tight for many doctors, and some relied on additional income, such as working as magistrates). Further, the convenience of the doctors' offices being in their homes is remembered in the light of late twentieth-century difficulties in getting a doctor for emergencies: "Dr. Donahue was in his own home there on King's Road and accessible after surgery hours. And he was more available to visit your home if you were not well enough to go to his office, and you put in a call, he'd come to your home" (Oral History Collection, Medical Communication Group, file 101).

19. J. C. Burnham, "American Medicine's Golden Age: What Happened to It," *Science,* 215(1982), 1478. Burnham emphasizes the relative lack of criticism, while recognizing that a continuum of concerns has existed throughout the history of medicine (e.g., practitioner greed). Burnham was concerned with the national picture, such that the undercurrent of concerns did not seem relevant. However, situations can differ locally as we suggest for Newfoundland.

20. Cf., A. F. Balis, "Miracle Medicine: The Impact of Sulfa Drugs on Medicine, the Pharmaceutical Industry and Government Regulation in the U.S. in the 1930s," unpublished doctoral thesis, City University of New York, 2000, pp. 76-142. The sense of ambivalence about medicine is well illustrated in several popular twentieth-century comic postcards; see J. K. Crellin and W. H. Helfand, "Learning from Medical Postcards" in N. D. Stevens (ed.), *Postcards in the Library: Invaluable Visual Resources,* Binghamton, NY: The Haworth Press, 1995, pp. 109-120.

21. I owe this view to discussions with Dr. Ian Rusted.

22. Recollections from senior physicians and Newfoundlanders, who often recollect deference to authority.

23. W. Grenfell, *Forty Years for Labrador,* Boston: Houghton Mifflin, 1932, p. 96.

24. The Oral History Collection, Medical Communication Group, offers many comments on costs. For example: "Dr. Kelly, he charged a dollar for what he used to call sounding you, using a stethoscope, and charge a dollar for a bottle of medicine. I remember going to him one time, and he sounded me alright, but he didn't give me any medicine because I had no money" (file 116); "I went to a doctor in St. John's, Dr. Scully. I had an infection in my ear. Dr. Scully. That's a long while ago and I didn't have very much money. I might spend 5 or 10 cents every weekend and I went down to him. He just looked at me and he said eczema. He wrote a prescription. 'Here,' he said, 'this will cost you $1.50.' I took the prescription and I started to go out. He said, 'aren't you going to pay me? I told you $1.50.' He said, 'what do you think I'm going to live on?' So I had to pay him $1.50" (file 009); "Doctors did an awful lot of calls they never ever got paid for. I know, for instance, Dr. Anderson became our family doctor and whether we had him one visit or two his standard fee for the year was $10.00" (file 107).

For an example of a last resort in Lancaster, England, see E. Roberts, "Oral History Investigations of Disease and Its Management for the Lancashire Working Class 1890-1939," in J. V. Pickstone, (ed.), *Health, Disease, and Medicine in Lancashire, 1750-1950, Four Papers on Sources, Problems, and Methods,* Manchester, UK: University of Manchester, Institute of Science and Technology (UMIST), 1980, pp. 33-51.

25. Oral History Collection, Medical Communication Group, file 101.

26. J. H. Cassedy, *Medicine in America: A Short History,* Baltimore: Johns Hopkins Press, 1991, p. 136.

27. J. S. Collings, "General Practice in England Today: A Reconnaisance," *The Lancet,* 258(1950), 555-585. The importance of the report is made clear by I. Loudon and M. Drury, "Some Aspects of Clinical Care in General Practice," in I. Loudon, J. Horder, and C. Webster (eds.), *General Practice Under the National Health Service,* London: Clarendon Press, 1998, pp. 92-127; Loudon and Drury outline contemporary criticisms of the report.

28. Oral History Collection, Medical Communication Group, file 004.

29. J. E. Candow, "An American Report on Newfoundland's Health Services in 1940," *Newfoundland Studies,* 5(1989), 236.

30. Oral History Collection, Medical Communication Group, file 008.

31. Oral History Collection, Medical Communication Group, file 009.

32. Oral History Collection, Medical Communication Group, file 004.

33. *The Globe and Mail,* July 5, 1923, p. 3.

34. *Twillingate Sun,* June 4, 1927, p. 2. Opium was in paregoric and some soothing powders; teething drops could contain mercury.

35. *The Daily News,* July 16, 1900, p. 2.

36. *The Daily News,* July 1, 1910, p. 2.

37. *The Daily News,* July 20, 1900, p. 2.

38. Quoted in P. I. Crellin and J. K. Crellin, *By the Patient and Not by the Book,* Durham, NC: Acorn Press, 1988, p. 44.

39. It is interesting to notice parallels with the situation in early modern Europe. Cf., M. Lindemann, *Medicine and Society in Early Modern Europe,* Cambridge, UK: Cambridge University Press, 1999, Chapter 7.

40. Oral History Collection, Medical Communication Group, file 109, referring to Charlie Tucker.

41. A distinctive feature of Newfoundland is the absence of a tradition of herbalists. Herbal knowledge was comparatively limited. Moreover, no evidence has been found that Newfoundland drugstores sold the commonplace packets of herbs that did much to sustain the herbal tradition elsewhere in North America up to the 1940s. Cf., J. K. Crellin, *Home Medicine: The Newfoundland Experience,* Montreal: McGill-Queen's University Press, 1994.

42. For British context, not irrelevant elsewhere, see O. Davies, "Cunning-Folk in the Medical Market-Place During the Nineteenth Century," *Medical History,* 43(1999), 55-73.

43. R. R. Andersen, J. K. Crellin, and B. O'Dwyer, *Healthways: Newfoundland Elders, Their Lifestyles and Values,* St. John's: Creative Publishers, 1998, p. 116.

44. Ibid., pp. 118-119.

45. Cf., S. Marks, "What Is Colonial About Colonial Medicine? And What Happened to Imperialism and Health?" *Social History of Medicine,* 10(1997), 205-219.

46. Such activities are well told in academic studies and memoirs—from C. M. Benoit, *Midwives in Passage: The Modernisation of Maternity Care,* St. John's: ISER, 1991, to H. G. Green, *Don't Have Your Baby in the Dory: A Biography of Myra Bennett,* Montreal: Harvest House, 1974.

47. R. M. Piercey, *True Tales of Rhoda Maude: Memoirs of an Outport Midwife,* St. John's: Faculty of Medicine, Memorial University of Newfoundland, 1992, p. 45.

48. The station, Battle Harbour, was in Labrador, then part of Newfoundland, although a similar pattern existed for the island. Anna Arklie manuscript in Lilian Stevenson Nursing Archives/Museum, St. John's. I am grateful to Janet Story for drawing my attention to the manuscript.

49. For a general account of Clinch, see K. B. Roberts, *Smallpox: An Historic Disease,* St. John's: Memorial University of Newfoundland, 1979, pp. 31-39. Vaccination in Newfoundland seemingly happened before July 1800, the month when Benjamin Waterhouse, the first vaccinator in the United States, vaccinated his children.

50. For memories of his clergyman father, N. Rusted, *Medicine in Newfoundland c. 1497 to the Early 20th Century: The Physicians and Surgeons Biographical Gleanings,* St. John's: Faculty of Medicine, Memorial University of Newfoundland, 1994, p. xv.

51. Andersen, Crellin, and O'Dwyer, *Healthways,* pp. 126-127.

52. D. G. Pitt, *E. J. Pratt: The Truant Years,* Toronto: University of Toronto Press, Volume 1, 1984, pp. 74-75, 78-79.

53. W. H. MacPherson, *The Evening Telegram,* December 16, 1922, p. 10. It is noteworthy that little other reference has been found to lay practitioners or health entrepreneurs in the local newspapers of Newfoundland.

54. *The Evening Telegram,* July 30, 1912, p. 3.

55. Quoted in M. B. Strauss (ed.), *Familiar Medical Quotations,* Boston: Little, Brown and Co., 1968, p. 125.

56. For review of some issues and trends in one set of English twentieth-century books and trends (e.g., gradual reduction of oral liquids and increase of oral solids as tablets) see S. Anderson and C. Homan, "Prescription Books As Historical Sources," *Pharmaceutical Historian,* 29(1999), 51-54. For some comments on early twentieth-century England see I. M. Slocombe, "A Bradford-on-Avon Pharmacy: Prescription Books, 1863-1918," *Pharmaceutical Historian,* 26(1996), 17-19; K. D. Richardson, "A Wartime Prescription Book," *Pharmaceutical Historian,* 25 (3) (1995), 1-2. Richardson notes more than 50 percent of tablets and capsules prescribed by proprietary names. Only nineteenth-century U.S. prescription books have been analyzed in publications.

The same basic trend toward simpler prescriptions and the prescribing of manufactured products is comparable to the prescriptions of two physicians, Isaac Henderson Lutterloh and I. Hayden Lutterloh, father and son, in North Carolina. Both prescribed many brand names. This could be linked with their ownership of a drugstore, though there is no evidence to suggest their prescriptions were geared toward profit margins. Few complex prescriptions were prescribed (prescriptions, author's collection). Unfortunately the formula of a favored prescription, Hospital Tonic, is not known. See also, P. I. Crellin and J. K. Crellin, *By the Patient, Not by the Book.*

57. For figures see H. C. Muldoon, *Lessons in Pharmaceutical Latin and Prescription Writing and Interpretation,* New York: John Wiley and Sons, 1925, p. 3.

58. Ibid., p. 2.

59. Even prescriptions that were legible to the patient (druggists even had deciphering problems with some) generally remained an enigma for them, though the nature of this changed when, from the 1960s onward, the English name of a dispensed medicine was written or typed on the container label.

60. Paregoric, as presented here, is the British formula: compound tincture of camphor, with tincture of opium (laudanum). The U.S. paregoric, camphorated tincture of opium, contains powdered opium. See *The British Pharmaceutical Codex,* London: The Pharmaceutical Press, 1923, pp. 790-791.

61. Similar prescriptions—omitting tincture of squill and including sodium bicarbonate, liquor calcii (calcium hydroxide), or elixir lactopepsin—were prescribed for stomach ailments.

62. Oral History Collection, Newfoundland Pharmaceutical Association, file John Stowe. Fourteen or fifteen ingredients were unusual, and memories can be misleading.

63. Macpherson prescription, dated January 6, 1922. History of Medicine collection, Faculty of Medicine, Memorial University of Newfoundland. For more on intestinal antiseptics used at the time of Macpherson's medical education see J. K. Crellin, "Internal Antisepsis or the Dawn of Chemotherapy," *Journal of the History of Medicine and Allied Sciences,* 36(1981), 9-18. Macpherson had other acidosis medicines, including an alkaline powder for gastric acid (see shop formula notebook, McMurdo drugstore, Newfoundland Pharmaceutical Association Archives).

64. D. W. Cathell, *The Physician Himself and What He Should Add to His Scientific Acquirements,* Baltimore: Cushings and Barkley, 1883, pp. 92, 127.

65. R. A. Hatcher and C. Eggleston, *Useful Drugs,* Chicago: American Medical Association, 1926, p. 3.

66. Cf., G. Sonnedecker, *Kremers and Urdang's History of Pharmacy,* Philadelphia: Lippincott, 1976, p. 282. After changing direction in 1958, publication of *New and Nonofficial Remedies* ceased in 1972. Approval for an entry included complying with specific "rules" that included no direct or indirect advertising to the public (with a few exceptions).

67. Cf., series of articles of "Favourite Prescriptions" published in *The Practitioner* from 1935 to 1936. The first was "The Pharmacopoeia of St. Bartholomew's Hospital," *The Practioner,* 134(1935), 96-108.

68. M. A. Bealle, *The Drug Story,* Washington, DC: Columbia Publishing Co., 1949, p. 20.

69. For background see J. R. McTavish, "What Did Bayer Do Before Aspirin? Early Pharmaceutical Marketing Practices in America," *Pharmacy in History,* 41(1999), 3-15.

70. Ibid.

71. For the development of research in companies and its influence with a focus on the United States, see J. Liebenau, *Medical Science and Medical Industry: The Formation of the American Pharmaceutical Industry,* Baltimore: Johns Hopkins University Press, 1987; J. P. Swann, *Academic Scientists and the Pharmaceutical Industry: Cooperative Research in Twentieth-Century America,* Baltimore: Johns Hopkins University Press, 1988.

72. For illustrative comments on the changing terminology of kidney disease see S. J. Peitzman, "From Bright's Disease to End-Stage Renal Disease," in C. E. Rosenberg and J. Golden (eds.), *Framing Disease: Studies in Cultural History,* New Brunswick, NJ: Rutgers University Press, 1992, pp. 3-19. Long-familiar conditions such as *liverishness* and *Bright's disease* also disappeared; new terminology such as *end-stage renal disease* displaced the latter, one shift to language that some would say symbolizes the coldness of science. *Psychoactive medications,* for example, are grouped in a mix of chemical and pharmacological language that includes "benzodiazepines" and "SSRIs."

73. Much has been said of symbolism; see cf., P. Davis, *Managing Medicines: Public Policy and Therapeutic Drugs,* Buckingham, UK: Open University Press, 1997, pp. 43-45, for terms such as *magic bullet.* See also S. van der Geest and S. R. Whyte, "The Charm of Medicines: Metaphors and Metonyms," *Medical Anthropological Quarterly,* 3(1989), 345-367; and M. Brown, "Anthropology Can Benefit Pharmacy," *Pharmaceutical Journal,* 268(2002), 543.

74. See V. Berridge and G. Edwards, *Opium and the People: Opiate Use in Nineteenth-Century England,* London: Allen Lane/St. Martins, 1981. The theme runs through the book but for example of specific comment, see pp. 241-242.

75. Other topics could be covered, such as the role of the adulteration of food and drugs. Cf., J. Abraham, *Science, Politics, and the Pharmaceutical Industry,* New York: St. Martin's Press, 1995, pp. 36-86.

76. For emphasis on this see M. P. Earles, "A History of the Society," *150 Years of a Science-Based Profession, Supplement to the Pharmaceutical Journal,* April 27, 1991, pp. S2-S17. See also P. Bartrip, "A 'Pennurth of Arsenic for Rat Poison': The Arsenic Act, 1851, and the Prevention of Secret Poisoning," *Medical History,* 36(1992), 53-69.

77. See M. P. Earles, "Jacob Bell and Poisons Legislation in Britain," in F. J. Puerto Sarmiento (ed.), *Farmacia e Industrializacion, Libro Homenje al Doctor*

Guillermo Folch Jou (Pharmacy and Industrialization: Festschrift to Doctor Guillermo Folch Jou), Madrid: Sociedad Española de Historia de la Farmacia, 1985, pp. 137-155. Cf., J. Bell and T. Redwood, *Historical Sketch of the Progress of Pharmacy in Great Britain,* London: Pharmaceutical Society of Great Britain, 1880, pp. 199-203.

78. Earles, "A History of the Society."

79. Ibid., p. S11.

80. Cf. Berridge and Edwards, *Opium and the People,* pp. 113-116.

81. S. W. F. Holloway, *Royal Pharmaceutical Society of Great Britain 1841-1991,* London: The Pharmaceutical Press, 1991, p. 239.

82. Discussed in S. W. F. Holloway, "The Regulation of the Supply of Drugs in Britain Before 1868," in R. Porter and M. Teich (eds.), *Drugs and Narcotics in History,* Cambridge, UK: Cambridge University Press, 1995, pp. 77-96.

83. Part 2 substances could be sold to anybody, in any amount, so long as containers in which they were dispensed were labeled "poison." In fact, the act had many loopholes in "protecting" the public. "Patent" medicines were exempt, fines for violating the act were small, and the pharmaceutical society did not have the resources to prosecute other than some token cases. Cf., T. M. Parssinen, *Secret Passions, Secret Remedies: Narcotic Drugs in British Society 1820-1930,* Philadelphia: Institute for the Study of Human Issues, 1983, pp. 68-78.

84. To the concern of many people, chloral hydrate was included only in Part 2 of the poison schedule. See M. J. Clarke, "Chloral Hydrate: Medicine or Poison?" *Pharmaceutical Historian,* 18(4)(1988), 2-4.

85. For more on the carbolic acid story and other suggested rejections by the Privy Council see Holloway, *The Royal Pharmaceutical Society,* pp. 285-294.

86. Cf., V. Berridge, "Professionalization and Narcotics: The Medical and Pharmaceutical Professions and British Narcotic Use 1868-1926," *Psychological Medicine,* 8(1978), 361-372.

87. Cf., L. Lewis, "Health and Health Care in the Progressive Era," in Cooter and Pickstone (eds.), *Medicine in the Twentieth Century,* pp. 81-95.

88. Quoted in L. G. Matthews, *History of Pharmacy in Britain,* Edinburgh: Livingstone, 1962, p. 371.

89. M. Hodges and G. E. Appelbe, "Control and Safety of Drugs, 1868-1968 (Part 1)," *Pharmaceutical Journal,* 239(1987), 119. Canadian legislation is also considered to have been centered on adulteration.

90. D. L. Cowen, personal communication; see also Cowen's "The Development of State Pharmaceutical Law," *Pharmacy in History,* 37(1995), 49-58.

91. See Sonnedecker, *Kremers and Urdang's History of Pharmacy,* p. 217.

92. For recognition of the equal importance of poisons in the story of pharmacy legislation see J. H. Beal, "The Evolution of Pharmacy Laws in the United States," *American Druggist and Pharmaceutical Record,* 36(1900), 179-180. See also J. H. Beal, "A General Form of Pharmacy Law Suitable for Enactment by the Several States of the United States," *Proceedings of the American Pharmaceutical Association,* 48(1900), 309-318. Poisons legislation remained within pharmacy laws, but adulteration became part of other legislation. I am grateful to D. L. Cowen for information on the Colorado 1872 control of poisons (Table 4.2).

93. Cowen, "The Development of State Pharmaceutical Law."

94. Newfoundland Statutes, Regulation of the Sale of Poisons Act, 49 Victoria, XII, 1886.

95. Chapter 49 of the Regulation of the Sale of Poisons Act. The country-wide Medical Society of Newfoundland, as distinct from the St. John's Society, was established in 1893.

96. Newfoundland Statutes, An Act Respecting the Pharmaceutical Society and the Sale of Drugs in this Colony, 10 Ed. VII, cap 4.

97. *Proceedings of the House of Assembly and Legislative Council During the Second Session of the 22nd General Assembly of Newfoundland, 1910,* St. John's: Robinson, p. 735. In fact, much of the original poisons legislation covering the household/agricultural use of poisons remained as separate legislation (*The Consolidated Statutes of Newfoundland* (Third Series), Vol. 1, St. John's: Robinson and Co., 1919, Chapter 48).

98. Minutes, January 12, 1910, Newfoundland Pharmaceutical Association Archives. The association's objectives were "the improvement of its members in pharmaceutical knowledge and skill, and the promotion of their material interests; the elevation of the standard of pharmaceutical practice throughout the Island, and the protection of the public against ignorant and incompetent dealers in drugs and poisons, and generally the advancement of pharmacy, and its connected science."

99. Unlike in Britain, the United States, and Canada, there was no formal education in addition to an apprenticeship, nor any formal pharmacy organization to focus attention on professional or even trade issues. Thus it was early in 1910 that a group of Newfoundland druggists felt reform was needed. Ten druggists met in St. John's on January 2, 1910, and decided to petition for a Pharmacy Act and to establish the Pharmaceutical Society of Newfoundland, a petition that was soon successful, as previously noted. Despite this significant development, when, in 1911, the Pharmaceutical Society of Great Britain wished to establish "reciprocal relationships," i.e., registration with "similar societies in other parts of the Empire," Newfoundland druggists recognized they could not meet the necessary educational criteria: "It was decided that under existing conditions at present, it is impossible for us to entertain any reciprocal relations whatever" (letter from Secretary M. Murphy, Newfoundland Pharmaceutical Society, to the colonial secretary, January 20, 1912, Newfoundland Pharmaceutical Association Archives. Later, this was elaborated: "We in this Colony are much in the position of the members of the Pharmaceutical Society of Gr. Britain in the years immediately succeeding 1867, and conditions in Newfoundland have not been such as to make a high standard of Pharmaceutical knowledge possible. For these reasons it seemed to the Society that any attempt to coordinate with the Pharmacy Societies of Gr. Britain, and the colonies who have had Pharmacy laws for a considerable number of years, would be out of the question with us for some years to come" (letter from Secretary M. J. Murphy, Newfoundland Pharmaceutical Secretary, January 27, 1913, Newfoundland Pharmaceutical Association Archives.)

100. One loophole in the act, that Newfoundlanders could import small quantities of "poisons into the Colony," was closed in 1912. See *Proceedings of the House of Assembly and the Legislative Council During the Fourth Session of the 22nd General Assembly of Newfoundland 1912,* St. John's: Robinson, pp. 288-289. The 1954 legislation, An Act to Establish the Pharmaceutical Association, changed the organization's name from Pharmaceutical Society to Pharmaceutical Association in keeping with the practice in other Canadian provinces.

101. *Proceedings of the House of Assembly and the Legislative Council During the Second Session of the 22nd General Assembly of Newfoundland 1910,* St. John's: Robinson, pp. 735-735.

102. Oral History Collection, Newfoundland Pharmaceutical Association, Bill O'Mara.

103. Although specific definitions of most terms can be found in the medical literature, in practice they have always been used somewhat indiscriminately, even within the medical profession. *True addiction* is generally diagnosed as the presence of an "abstinence syndrome," with marked physiological effects on withdrawal of a narcotic; *drug dependence* can have an analogous spectrum of symptoms, but with less severe withdrawal symptoms than an abstinence syndrome. *Habituation* commonly refers to the need for increasing dosage to maintain a desired effect; however, withdrawal symptoms can also occur.

104. For more on addiction in Britain see V. Berridge, *Opium and the People: Opiate Use and Drug Control Policy in Nineteenth- and Early Twentieth-Century England,* London: Free Association Books, 1999, pp. 264-278; for United States, E. Benoit, "Controlling Drugs in the Welfare State: U.S. Drug Policy in Comparative and Historical Perspective," doctoral thesis, New York University, 2000, e.g., p. 37.

105. See Benoit, "Controlling Drugs in the Welfare State," pp. 90, 170-172, 217-218.

106. Exceptions exist. D. F. Musto points out "state laws designed to curb the abuse of morphine and cocaine came mostly in the last decade of the nineteenth century." D. F. Musto, *The American Disease: Origins of Narcotic Control,* New York: Oxford University Press, 1987, pp. 8-9.

107. For more on opium in the United States see Musto, *The American Disease,* pp. 5-6. For relevant British background see Berridge, *Opium and the People,* 2000, pp. 235-257; and D. Peters, "The British Response to Opiate Addiction in the Nineteenth Century," *Journal of the History of Medicine and Allied Sciences,* 36(1981), 455-488.

For local concerns, a campaign for Chinese exclusion in Canada, concurrent with a moral panic over drug use, was probably very relevant to the severity of the Canadian law. Opium was associated with Chinese Canadians, prostitutes, and dissolute young men. See C. Carstairs, "'Hop Heads' and 'Hypes': Drug Use, Regulation, and Resistance in Canada, 1920-1961," doctoral thesis, University of Toronto, 2000, pp. 6, 123-166, and C. Carstairs, "Deporting 'Ah Sin' to Save the White Race: Moral Panic, Racialization, and the Extension of Canadian Drug Laws in the 1920s," *Canadian Bulletin Medical History,* 16(1999), 65-88. Carstairs also points out different scholarly views about the precise impact of the hostility on controls. For helpful discussion on panics in the United States in the second half of the twentieth century see P. Jenkins, *Synthetic Panics: The Symbolic Politics of Designer Drugs,* New York: New York University Press, 1999.

108. D. R. Gordon, *The Return of the Dangerous Classes: Drug Prohibition and Policy Politics,* New York: Norton, 1994.

109. See Musto, *The American Disease,* pp. 54-68; D. T. Courtwright, *Dark Paradise: Opiate Addiction in America Before 1940,* Cambridge, MA: Harvard University Press, 1982, pp. 104-106; and Berridge, *Opium and the People,* pp. 262-264. Britain, under a regulation of the Defence of the Realm Act in 1916, made it illegal for anyone except physicians, pharmacists, and veterinarians to be in possession of

cocaine, to sell it, or to give it away. It could be supplied only on physicians' prescriptions.

110. See C. J. Acker, "From All-Purpose Anodyne to Marker of Deviance: Physicians' Attitudes Toward Opiates in the US from 1890 to 1940," in Porter and Teich (eds.), *Drugs and Narcotics in History,* 1995, pp. 114-132.

111. Musto, *The American Disease,* p. 14, makes the point for the nineteenth century, but the sentiment persisted.

112. See Musto, *The American Disease,* for various references to "dope doctors"; unprofessional behavior was, seemingly, not uncommon. In Canada, with similar policies, new regulations certainly precipitated a constant hunt for forged prescriptions, overprescribing by doctors, and addicts or dealers who visited multiple doctors. For more on the Canadian scene see Carstairs, "'Hop Heads' and 'Hypes': Drug Use, Regulation, and Resistance in Canada, 1920-1961," pp. 67-104. Canadian controls included limiting the monthly amount of paregoric used by drugstores (p. 95).

113. "Health and Public Welfare Act, 1931," *Acts of the General Assembly of Newfoundland,* St. John's: King's Printer, 1931, p. 252. (22 Geo V cap 12.) The narcotics were cocaine, eucaine, codeine, opium, morphine, and heroin, as well as any salts, compounds, or preparations. The 1936 Act Relating to Dangerous Drugs dealt only with matters of trade and possession. Medicines control under the Health and Public Welfare Act was unique in comparison with provinces in mainland Canada, but various differences existed between provinces; cf., G. L. Kalbfleisch, "Prescription Drug Legislation," *Canadian Pharmaceutical Journal,* 85(1952), 88-90, 99. Newfoundland's later Dangerous Drug Act of 1936 dealt only with importation, exportation, production, and dealing.

114. See "An Act Further to Amend the Health and Public Welfare Act, 1931," *Acts of the Honourable Commission of Government of Newfoundland, 1945,* St. John's: King's Printer, 1945, pp. 11-15. The sulfonamides were sulfanilamide, sulfapyridine, sulfathiazole, and sulfaguanidine. Provisions were made to add other substances, though none was added by the time the revised statutes were published in 1952. In 1946 repeat prescribing of certain narcotics was made easier (*Newfoundland Gazette,* October 22, 1946, p. 1).

115. Musto, *The American Disease,* pp. 65-68.

116. Prior to the Newfoundland legislation (1915 for 1917 commencement), Newfoundland, as in Canada, had enacted a law allowing communities to vote for local prohibition. By 1915 most communities were dry. See J. Noel, *Canada Dry: Temperance Crusades Before Confederation,* Toronto: University of Toronto Press, 1995, especially pp. 46, 53, 217-226. See also W. G. Bartlett, "Prohibition Era in Newfoundland 1915-1924," history paper (1971), Centre for Newfoundland Studies, Queen Elizabeth II Library, Memorial University of Newfoundland, for detailed background.

117. Rules and Regulations under the Act Respecting the Prohibition of the Importation, Manufacture and Sale of Intoxicating Liquors, October 23, 1917, published in *The Newfoundland Quarterly.*

118. Cf., G. Griffenhagen, "Medicinal Liquor in the United States," *Pharmacy in History,* 29(1987), 29-34.

119. C. T. Fitz-Gerald, *The 'Albatross:' Being the Biography of Conrad Fitz-Gerald 1847-1933,* Bristol: Arrowsmith, 1935, p. 144.

120. Although the druggists' objections to new responsibilities were seemingly at odds with efforts to improve their professional standing, the business/professional dichotomy of pharmacy has to be remembered, as well as the fact that no one wanted more record-keeping duties. Moreover, Newfoundland druggists may have been strong supporters of temperance. A letter to the governor in council (undated, Newfoundland Pharmaceutical Association Archives) requested that the act "be amended so that licensed druggists shall not be in a position to obtain a license to sell intoxicating liquors for medicinal purposes. . . . Our reason for asking this amendment is that we fear that if the law is allowed to stand as at present it will be a source of very great annoyance to us in business, and in any event is quite unnecessary" (Newfoundland Pharmaceutical Association Archives). The outcome is unclear, but some druggists did not sell intoxicating substances. See R. E. Spence, *Prohibition in Canada*, Toronto: The Ontario Branch of the Dominion Alliance, 1919. Spence says that "druggists, not wishing to have the reputation not being strict in the observance of the law, refused to carry any liquor" (p. 499).

121. Cf., a series of papers on the theme of "Use and Abuse of Drugs and Preparations," in *The Practitioner,* 138(1937), 337-528.

The blurring between narcotics and certain medicines has been noted for Britain, although it was still concluded in 1999 that "narcotics have . . . retained the status of 'medicines' in British society through continuing medical ownership (and a much lesser degree of pharmaceutical control). This conceptualisation has been a powerful driving force behind policy by comparison with the United States where medical ownership was never so strongly established" (V. Berridge, *Opium and the People,* 2000, p. 289). It is of interest, too, that Britain made efforts to sharpen the boundaries when it enacted the 1968 *Medicines* Act, the *Medicines* Control Agency, and, in 1964, the Committee on Safety of Drugs (later Medicines) (Ibid., p. 288).

122. For a sense of the proliferation of barbiturates see J. W. Dundee and P. D. A. McIlroy, "The History of the Barbiturates,"*Anaesthesia,* 37(1982), 726-734.

123. See R. D. Gillespie, "On the Alleged Dangers of the Barbiturates," *Lancet,* 1(1934), 337-345. For the perspectives of a consumer advocate see C. Medawar, *Power and Dependence: Social Audit on the Safety of Medicines,* London: Social Audit, 1992, pp. 56-69.

124. "Medical Notes in Parliament," *British Medical Journal,* 1(1931), 519. See also *British Medical Journal,* 1(1934), 340. For Willcox's concerns see W. Willcox, "Toxic Drugs Their Use and Misuse," *The Practitioner,* 135(1935), 97-108.

125. See "Report of the Poisons Board," *British Medical Journal,* 1(1935), 1269-1270; "The Recommendations of the Poisons Board," *British Medical Journal,* 2(1935), 32. Prescription-only medicines were ultimately listed in a fourth schedule. See "Poison Rules: An Explanatory Leaflet," *British Medical Journal,* 2(1936), 770.

126. W. Willcox, "Toxic Drugs: Their Use and Misuse," *The Practitioner,* 135 (1935), 108. Holloway, *Royal Pharmaceutical Society of Great Britain, 1841-1991,* 1991, p. 395, attributes the controls to physician Sir William Willcox. Holloway notes (but does not document) that it was impossible to control barbiturates under the Dangerous Drug Act of 1920, so they were accommodated into a new schedule of prescription-only medicines in the 1933 Act.

127. Anonymous, "Regulation of the Sale of Barbiturates by Statute," *Journal of the American Medical Association,* 114(1940), 2029-2036. The number of states

with controls had increased to thirty-six in 1945 (J. P. Swann, "FDA and the Practice of Pharmacy: Prescription Drug Regulation Before the Durham-Humphrey Amendment of 1951," *Pharmacy in History,* 36[1994], 55-70). For national sensitivities, a 1940 editorial titled "Barbital and Its Derivatives," Journal of the American Medical Association, 114(1940), 2020-2021, noted Willcox's activity.

128. Editorial, "The Barbiturates," *Lancet,* 253(1947), 583. Problems tended to be blamed on patients.

129. P. J. Giffen, S. Endicott, and S. Lambert, *Panic and Indifference: The Politics of Canada's Drug Laws,* Ottawa: Canadian Centre on Substance Abuse, 1991, pp. 2-3.

130. E. L. Abel, *Marihuana: The First Twelve Thousand Years,* New York: Plenum Press, 1980, pp. 231-234. For a discussion on availability see editorial, "Marijuana," *Canadian Medical Association Journal,* 31(1934), 544-546. For perspectives on the U.S. scene see J. H. Young, "Federal Drug and Narcotic Legislation," *Pharmacy in History,* 37(1995), 59-67. Young notes that under the 1906 Federal Pure Food and Drugs Act the quantity of cannabis in an over-the-counter preparation had to be noted on the label.

131. Other substances fell into the category, but for emphasis on amphetamines and barbiturates see D. E. Smith and D. R. Wesson, *Uppers and Downers,* Englewood Cliffs, NJ: Prentice-Hall, 1973.

132. See Working Party of the Royal College of Psychiatrists and the Royal College of Physicians, *Drugs, Dilemmas, and Choices,* London: Gaskell, 2000, p. 46. With regards to amphetamine and some context to their use see D. T. Courtwright, *Forces of Habit: Drugs and the Making of the Modern World,* Cambridge, MA: Harvard University Press, 2001, pp. 78-79.

133. See R. Davenport-Hines, *The Pursuit of Oblivion: A Global History of Narcotics 1500-2000,* London: Weidenfeld and Nicolson, 2001, p. 307.

134. For discussion and comparison of U.S. and Canadian trends see E. Benoit, "Controlling Drugs in the Welfare State: U.S. Drug Policy in Comparative and Historical Perspective," doctoral thesis, New York University, 2000.

135. See H. M. Marks, "Revisiting 'The Origins of Compulsory Drug Prescriptions,'" *American Journal of Public Health,* 85(1995), 109-115.

136. See Swann, "FDA and the Practice of Pharmacy." Included for prescription-only were sulfa drugs, aminopyrine (and related products), and cinchophen and similar products. It is noteworthy that Canada acted at the same time. A 1941 amendment to the Food and Drugs Act added the following substances (including any related salts and derivatives) as prescription only: aminopyrine, barbituric acid, any ureide possessing a distinctly hypnotic action, Benzedrine (except inhalers, added in 1943), cinchophen and neocinchophen, ortho-dinitrophenol, sulfa drugs, thyroid preparations, and phenytoin sodium. See L. I. Pugsley, "The Administration and Development of Federal Statutes on Foods and Drugs in Canada," *Medical Services Journal,* 23(1967), 387-449; a more detailed account: A. S. Davidson, *Genesis and Growth of Food and Drug Administration in Canada,* manuscript 1949, McGill Medical Library; see also Kalbfleisch, "Prescription Drug Legislation"; and D. R. Kennedy, "One Hundred Years of Pharmacy Legislation," in *One Hundred Years of Pharmacy in Canada,* Toronto: Canadian Academy of the History of Pharmacy, 1969, pp. 25-37.

137. Swann, "FDA and the Practice of Pharmacy."

138. See Marks, "Revisiting 'The Origins of Compulsory Drug Prescriptions'"; and Swann, "FDA and the Practice of Pharmacy."

139. See J. H. Young, *The Medical Messiahs: A Social History of Health Quackery in Twentieth-Century America,* Princeton, NJ: Princeton University Press, 1967, pp. 44-50 and 53, for reference to increased numbers.

140. See G. Kay, "Healthy Public Relations: The FDA's 1930s Legislative Campaign," *Bulletin of the History of Medicine,* 75(2001), 446-487.

141. For relevant comments on opium preparations see S. Anderson and V. Berridge, "Opium in 20th-Century Britain: Pharmacists, Regulation, and the People," *Addiction,* 95(2000), 23-36.

142. L. I. Pugsley, "The Administration and Development of Federal Statutes on Foods and Drugs in Canada"; A. S. Davidson, *Genesis and Growth of Food and Drug Administration in Canada.*

143. "An Act Respecting Proprietary or Patent Medicines," British North American Acts, 1867-1919, Ottawa: King's Printer, 1919, pp. 457-462. Thirty-one substances were listed for labeling; for substances listed in the U.S. Pure Food and Drug Act see 59th Congress, Session 1, Chp. 3915, pp. 768-772; see also J. H. Young, "Federal Drug and Narcotic Legislation," *Pharmacy in History,* 37(1995), 59-67.

144. The figure, which must be an estimate, appears in C. A. Morell, "Government Control of Food and Drugs," *Canadian Pharmaceutical Journal,* May (1957), 27-31.

145. A. S. Davidson, *Genesis and Growth of Food and Drug Administration in Canada,* p. 75.

146. M. C. Smith, *Pharmacy and Medicine on the Air,* p. 1.

147. A. Buerki, "The Public Image of the American Pharmacist in the Popular Press," *Pharmacy in History,* 38(1996), 72.

148. See S. Anderson and V. Berridge, "The Role of the Community Pharmacist in Health and Welfare, 1911-1986," in Bornat et al. (eds.), *Oral History, Health, and Welfare,* pp. 48-74. There were also commercial practices in such diverse areas as veterinary medicine, tobacconist, off-license (spirits, wine, and beer), and housing a post office.

149. J. Bell, "On the Professional Character of the Pharmaceutical Chemist," *Pharmaceutical Journal and Transactions,* 2(1842-1843), 1-7.

150. In the context of chain pharmacies in the United States, it has been said that "the degree to which pharmacy has been exploited commercially in the United States is perhaps unique historically among highly civilized nations" (Sonnedecker, *Kremers and Urdang's History of Pharmacy,* p. 304). The "middle road" of the Newfoundland scene is reflected in photographs in the possession of the Newfoundland Pharmaceutical Association.

151. In 1911, of forty-one pharmacists registered in consequence of the 1910 Pharmacy Act, twenty-six were in St. John's. The numbers and ratios changed only slowly up to 1950. Cooperation among druggists was well known in Britain in the 1950s and 1960s and beyond.

152. A peak advertising time was Christmas, which brought out intensive promotion of nonmedicinal products. Nevertheless, emphasis during the pre-1950s remained on personal hygiene, perfumes, and toiletries, a reminder of the relationship between health and beauty, noted earlier. A typical large advertisement (1915, for example) for "McMurdo's Christmas Goods" competed with other druggists pro-

moting dressing cases, hairbrushes, bath salts, and perfumes (*The Daily News,* December 18, 1915, p. 6). Stiff Christmas competition led to various inducements among drugstores, such as a raffle ticket for every purchase of 25 cents and over (*The Daily News,* December 14, 1915, p. 1; *The Evening Telegram,* July 12, 1917, p. 6 advertisements of Peter O'Mara).

153. G. L. Saunders, *Rattles and Steadies: Memoirs of a Gander River Man Retold,* St. John's: Breakwater, 1986, p. 138.

154. Smith, *Pharmacy and Medicine on the Air,* pp. 125-136.

155. From a 1950s' Bulletin MUNFLA-NAC tapes 83B/C by kind permission of Canadian Broadcasting Corporation. Information on the Doyle bulletins and the humor in some of the messages can be found in P. Hiscock, *Folklore and Popular Culture in Early Newfoundland Radio Broadcasting: An Analysis of Occupational Narrative, Oral History, and Song Repertoire,* master's thesis, Memorial University of Newfoundland, 1987. See also the Oral History Collection, Newfoundland Pharmaceutical Association, Tom Doyle.

156. List from Oral History Collection, Newfoundland Pharmaceutical Association, Tom Doyle.

157. Another noteworthy feature of Doyle was his early enthusiasm for vitamins, viewed as important constituents in the oil. His enthusiasm was fostered by his father-in-law, Robert H. Mershon, an American chemist who published on the benefits of vitamins in the 1920s (Oral History Collection, Newfoundland Pharmaceutical Association, Tom Doyle). Around 1950, Doyle added to his Royal Blue Line: his gelatin capsules (to help overcome the taste) were packaged in blue and gold and clearly indicated that the oil in the capsules was Newfoundland oil.

158. *Newfoundland Quarterly,* 14(1)(1914), 23.

159. Oral History Collection, Newfoundland Pharmaceutical Association, Robert McGraw.

160. W.D. Parsons, personal communication.

161. Oral History Collection, Newfoundland Pharmaceutical Association, Bill O'Mara.

162. Oral History Collection, Medical Communication Group, files 104 and 106.

163. For dispensing of family recipes in England see P. Schweitzer (ed.), *Can We Afford the Doctor?* London: Age Exchange, 1985, pp. 19, 22.

164. Oral History Collection, Medical Communication Group, files 001 and 002.

165. Oral History Collection, Medical Communication Group, file 104.

166. Ibid.

167. Oral History Collection, Newfoundland Pharmaceutical Association, Cecil Burke. The toxic effect of side effects of the mercury preparation calomel and contributions to "pink disease" in children were noted in Chapter 3. Mercury head-lice treatment was another potential problem.

168. The actual prescription reads "Chlorodyne, dram iv, Tr. Camph. Co., dram iv, Tr. Scillae, dram i, Tr. Ipecac, dram i, Spt. Aether Nit, dram iv, Spts. Chloroformi, minum xv, Syrup, q.s. ad ounces viii. Sig, dram i q.4.h" (McMurdo's shop recipe notebook, Newfoundland Pharmaceutical Association Archives).

169. Oral History Collection, Medical Communication Group, file 106.

170. Oral History Collection, Newfoundland Pharmaceutical Association, John Stowe.

171. For reference to sales in St. John's see W. D. Parsons, "The Spanish Lady and the Newfoundland Regiment" available online at <http://raven.cc.ukans.edu/~kansite/ww_one/medical/parsons.htm>.

172. Anderson and Berridge, "Opium in 20th-Century Britain."

173. Oral History Collection, Newfoundland Pharmaceutical Association, John Stowe.

174. Ibid.

175. Ibid.

176. J. J. Dearin, "St. John's Medical Hall," *Hutchinson's Newfoundland Directory 1864-65*, St. John's: McConnan, 1864, p. 99.

177. M. Connors, "True and Honest Dispensing," *The Daily News,* July 9, 1900.

178. From advertisement of "J. J. Kielley, Successor to Kavanagh's Drug Store," St. Johns, *The Newfoundland Directory*, St. John's: Newfoundland Directories, 1928, p. 219.

179. I. H. Lutterloh et al. personal communications.

180. Oral History Collection, Newfoundland Pharmaceutical Association, Bob O'Mara. For some interesting reminiscences on Evans Medical see C. W. Robinson, *Twentieth-Century Druggist*, Beverley, UK: Galen Press, 1983, pp. 167-186.
That crude drugs and chemicals were mostly obtained from Britain is evident from museum collections in Newfoundland. Surviving stock bottles came from a striking range of British companies, such as Allen and Hanburys, Armour and Co., Ayrton Saunders and Co., British Drug Houses, W. J. Bush and Co., Burroughs Wellcome, Giles Schact and Co., Potter and Clarke, Smith and Co., Southall Bros and Barclay, and Evans Lescher and Webb (Evans Medical). Further, one pharmacist recollected: "A lot of the drugs in my early days at McMurdo's all came from England. [It seems] practically everything on the shelves, the bottles, the powders, had British Drug Houses written on them, so a lot of our early years in pharmacy was using British medications and drugs. It was later, when we became a province of Canada, that the wholesalers were closed up because of the thousands of dollars that we needed to check and test everything which couldn't be done here, so a lot of our business ended up in Toronto where the multinationals up there were able to abide by the Food and Drug regulations in that regard. Back in the early days, I think we all thought British" (Oral History Collection, Newfoundland Pharmaceutical Association, Robert McGraw).

181. For example, "Export/An Evans Product/Belladonna Plaster" (Oral History Collection, Newfoundland Pharmaceutical Association, Hugh Conroy and John Stowe). Others remember the much-used Martindale's *Extra Pharmacopoeia*. However, for many years, the British Union Jack over the "American" soda fountain in the McMurdo store, beyond a mark of respect to the British Empire, seemed to symbolize an accepted mix of commercialism and professionalism.

182. Oral History Collection, Newfoundland Pharmaceutical Association, John Stowe.

183. C. Eggleston, *Essentials of Prescription Writing*, Philadelphia: W. B. Saunders, 1913; F. A. Colbeck and A. Chaplin, *The Science and Art of Prescribing*, London: Henry Kimpton, 1919; W. J. Robinson, *A Treatise on Prescription Incompatibilities and Difficulties: Including Prescription Oddities and Curiosities,* New York: Critic and Guide Company, 1919; D. M. Macdonald, *The Students' Pocket Prescriber and Guide to Prescription Writing,* Edinburgh: E. and S. Livingstone,

1941. For discussion of some of the issues involved see J. S. Haller Jr., "With a Spoonful of Sugar: The Art of Prescription Writing in the Late 19th and Early 20th Century," *Pharmacy in History,* 26(1884), 171-178.

184. Oral History Collection, Newfoundland Pharmaceutical Association, Cecil Burke.

Chapter 5

1. G. W. Thomas, *From Sled to Satellite: My Years with the Grenfell Mission,* [Toronto]: Irwin Publishing, 1987, p. 17.

2. T. Mahoney, *The Merchants of Life: An Account of the American Pharmaceutical Industry,* New York: Harper and Brothers, 1959, p. 1. Skeptics such as R. J. Dubos (*Medical Utopias,* New York: Rockefeller Press, 1959) were overshadowed.

3. For a helpful review of the many challenges facing medicine with special reference to Britain see J. Gabe, D. Kelleher, and G. Williams (eds.), *Challenging Medicine,* London: Routledge, 1994. For some relevant contemporary accounts of the 1970s see J. D. Williamson and K. Danaher, *Self-Care in Health,* London: Croom Helm, 1978.

4. D. Coburn, "Canadian Medicine: Dominance or Proletarianization," *The Milbank Quarterly,* 66 (Suppl. 2)(1988), 92-116.

5. The levels of uncertainty were heightened in the second half of the century as new areas emerged; cf., a review by R. C. Fox, "Medical Uncertainty Revisited," in G. L. Albrecht, R. Fitzpatrick, and S. C. Scrimshaw, *Handbook of Social Studies in Health and Medicine,* London: Sage Publications, 2000, pp. 408-425. One issue constantly recurring in the medicines story is uncertainty over the limits to medical intervention; cf., such books as S. G. Wolf and B. B. Berle (eds.), *Limits of Medicine: The Doctor's Job in the Coming Era,* New York: Plenum Press, 1976; see also I. Illich, *Limits to Medicine: Medical Nemesis: The Expropriation of Health,* Toronto: McClelland and Stewart, 1976.

6. J. Le Fanu, *The Rise and Fall of Modern Medicine,* New York: Carroll and Gref, 1999, pp. 215-220. For one of the latest of a growing number of books examining aspects of pharmaceutical innovation, a sense of the innovation issue, but with an historical view see R. Landau, A. B. Achilladelis, and A. Scriabone (eds.), *Pharmaceutical Innovation: Revolutionizing Human Health,* Philadelphia: Chemical Heritage Press, 1999.

7. The story embraces the issue whether the thalidomide tragedy could have been foreseen or the drug withdrawn more promptly. Cf., A. Dally, "Thalidomide: Was the Tragedy Preventable?" *Lancet,* 351(1998), 1197-1199; see also correspondence, Ibid., p. 1591. Thalidomide was taken as a sedative/morning-sickness treatment during early pregnancy. For a listing of major catastrophes see M. L. Burstall and B. G. Reuben, *Critics of the Pharmaceutical Industry,* London: REMIT Consultants, 1990, pp. 20-24. For more on amphetamines and barbiturates see C. O. Jackson, "Before the Drug Culture: Barbiturate/Amphetamine Abuse in our American Society," *Clio Medica,* 11(1976), 47-58.

8. See J. Mayer, "Cheese and Monoamine Oxidase Inhibitors," *Postgraduate Medicine,* 44(1968), 185-186.

9. J. Goodman, "Pharmaceutical Industry," in R. Cooter and J. Pickstone (eds.), *Medicine in the Twentieth Century,* Amsterdam, Netherlands: Harwood Academic, 2000, pp. 141-154.

10. Quote from a Newfoundlander senior, Oral History Collection, Medical Communication Group, English Department, Memorial University of Newfoundland, file 005.

11. Oral History Collection, Medical Communication Group, file 002.

12. See D. Healy, *The Antidepressant Era,* Cambridge, MA: Harvard University Press, 1997, p. 2.

13. Risk/benefit information can be difficult to interpret, especially if percentages only are given. Interest in risk/benefit determinations with medicines first emerged in the 1970s, though a focus on risk factors and disease occurred much earlier; for example, see P. Jasen, "Breast Cancer and the Language of Risk, 1750-1950," *Social History of Medicine,* 15(2002), 17-43.

14. For more on issues regarding early kidney transplantation that fostered challenges to medicine see R. C. Fox and J. P. Swazey, *The Courage to Fail: A Social View of Organ Transplants and Dialysis,* Chicago: University of Chicago Press, 1974, pp. 60-83.

15. For discussion from a number of individuals see Wolf and Berle (eds.), *Limits of Medicine: The Doctor's Job in the Coming Era,* pp. 23-66.

16. The 1950s saw adoption of the Children's Health Plan (1957), which provided free medical (including doctors' prescriptions) and dental care for all children up to their sixteenth birthday. Further, the Federal-Provincial Hospital Plan of 1958 covered limited hospital services, including medicines for adults (physicians' fees were excluded). See J. Martin, *Leonard Albert Miller: Public Servant,* Markham, Canada: Fitzhenry and Whiteside, 1998, pp. 59-64.

17. *The Evening Telegram,* April 1, 1969, p. 6. For some background, C. H. Shillington, *The Road to Medicare in Canada,* Toronto: Del Graphics, 1972; other context: H.E. Macdermott, *One Hundred Years of Medicine in Canada,* Toronto: McClelland and Stewart, 1967, pp. 80-94.

18. Editorial, *Newsletter Newfoundland Medical Association,* 1(1)(1958), 1.

19. J. F. Janes, "Pharmaceutical Contribution," *Newsletter of the Newfoundland Medical Association,* 1(7)(1959), 5. The president added, besides teaching students how to prepare "emulsions, suspensions, intricate mixtures, ointments and creams, eye and ear preparations, solutions," education had expanded to teaching about hormones, antibiotics, tranquilizers, anti-hypertensives, etc. and "each new product as it appears on the market," along with physiology.

20. Newspaper reports, *The Evening Telegram,* July 10 and 14, 1959, pp. 4 and 3 respectively.

21. For insights into specialist power and pervasive influence see R. Stevens, *Medical Practice in Modern England: The Impact of Specialization and State Medicine,* New Haven: Yale University Press, 1966; R. Stevens, *American Medicine and the Public Interest,* New Haven: Yale University Press, 1971.

22. One example occurred in the 1960s, when an ophthalmologist observed the high incidence of pterygium (growth of conjunctiva across the cornea). Various genetic traits also became clearer at the time, evidence in the many sufferers of genetically linked conditions, especially in isolated Newfoundland communities. See J. G.

Gillan, *Through Northern Eyes,* Calgary: University of Calgary Press, 1991, pp. 51-54.

23. It is noteworthy that the views on fading values now parallel others that link "progress" with the "poisoning" of the environment (e.g., with hormones in the water supply) and increasing risks to health. Traditional values are said to have virtually disappeared from North American self-care, apart from among some disadvantaged groups (e.g., the uninsured in the United States). For some issues among the uninsured see N. Vuckovic, "Self-Care Among the Uninsured: 'You Do What You Can,'" *Health Affairs,* 19(4)(2000), 197-199.

24. Health care as a right is attributed to Monique Bégin, Canadian minister of health, who piloted the act through parliament (M. Bégin, *Medicare—Canada's Right to Health,* Montreal: Optimum Publishing International, 1988). For more current thinking see M. E. Aubrey, "Canada's Fatal Error—Health Care and a Right (Part 1)," *Medical Sentinel,* 6(1)(2001), 26-28, available online at <http://www.haciendapub.com/aubrey.html>, accessed March 2002.

25. For background see J. Z. Bowers and E. Purcell (eds.), *New Medical Schools at Home and Abroad,* New York: Josiah Macy Jr. Foundation, 1978, p. vii. The Faculty of Medicine, Memorial University of Newfoundland, is included.

26. For an overview see I. Rusted, "Faculty of Medicine, Memorial University of Newfoundland," in Bowers and Purcell (eds.), *New Medical Schools at Home and Abroad,* pp. 219-259. The topic of *quality,* very much a hallmark of medicine in the last decades of the twentieth century, infused the foundation and early years of the school. As a key founder of the medical school and as its first dean, Ian Rusted constantly emphasized quality by acquiring "top faculty" and developing a "first-rate medical school"—views widely reported in local newspapers. Perhaps the first reference to quality was in *The Evening Telegram,* December 12, 1967. A newspaper cuttings file reveals the repetition of this concept of quality (Faculty of Medicine Founders' Archives, Memorial University of Newfoundland, collection 005). Other physicians promoted similar messages. Lord Taylor, a physician and president and vice-chancellor of Memorial University of Newfoundland, said: "Building a medical school at the University was the only hope for Newfoundland to have a first class medical service" (*The Evening Telegram,* October 13, 1971). Cloid Green stated that "foreign doctors could always be recruited to come to Newfoundland," but that a higher level of care would result from the medical school ("Doctor Claims MUN Medical School Will Improve Health Care in Province," *The Evening Telegram,* February 9, 1972). One noteworthy development in the province was the announcement in 1976 of the first kidney transplant in Newfoundland, long after transplants had become commonplace (*The Evening Telegram,* February 4, 1976). The short life of this program is just one instance of many disappointments on the island: a project so often "almost there," only to collapse and encourage a sense of inferiority. For more on Newfoundland's inferiority complex see I. Rusted, "Address to Convocation," *Gazette,* 34(November 1, 2001), 7. I add a note on Ian Rusted to illustrate how he, like Gerald Doyle (Chapter 4), was able to catalyze change in health care. After three years (1949-1952) post-MD experience at the Mayo Clinic in Minnesota and the offer of a position there, Rusted surprised many colleagues by returning to his homeland. As the first medical consultant for the Newfoundland Department of Health (full-time 1952-1953, and then part-time until 1967), he was the first recognized specialist in internal medicine on the island.

27. The term *center* had in fact been used in North America for medical complexes since the 1930s. For an interesting discussion focusing on academic health centers see G. B. Risse, *Mending Bodies, Saving Souls: A History of Hospitals*, New York: Oxford University, 1999, pp. 569-618.

28. G. Fodor, "Epidemiological Studies of Hypertension in Newfoundland 1967-1983," unpublished typescript, 1982, p. 1, Faculty of Medicine Founders Archives file no. 5.06.002. See also E. C. Abbott, "The Epidemiology of Hypertension in Newfoundland," *Newsletter Newfoundland Medical Association*, 10(2)(1968), 11-12. The latter study was noted in "Studying Blood Pressure in Newfoundland Towns," *The Evening Telegram*, November 8, 1967, p. 6, and reported researcher Dr. Abbott as saying that "as far as he [k]new it was the first study of this type in Canada." See also, J. M. Gray, "Internal Medicine—Problems and Progress," *Newsletter Newfoundland Medical Association*, 18(4)(1968), 11.

29. J. Sheldon, "Changing Patterns of Medical Practice in an Outport," a first-hand account by a physician, unpublished, typescript 1982, p. 3, Faculty of Medicine Founders Archives, file no. 5.16.002.

30. Cf., I. Kawachi and P. Conrad, "Medicalization and the Pharmacological Treatment of Blood Pressure," in P. Davis (ed.), *Contested Ground: Public Purpose and Private Interest in the Regulation of Prescription Drugs*, New York: Oxford University Press, 1996, pp. 26-56. It eventually became clear that the correlation between salt intake and hypertension was not straightforward. Cf., L. Goldman and J. C. Bennett (eds.), *Cecil Textbook of Medicine*, Philadelphia: W. B. Saunders, 2000, p. 264.

31. Hugh Twomey papers, History of Medicine Collection, Faculty of Medicine, Memorial University of Newfoundland.

32. Cf., C. W. M. Wilson, J. B. Banks, R. E. A. Mapes, and S. M. T. Korte, "The Assessment of Prescribing: A Study of Operational Research," in G. McLachlan (ed.), *Problems and Progress in Medical Care*, Oxford: Nuffield Provincial Hospitals Trust, 1964, pp. 171-201, which emphasizes the "considerable increase in the number of proprietary drugs prescribed in the National Health Service" (p. 3).

33. The tonic is widely remembered by senior physicians and members of the public.

34. Whitbourne case records, 1958-1960 (November 22, 1958), History of Medicine Collection, Faculty of Medicine, Memorial University of Newfoundland.

35. In the early decades of vitamins, references to tonics were commonplace; cf., A. B. C. and D. Pearls in *Davis and Lawrence Co., Montreal, Price Product List*, n.d. (c. 1940), p. 9. For a general account of vitamins see R. D. Apple, *Vitamania: Vitamins in American Culture*, New Brunswick, NJ: Rutgers University Press, 1996.

36. A. H. Douthwaite, "The Use and Abuse of Multivitamin Preparations," *The Practitioner*, 182(1959), 74-76.

37. John Sheldon, personal communication, 2002.

38. See *The Evening Telegram*, December 4, 1954, p. 16. Formula from the label on a tonic wine in 2001, which now contains the statement, "The name Tonic Wine does not imply health giving or medicinal properties."

39. *The Evening Telegram*, December 24, 1954, p. 14. It competed, with much advertising, with other tonic wines such as Emu Tonic Wine.

40. *The Evening Telegram*, December 21, 1954, p. 7.

41. *The Evening Telegram*, December 14, 1954, p. 23.

42. *The Evening Telegram,* December 17, 1954, p. 10. The equally well-known Wampole's Extract of Cod Liver was an "ideal year-round tonic for all ages. . . . It helps build sturdy health and energy. Try it" (*The Evening Telegram,* December 6, 1954, p. 8).

43. *The Evening Telegram,* December 14, 1954, p. 5.

44. *The Evening Telegram,* December 24, 1954, p. 9.

45. *The Evening Telegram,* December 2, 1954, p. 17.

46. Dr. Nigel Rusted, personal communication, 2002.

47. *The Evening Telegram,* December 11, 1954, p. 23.

48. *The Evening Telegram,* December 16, 1954, p. 7.

49. *The Evening Telegram,* December 2, 1954, p. 10.

50. Oral History Collection, Medical Communication Group, file 005. One druggist vouched in 1992, "Eno's is the best, you can get the little tablets now," Ibid., file 007.

51. *Time* (Canadian edition), 75(February 22, 1960), 53.

52. See J. H. Young, *The Medical Messiahs: A Social History of Health Quackery in Twentieth-Century America,* Princeton: Princeton University Press, 1967, pp. 309-315. Oral History Collection, Newfoundland Pharmaceutical Association, James Aylward. *Time* (Canadian edition), 99(May 1, 1972), p. 34, carried a report that complaints had been laid against three firms for "misleading and unfair advertising," including statements that their products relieve "nervous tension."

53. See G. L. Kalbfleisch, "Pharmaceutical Legislation 1907-1957," *Canadian Pharmaceutical Journal,* 90(1957), 726-728.

54. Oral History Collection, Medical Communication Group, file 002.

55. See J. Coleman, H. Menzel, and E. Katz, "Social Processes in Physicians' Adoption of a New Drug," *Journal of Chronic Diseases,* 9(1959), 1-19. The authors indicated that physicians who quickly introduced the new compound had been frequently exposed to information on the product or maintained a variety of contacts with a large number of colleagues. However, although professional support in decision making was important, the many possible variables suggest that decisions were dependent on the individual physician and the context of his or her practice. A 1964 British report indicated that responses to medicines were shaped by such considerations as medical training, pharmaceutical company advertising, the use of standard medical books (e.g., *British National Formulary*), consultant advice, and discussions with colleagues (See Wilson et al., "The Assessment of Prescribing").

56. One Newfoundland physician remembers well the lesson learned with sulfonamides and the need to give sufficient fluids when administering them. Nigel Rusted, personal communication, 2002.

57. A generally conservative practice is remembered by physicians and patients. See also Whitbourne case records, 1958-1960, History of Medicine Collection, Faculty of Medicine. General pains such as "Pain in knee"; "Lumbago"; "Pain in neck"; or "Pain under ribs" were commonly prescribed treatment with liniments (e.g., Liniment of Gaultheria) and analgesics (e.g., aspirin).

58. M. D. Rawlins, "Doctors and Drug Makers," *The Lancet,* 2(1984), 276-278.

59. J. Horder, "Long-Term Tranquilliser Use: A General Practitioner's View," in J. Gabe (ed.), *Understanding Tranquilliser Use: The Role of the Social Sciences,* London: Tavistock/Routledge, 1991, pp. 165-166. It is noteworthy that the physicians seemingly lumped antidepressants and tranquilizers together. Difficulties arose

in stopping preparations such as benzodiazepines and amphetamines, widely used in the 1960s and earlier. See Ibid., p. 229, for benzodiazepines; see also P. H. Connell, "Drug Addiction," in R. Daley and H. Miller (eds.), *Progress in Clinical Medicine,* Edinburgh: Churchill Livingstone, 1971, pp. 543-578.

60. See J. P. Griffin, "Therapeutic Conservatism: More Costly in the Long Term," *PharmacoEconomics,* 7(1995), 378-387; and J. P. Griffin, "Therapeutic Conservatism or Therapeutic Fossilization?" *International Pharmacy Journal,* 9(January-February 1995), 19-26. Griffin indicates that the average physician in Britain takes care of two or three times as many patients as his or her counterparts in Europe but prescribes fewer items per patient per year than in most other developed countries. The British doctor is also much less likely to prescribe a new medicine than his or her European counterparts. See also meeting report: P. Mason, "Is UK Prescribing Too Conservative?" *Pharmaceutical Journal,* 268(2002), 881.

61. H. Miller, *Medicine and Society,* London: Oxford University Press, 1973, p. 9.

62. Quoted from the far-reaching U.S. congressional hearings on exposure of high prescription drug prices (beginning 1959) under the chairmanship of Senator Estes Kefauver (*Report of the Royal Commission on Food and Drug Prices,* St. John's: The Royal Commission on Food and Drug Prices, 1968, p. 86. Although the commission found that drugstore prices were lower than on the mainland, it also found that "some people cannot afford—or at least find it a hardship—to purchase drugs which are constantly and vitally necessary and without which their health would be in danger," Ibid., p. 8).

63. Cf., Wolf and Berle (eds.), *Limits of Medicine,* p. 42.

64. Quoted in C. Webster, *The Health Services Since the War,* Volume 1, *Problems of Health Care: The National Health Service before 1957,* London: Her Majesty's Stationary Office, 1988, p. 223.

65. Ibid., p. 222.

66. See J. P. Griffin, "An Historical Survey of UK Government Measures to Control the NHS Medicines Expenditure from 1948 to 1996," *PharmacoEconomics,* 10 (1996), 210-224. For context see P. Davis, *Managing Medicines: Public Policy and Therapeutic Drugs,* Buckingham: Open University Press, 1997.

67. In Newfoundland, for example, the average prescription cost in 1963 was CD$1.95. The Newfoundland drug bill in 1975 was CD$43.2 million and in 1997 it was CD$143.3 million (available online at <http:/www.cihi.ca/facts/nhex/tab-nfd. shtml>, accessed July 22, 2001).

68. Letter dated April 13, 1955. I am grateful to Dr. Rusted for sharing his correspondence with me.

69. For more on cortisone's use in Britain see J. Glynn, "The Discovery and Early Use of Cortisone," *Journal of the Royal Society of Medicine,* 91(1998), 513-517.

70. D. Cantor, "Cortisone and the Politics of Drama, 1949-55," in J. V. Pickstone (ed.), *Medical Innovations in Historical Perspective,* New York: St. Martin's Press, 1992, pp. 165-184. For initial overemphasis in the popular press see also G. Hetenyi and J. Karsh, "Cortisone Therapy: A Challenge to Academic Medicine in 1949-1952," *Perspectives in Biology and Medicine,* 40(1997), 426-439.

71. I am especially grateful to Dr. J. Martin for discussion on this point.

72. Glynn, "The Discovery and Early Use of Cortisone."

73. For background see R. Hoffenberg, *Clinical Freedom*, London: The Nuffield Provincial Hospital Trust, 1987.

74. Ibid., p. 14. See also disagreement with the view that "amphetamines should be removed from doctors in general and confined to certain consultants" (W. O. McCormick, "Amphetamine Prescribing," *British Medical Journal*, 2(1967), 445). An interesting exchange took place in the British parliament in 1955 when the minister of health indicated that doctors had a right to prescribe what they thought best for their patients. See "Medical Notes in Parliament. Doctors Right to Prescribe," *British Medical Journal*, 1(1955), 1226-1227.

75. A. Melville and R. Mapes, "Anatomy of a Disaster: The Case of Practalol," in R. Mapes (ed.), *Prescribing Practice and Drug Use*, London: Croom Helm, 1980, pp. 121-144.

76. A. Williams, "Health Economics: The End of Clinical Freedom?" *British Medical Journal*, 297(1998), 1183-1186.

77. T. Caulfield and K. Siminoski, "Physicians' Liability and Drug Formulary Restrictions," *Canadian Medical Association Journal*, 166(2002), 460.

78. Supplies were also sent to the mental hospital in St. John's, to nurses and nursing stations around the province, and to welfare patients in St. John's.

79. The history of formularies even precedes the printed examples of the seventeenth century. See G. Sonnedecker, *Kremers and Urdang's History of Pharmacy*, Philadelphia: Lippincott, 1976, pp. 258-260, for an outline of formularies in the United States.

80. The Canadian Committee on Pharmaceutical Standards, *The Canadian Formulary with Which Is Bound the Reference Companion*, Toronto: University of Toronto Press, 1935, p. 7. For a history of the Canadian Formulary see E. W. Stieb, "The AFPC Comes of Age, 1951-1969," in B. E. Riedel and E. W. Stieb (eds.), *A History of the Association of Faculties of Pharmacy of Canada: The First Fifty Years 1944-1954*, Saskatoon: Association of Faculties of Pharmacy of Canada, 2001, pp. 75-76.

81. *The British National Formulary* was for use within the National Health Service. Antecedents were the *National Formulary for National Health Insurance* and the *National War Formulary;* for information on formularies in the United States see D. E. Francke, "Origin and Development of the American Hospital Formulary Service," *Drug Intelligence and Clinical Pharmacy*, 6(1972), 448-456. Neither is remembered as having any impact in Newfoundland, though the American Hospital Formulary Service—described as a "master formulary" with the expectation that hospitals would "select" the monographs according to their own needs—attracted interest in Canada.

82. The 1955 *General Hospital Formulary, St. John's: General Hospital*, may have been the hospital's first; no earlier one has been located. For quotes, (1955) unpaginated introduction; (1965) unpaginated introduction.

83. The views of Dr. Nigel Rusted, senior surgeon at the time, on physician authority (personal communication, 2000). It is noteworthy that only eight "old-time" mixtures present in the 1955 version of the *General Hospital Formulary* reflected what was happening at the central pharmacy: carminative potassium citrate, iron ammonium citrate, ammonium carbonate, codeine phosphate, kadlin with opium, ammonium carbonate and tincture of stramonium, phenobarbiturate, and sodium

bromide. The next edition (1965) contained only six mixtures, which survived into the 1971-1972 edition.

84. For example, see L. Furness, "Formularies in Primary Care," *Primary Care Pharmacy,* 1(2000), 37-39.

85. H. Grabowsky and C. D. Mullins, "Pharmacy Benefit Management, Cost-Effectiveness Analysis, and Drug Formulary Decisions," *Social Science and Medicine,* 45(1997), 535-544. For a sense of direction see H. Meyer, "The Pills That Ate Your Profit," *Hospitals Health Networks,* (February 5, 1998), pp. 19-22. Emerging from PBMs in the 2000s are disease management programs, in which patients enroll in a program (therapeutic service) managed under the auspices of a PBM. These programs include nurse educators, educational mailings to patients, and the patients' physicians. Team care is promoted, but the primary goal is overall cost cutting. For more on these programs, visit the Web site of Pharmacy Benefit Management Institute, Inc. at <http://www.pbmi.com>, accessed August 2003. For issues in 2000 see H. L. Lipton, D. J. Gross, M. R. Stebbins, and L. H. Syed, "Managing the Pharmacy Benefit in Medicare HMOs: What Do We Really Know?" *Health Affairs,* 19(2)(2000), 42-58.

86. I. Starr, "The Use and Abuse of Mixtures of Active Drugs. Requirements of Modern Drug Therapy," *Journal of the American Pharmaceutical Association,* 181(1962), 126-130.

87. I. Rusted, letter dated March 3, 1955.

88. Homer company letter dated February 23, 1955, in possession of Dr. Ian Rusted.

89. P. Warwick, personal communication, 2002.

90. Advertisement for Dr. Hamilton's Pills, *The Evening Telegram,* July 6, 1907, p. 5.

91. See J. H. Warner, *The Therapeutic Perspective: Medical Practice, Knowledge, and Identity in America, 1820-1885,* Cambridge: Harvard University Press, 1986, pp. 250-252.

92. See A. Berman and M. A. Flannery, *America's Botanico-Medical Movements: Vox Populi,* Binghamton, NY: The Haworth Press, 2001, pp. 135-137.

93. See Warner, *The Therapeutic Perspective,* pp. 58-80.

94. W. T. Slater, "Therapeutics and Toxicology," *Annual Review of Medicine,* 1(1950), 391.

95. W. Alvarez, "How We Get New Drugs," *The Evening Telegram,* December 29, 1959, p. 13.

96. See D. Healy, "Good Science or Good Business?" *Hastings Center Report,* 30(2)(2000), 19-22; the same view is presented in other Healy writings, e.g., *The Antidepressant Era,* p. 257. R. S. Sobel raises further debate in "Public Health and the Placebo: The Legacy of the 1906 Pure Food and Drugs Act," *The Cato Journal,* 21(3)(2002), 463-450. Sobel argues that the "proven" placebo became unacceptable with the 1962 FDA policy.

97. E. D. Pellegrino, "The Sociocultural Impact of Twentieth-Century Therapeutics," in M. J. Vogel and C. E. Rosenberg (eds.), *The Therapeutic Revolution: Essays in the Social History of American Medicine,* Philadelphia: University of Pennsylvania Press, 1979, p. 255.

98. See Ibid., pp. 185-186; see also D. Healy, "The Case for an Individual Approach to the Treatment of Depression," *Journal of Clinical Psychiatry,* 61 (Suppl.) (2000), 618-623.

99. I. Marks, "Drugs in Psychiatric Practice," in E. M. Tansey, D. A. Christie, and L. A. Reynolds (eds.), *Wellcome Witnesses to Twentieth Century Medicine,* Volume 2, London: Wellcome Trust, 1998, p. 185.

100. L. Marks, " 'Not Just a Statistic': The history of USA and UK Policy over Thrombotic Disease and the Oral Contraceptive Pill, 1960s-1970s," *Social Science and Medicine,* 49(1999), 1139-1155.

101. See "Interim Report of the Special Advisory Committee on Oral Contraception and Response from Canadian Medical Association," *Canadian Medical Association Journal,* 102(1970), 1206-1207.

102. It is noteworthy that in Britain, with the introduction of the National Health Service (1948), state prescriptions virtually quadrupled overnight from about 70 million a year to around 250 million (S. Anderson, "The Changing Role of the Community Pharmacist in Health Promotion in Great Britain 1930-1995," *Pharmaceutical Historian,* 32(2002), 7-10).

103. Newfoundland Pharmaceutical Association Minutes, November 14, 1961, Newfoundland Pharmaceutical Association Archives. Federal legislation in Canada was (and is) concerned with guaranteeing that the drugs purchased by pharmacists for resale or use in dispensed prescriptions are pure, safe, and properly described and advertised. Provincial regulations, on the other hand, deal with licensing and what manner drugs can reach the market (e.g., as prescription only, as generics, or for general sale).

104. *The Evening Telegram,* December 22, 1954, p. 2. In 1949, Canadian federal legislation conferred prescription-only status on a number of products that include amphetamine, barbiturates, and sulpha drugs (see D. R. Kennedy, "One Hundred Years of Pharmacy Legislation" in *One Hundred Years of Pharmacy in Canada 1867-1967,* Toronto: Canadian Academy of the History of Pharmacy, 1969, pp. 25-37).

105. "Control of Drugs," *British Medical Journal,* 1(1960), 659. Remarks expressed in the British Parliament. For evidence of the U.S. FDA wishing to tighten regulations on new drugs in 1952 see P. Talalay (ed.), *Drugs in Our Society,* Baltimore: Johns Hopkins University Press, 1964, p. 286. See also comments by L. N. Cutler, "Practical Aspects of Drug Legislation," Ibid., p. 150, that "the public, the medical profession, and the pharmaceutical industry have all accepted the proposition that the government can and should have the power to bar a drug from reaching the market."

106. For helpful comments see A. Daemmrich, "A Tale of Two Experts: Thalidomide and Political Engagement in the United States and West Germany," *Social History of Medicine,* 15(2002), 137-158. For Canadian chronology and rapid acceptance of the product see J. D. Theoret, "Chronology of the Thalidomide Story," *Canadian Medical Association Journal,* 87(1962), 981-982.

107. *House of Commons Debates, Dominion of Canada Session 1962-63,* Volume 1, Ottawa: Queen's Printer, p. 979 (October 26, 1962). Another opposition speaker said the companies withdrew the product in March and that the government officially banned the product in April (p. 983). It was ironic that Frances Kelsey was Canadian born. It is noteworthy that the debate in the 1962 Canadian legislation

was almost entirely consumed with thalidomide, and that the drug was placed, along with LSD, in a new drug schedule that banned its sale. The mind-set of control was influenced by the growth of recreational drug use/abuse in the 1960s, much of it with prescription products (e.g., amphetamines, barbiturates); these became the "enemy" in the war on drugs.

108. See J. Swann, "Sure Cure: Public Policy on Drug Efficacy Before 1962," in G. J. Higby and E. C. Stroud (eds.), *The Inside Story of Medicines: A Symposium*, Madison, WI: American Institute History of Pharmacy, 1997, pp. 223-261.

109. J. Abraham, *Science, Politics, and the Pharmaceutical Industry: Controversy and Bias in Drug Regulation*, New York: St. Martin's Press, 1995, p. 57.

110. See Ibid., p. 59.

111. See Ibid., pp. 59-64.

112. For discussion on this period, without a clear distinction between efficacy and effectiveness, see L. N. Cutler, "Practical Aspects of Drug Legislation," in Talalay (ed.), *Drugs in Our Society*, pp. 149-159.

113. P. Talalay, "A Summary of Comments," in P. Talalay (ed.), *Drugs in our Society*, p. 272.

114. See J. Gabe and M. Bury, "Anxious Times: The Benzodiazepine Controversy and the Fracturing of Expert Authority," in Davis, *Contested Ground*, pp. 42-56.

115. For the context of uncertainty see R. C. Fox, "Medical Uncertainty Revisited," in Albrecht, Fitzpatrick, and Scrimshaw (eds.), *Handbook of Social Studies in Health and Medicine*, pp. 409-425.

116. See R. Davenport-Hines, *The Pursuit of Oblivion: A Global History of Narcotics 1500-2000*, London: Weidenfeld and Nicolson, 2001, p. 307.

117. I. Weisstub, "Back to the Old Treatment of Gonorrhoea," *Canadian Medical Association Journal*, 40(193), 389.

118. For history in the United States see J. P. Swann, "FDA and the Practice of Pharmacy: Prescription Drug Regulation Before the Durham-Humphrey Amendment of 1951," *Pharmacy in History*, 36(1994), 55-70.

119. "The D-H Amendment—an Indictment of Pharmacy," *American Journal of Pharmacy*, 124(1952), 41-42.

120. J. P. Swann, "A Perspective on FDA Oral Histories," available online at <http://www.fda.gov/oc/history/oralhistories/overview.html>, accessed August 2003.

121. On November 28, 1949, the minutes of the Newfoundland Pharmacy Board reported agreement that "consideration be given to strengthening the Pharmaceutical Act and bringing it in line with the other Provincial Acts" (Newfoundland Pharmaceutical Association Archives).

122. Newfoundland Pharmacy Board minutes, November 10, 1948.

123. The Newfoundland Pharmacy Board minutes, May 13, 1954, noted that nothing could be done under the old Pharmacy Act, but when a new act came into effect, action would be taken immediately.

124. Newfoundland Pharmaceutical Association Annual Meeting November 17, 1960.

125. Newfoundland Pharmaceutical Association minutes, November 14, 1961.

126. Newfoundland Pharmaceutical Association Annual General Meeting, November 20, 1958.

127. For background see A. R. Jonsen, *The Birth of Bioethics*, New York: Oxford University Press, 1998.

128. A large volume of commentary emerged on the topic of drug lag. As an example, of interest for underscoring congressional interest, see G. F. Roll, "Of Politics and Drug Regulation," *Medical Marketing and Media,* 12 (April) (1977), 17-18, 20, 22, 24-26, 28-31.

129. W. M. Wardell, "Introduction of New Therapeutic Drugs in the United States and Great Britain: An International Comparison," *Clinical Pharmacology and Therapeutics,* 14(1973), 773. Wardwell, with colleagues, became a vigorous critic of drug lag.

130. For one discussion on AIDS see S. Epstein, *AIDS, Activism, and the Politics of Knowledge,* Berkeley: University of California Press, 1996, pp. 208-234.

131. See J. Goodman, "Pharmaceutical Industry," in Cooter and Pickstone (eds.), *Medicine in the Twentieth Century,* pp. 141-154.

132. A. F. Balis, "Miracle Medicine: The Impact of Sulfa Drugs on Medicine, the Pharmaceutical Industry, and Government Regulation in the U.S. in the 1930s," doctoral thesis, The City University of New York, 2000, p. 18.

133. By the 1990s it had become customary to refer to sulfonamides as antibiotics rather than chemotherapeutic agents distinct from antibiotics.

134. For more on emergence of the concept of antibiosis see J. K. Crellin, "Antibiosis in the 19th Century," in J. Parascandola (ed.), *The History of Antibiotics: A Symposium,* Madison, WI: American Institute History of Pharmacy, 1980, pp. 5-13. For the beginning of the sulfonamide story see I. Loudon, "Puerperal Fever, the Streptococcus, and the Sulphonamides, 1911-1945," *British Medical Journal,* 2(1987), 485-490; I. Loudon, *Death in Childbirth: An International Study of Maternal Care and Maternal Mortality 1800-1850,* Oxford: Clarendon Press, 1992, pp. 254-261.

135. See Balis, "Miracle Medicine," pp. 114-115.

136. E. C. Dodds, "A Review of Recent Progress in the Chemotherapy Septicaemia," *The Practitioner,* 137(1936), 719-724.

137. Loudon, "Puerperal Fever, the Streptococcus, and the Sulphonamides." For Newfoundland information I am grateful to Dr. Nigel Rusted.

138. For some details of the sulfanilamide disaster, see J. H. Young, "Sulfanilamide and Diethylene Glycol" in J. Parascandola and J. C. Whorton (eds.), *Chemistry in Modern Society: Historical Essays in Honor of Aaron J. Ihde,* ACS Symposium Series 228, Washington, DC: American Chemical Society, 1983, pp. 104-125.

139. Abraham, *Science, Politics and the Pharmaceutical Industry,* p. 83. There was, even after the tragedy made headlines, no trace of regulatory reform activity in the Ministry of Health in Britain.

140. The comment about the attitude of U.S. physicians was made by A. F. Balis, "Miracle Medicine," pp. 18 and 114.

141. Cf., H. M. Marks, *The Progress of Experiment: Science and Therapeutic Reform in the United States 1900-1990,* Cambridge: Cambridge University Press, 1997.

142. W. Osler, *Principles and Practice of Medicine,* New York: Appleton, 1907, p. 165. Osler notes that the "Men of Death" phrase was first used for tuberculosis.

143. A. W. Policoff, "M. and B. 693," typescript, History of Medicine collection, Faculty of Medicine.

144. One recollection of boils in Newfoundland before World War II stated: "an awful lot of people had festers and boils and sore hands. I suppose things weren't very hygienic in fishing then, your arm or fingers got rubbed, and necks got rubbed

with oil jackets. You had boils, big old sores" (Oral History Collection, Medical Communication Group, file 009). Boils were commonplace even outside the fishery; Newfoundland seniors remember often having a "plague" of them when they were in their teens, and often sties as well. A fascinating diversity of poultices were used in treatment, from chickweed to dragon's blood (Oral History Collection, Medical Communication Group, file 114, and Crellin, *Home Medicine*, p. 137). It is appropriate to add that for small infected cuts, antiseptics such as iodine and mercurochrome competed with the popular Mecca ointment, all of which were readily available in local stores or pharmacies. Less expensive, of course, were the application of turpentine bladders (from pine), universally known on the island. Some Newfoundlanders felt this treatment had anti-infection properties. Aside from the ubiquitous "soft bread" poultice—"there was nothing to beat it for infection" (Oral History Collection, Medical Communication Group, file 006).

145. N. Rusted "Sulfapyridine or M and B 693," June 22, 1939, typescript, History of Medicine Collection, Faculty of Medicine.

146. For some context see the letter to the editor of the *New England Journal of Medicine,* 216(1937), 711: "There is no question about the over-enthusiasm of the medical profession for 'sure-cure' remedies. I do not see how this remedy gained such quick recognition, but it goes to show that doctors are just as gullible to exploitation of cures as the laity" (Quoted in Balis, "Miracle Medicine," p. 118).

147. For more on Britain's chief medical officer see A. Hardy, *Health and Medicine in Britain,* Basingstoke: Palgrave, 2001, p. 120. For information on Newfoundland see J. E. Candow, "An American Report on Newfoundland's Health Services in 1940," *Newfoundland Studies,* 5(1989), 221-239; P. Neary, "And Gave Just As Much As They Got: A 1941 American Perspective on Public Health in Newfoundland," *Newfoundland Studies,* 14(1998), 50-70; P. Neary, " 'A Grave Problem Which Needs Immediate Attention': An American Report on Venereal Disease and other Health Problems in Newfoundland, 1942," *Newfoundland Studies,* 15(1999), 79-103.

148. Arrangements were in place for special government payments to physicians to treat venereal disease free of charge. See P. Neary, "Venereal Disease and Public Health Administration in Newfoundland in the 1930s and 1940s," *Canadian Bulletin of Medical History,* 15(1998), 129-151. A 1940 report stated that Newfoundland physicians treating syphilis were paid by the government three dollars for each injection of arsphenamine, bismuth, or mercury. Two years later (November 1942) the same fee structure was reported, as well as the use of "arsenicals and bismuth" and sulfathiazole.

149. I. Weisstub, "Back to the Old Treatment of Gonorrhoea." For comments see J. Dicken McGinness, "From Salvarsan to Penicillin: Medical Science and VD Control in Canada," in W. Mitchinson and J. Dickin McGinnis (eds.), *Essays in the History of Canadian Medicine,* Toronto: McClelland and Stewart, 1988, pp. 126-147.

150. L. A. Miller, "A Plea for Public Health," lecture delivered to St. John's Clinical Society, February 13, 1941, History of Medicine Collection, Faculty of Medicine.

151. For reforms see Neary, "Venereal Disease and Public Health Administration in Newfoundland in the 1930s and 1940s."

152. See J. Parascandola, "John Mahoney and the Introduction of Penicillin to Treat Syphilis," *Pharmacy in History,* 43(2001), 3-22.

153. See P. S. Ward, "Antibiotics and International Relations at the Close of World War II," in J. Parascandola (ed.), *The History of Antibiotics: A Symposium,* Madison, WI: American Institute of the History of Pharmacy, 1980, pp. 101-112.

154. For an account of the case see Neary, "Venereal Disease and Public Health Administration in Newfoundland in the 1930s and 1940s," pp. 147-148.

155. *Newfoundland Gazette,* January 9, 1945, p. 13. For an account of treatment at the Mayo Clinic, which illustrates why the introduction of arsenicals did not replace existing treatments (or prevent the introduction of new ones, such as fever therapy) for specific clinical situations, see J. S. Sartin and H. O. Perry, "From Mercury to Malaria to Penicillin: The History of the Treatment of Syphilis at the Mayo Clinic, 1916-1955," *Journal of the American Academy of Dermatology,* 32(1995), 255-261. The four approved methods for the treatment of gonorrhea follow: (1) sulphonamide compounds, or other approved biological therapy; (2) local treatment by instillations, irrigations, and topical applications; (3) fever therapy; and (4) penicillin or other approved biologicals.

156. For discussion of the American scene, D. P. Adams, *"The Greatest Good to the Greatest Number": Penicillin Rationing on the American Home Front, 1940-1945,* New York: Peter Lang, 1991. Dr. Ian Rusted was the first person officially to prescribe the antibiotic to a civilian in Newfoundland, in the spring of 1945.

157. *Dominion of Canada. Official Report of Debates House of Commons, 10 George VI, 1946, Vol. IV, 1946,* Ottawa: King's Printer, 1947, p. 361.

158. N. Britten, "Patients' Ideas about Medicines: A Qualitative Study in a General Practice Population," *British Journal of General Practice,* 44(1994), 465-468.

159. Whitbourne case records, 1968-1960, History of Medicine Collection, Faculty of Medicine.

160. Oral History Collection, Newfoundland Pharmaceutical Association, Cecil Burke, July 22, 1999. Sales of the lozenges continued despite warnings in Newfoundland and elsewhere that, because they contained inadequate doses, they were likely to promote penicillin-resistant organisms. In 1963, a question in the British House of Commons received a reply that the Ministry of Health had no evidence of tolerance created by such self-medication. See "Self-Medication with Antibiotic Lozenges," *British Medical Journal,* 1(1963), 960.

161. Streptomycin was, in fact, soon used in conjunction with other products (e.g., PAS, para-aminosalicylic acid), a stategy to reduce the development of resistant organisms. For an interesting account, including the controversy over who "discovered" streptomycin see M. Wainwright, *Miracle Cure: The Story of Penicillin and the Golden Age of Antibiotics,* Oxford: Blackwell, pp. 118-140.

162. See Thomas, *From Sled to Satellite,* pp. 66-67. Thomas suggests this was the first use of streptomycin in Newfoundland, but that was not so.

163. "Streptomycin and T.B. Meningitis," *British Medical Journal,* 1(1947), 814.

164. The decline of tuberculosis has occasioned a vast literature and much controversy. For a review of the questioning of the relevance of lifestyle see L. G. Wilson, "The Historical Decline of Tuberculosis in Europe and America: Its Causes and Significance," *Journal of the History of Medicine and Allied Sciences,* 45(1990), 366-396. A detailed study of tuberculosis in Newfoundland might contribute to the

controversy, including consideration of multiple factors. It is still believed by many historians that lifestyle changes were especially important in controlling the disease, but physicians in Newfoundland looking back to the 1950s hardly feel this is relevant.

The saga of BCG vaccination and resistance to it, especially in the United States, is considered by G. D. Feldberg, *Disease and Class: Tuberculosis and the Shaping of Modern North American Society,* New Brunswick, NJ: Rutgers University Press, 1995; for a discussion of BCG vaccinations in Newfoundland see E. House, *Light at Last: Triumph over Tuberculosis in Newfoundland and Labrador,* St. John's: Jesperson Press, 1981, pp. 162-167.

165. Of course, that does not discount possible change in the virulence of the organism.

166. J. G. Kidney and E. MacLaughlin, "Streptomycin in the Treatment of Pulmonary tuberculosis," *Journal of the Medical Association of Eire,* 22(1948), 3-8.

167. E. Shorter, *A History of Psychiatry from the Era of the Asylum to the Age of Prozac,* New York: Wiley and Sons, 1997, p. 317. Shorter recognizes D. Healy for this view, expressed by Healy in various writings. Healy has repeatedly expressed concern with channeling a diversity of clinical situations into one diagnosis. A related concern of Healy's is that the diversity of actions of antidepressives (e.g., reducing emotional responses or promoting "get-up-and-go") is often overlooked and not tailored to the particular needs of a patient. See D. Healy, "The Case for an Individual Approach to the Treatment of Depression," *Journal of Clinical Psychiatry,* 61(Suppl. 6) (2000), 18-23.

168. I. Tait, "Drugs in Psychiatric Practice," in Tansey, Christie, and Reynolds (eds.), *Wellcome Witnesses to Twentieth Century Medicine,* Volume 2, p. 169. The Green Medicine was also known to physicians in Newfoundland.

169. See Whitbourne case records, History of Medicine Collection, Faculty of Medicine. Other prescription information in this section is from same source.

170. Although meprobamate is commonly seen as the "first" minor tranquilizer Mephensin was being promoted in 1950, though of limited clinical use because of its short action. See F. M. Berger, "The Tranquilizer Decade," *Journal of Neuropsychiatry,* 5(1964), 403-410. Berger also notes the atmosphere of excitement at the time "rarely matched in contemporary history, but reminiscent of great discoveries of the past" (p. 403).

171. E. Shorter, *A History of Psychiatry from the Era of the Asylum to the Age of Prozac,* pp. 315-316.

172. "Let down for Miltown," *Time* (Canadian edition), 85(April 30) (1965), 47.

173. Whitbourne case records, 1958-1960, History of Medicine Collection, Faculty of Medicine; also derived from personal recollections of physicians.

174. M. Weatherall, "Tranquillizers," *British Medical Journal,* 1(1962), 1221.

175. For one of many references to these books see Berger, "The Tranquilizer Decade."

176. For accounts see Healy, *The Antidepressant Era;* for a synopsis see Shorter, *A History of Psychiatry from the Era of the Asylum to the Age of Prozac,* pp. 320-325.

177. For comments on the rise of antidepressives see D. Healy, "The Three Faces of the Antidepressants: A Critical Commentary on the Clinical-Economic Context

of Diagnosis," *Journal of Nervous and Mental Disease,* 187(1999), 174-180; for illustration of other scares see "Valium Alarm," *Time,* 117(January 19) (1981), 74.

178. At the time "fuzzy borders and overlap" existed between agitated depression and anxious depression. See D. Healy (ed.), *The Psychopharmacologists II,* London: Altman, 1998, p. 126 (interview with Max Lurie).

179. See interesting perspectives on usefulness from G. Beaumont, "Drugs in Psychiatric Practice," in Tansey, Christie, and Reynolds (eds.), *Wellcome Witnesses to Twentieth Century Medicine,* Volume 2, p. 159; see also I. Marks, Ibid., p. 162.

180. The abuse of barbiturates and amphetamines has been noted in Chapter 4, but for specific information on Drinamyl in Britain see T. Bewley, "Recent Changes in the Pattern of Drug Abuse in the United Kingdom," *Bulletin of Narcotics,* 4(1966), 1-14.

181. For recent general discussions see L. Payer, *Disease-Mongers: How Doctors, Drug Companies, and Insurers Are Making You Feel Sick,* New York: Wiley and Sons, 1992; see also R. Moynihan, I. Heath, and D. Henry, "Selling Sickness: The Pharmaceutical Industry and Disease Mongering," *British Medical Journal,* 324(2002), 886-891. In the context of mental health and "drugs looking for markets," social phobia is an issue: "now [1997] we are supposed to have drugs for social phobia, but before we can get anyone to prescribe them, we have to teach the general practitioners what social phobia is" (comments by G. Beaumont in "Drugs in Psychiatric Practice," p. 160).

182. D. Healy, "The Three Faces of the Antidepressants: A Critical Commentary on the Clinical-Economic Context of Diagnosis," *The Journal of Nervous and Mental Disease,* 187(1999), 176. Healy notes companies such as Roche were slow to appreciate a market for antidepressants in the 1950s (Ibid. and Beaumont, "Drugs in Psychiatric Practice," p. 142.) The term *antidepressant* was seemingly introduced by Max Lurie (D. Healy, *The Psychopharmacologists II,* London: Altman, 1998, pp. 128-129, interview with Max Lurie, "The Enigma of Isoniazid"). Upon its introduction Tofranil was for a while called a thymoleptic rather than an antidepressant. Iproniazid was called a "psychic energizer." Healy considers that at the time depression was not a widespread issue in general practice.

183. D. L. Davis, "Medical Misinformation: Communication Between Outport Newfoundland Women and Their Physicians," *Social Science and Medicine,* 18(1984), 273-278. See also P. S. Dinham, *You Never Know What They Might Do: Mental Illness in Outport Newfoundland,* St. John's: Institute of Social and Economic Research, Memorial University of Newfoundland, 1977, pp. 50-54. Dinham makes clear that "just nerves" identifies a person as not mentally ill.

184. As elsewhere, Newfoundland women were also being prescribed hormone replacement therapy.

185. I am especially grateful to Dr. Paddy Warwick for alerting me to this phrase.

186. D. L. Davis, "The Variable Character of Nerves in a Newfoundland Fishing Village," *Medical Anthropology,* 11(1989), 63-78. One might have expected that "nerves" would have been described as "anxiety," since minor tranquilizers were still more widely prescribed than antidepressants. (See, for example, M. C. Smith, *A Social History of the Minor Tranquilizers,* Binghamton, NY: Pharmaceutical Products Press, 1991, p. 33.) However, depression was widespread and antidepressants were well known.

187. IMS health data: <http://www.imshealthcanada.com>.

188. Ibid.

189. For some review of this see S. L. Speaker, "From 'Happiness Pills' to 'National Nightmare': Changing Cultural Assessment of Minor Tranquilizers in America, 1955-1980," *Journal of the History of Medicine and Allied Sciences,* 52(1997), 338-376; see also M. C. Smith, *Small Comfort: A History of the Minor Tranquilizers.*

190. Fox notes a more pervasive societal interest in uncertainty in the 1960s and 1970s; Fox, "Medical Uncertainty Revisited."

191. H. P. G., "The Pill," *Canadian Medical Association Journal,* 94(1966), 1015.

192. See G. P. R. Tallin, "The Legal Implications of the Non-Therapeutic Practices of Doctors," *Canadian Medical Association Journal,* 87(1962), 207-215.

193. For discussion of the Canadian scene see A. McLaren and A. T. McLaren, *The Bedroom and the State,* Toronto: McClelland and Stewart, 1886, pp. 134-136.

194. See E. S. Watkins, *On the Pill, A Social History of Oral Contraceptives 1950-1970,* Baltimore: Johns Hopkins University, 1998, especially pp. 73-102; See also L. Marks, "'Andromeda Freed from Her Chains': Attitudes Toward Women and the Oral Contraceptive Pill, 1950-1970," in L. Conrad and A. Hardy (eds.), *Women and Modern Medicine,* Amsterdam, Netherlands: Rodopi, 2001, pp. 217-244; A. Tone, *Devices and Desires: A History of Contraceptives in America,* New York: Hill and Wang, 2001, pp. 242-249; L. V. Marks, *Sexual Chemistry: A History of the Contraceptive Pill,* New Haven, CT: Yale University Press, 2001.

195. There has been much interest in Catholic usage, for example, see B. Asbell, *The Pill: A Biography of the Drug That Changed the World,* New York: Random House, 1995 and other references cited in this discussion. The demand for the Pill in the early years was variable. The Newfoundland scene matches the view that the 1960s was not the "sexual revolution" it was made out to be. For example, economics was an additional issue (the Pill was relatively expensive), and about 50 percent of Newfoundlanders were Roman Catholic. Moreover, for most of the 1960s the Pill was used almost entirely by married women with large families, including some Catholics after hearing of the support some Catholic doctors gave to the Pill. Some women still visited their doctors with some degree of stealth concerning contraception, a holdover of the desperation that earlier had led a few women to try an extreme form of birth control, namely to convince their doctors that they needed hysterectomies because of excessive menstrual bleeding. However, their hemoglobin levels rarely bore this out. By the end of the 1960s a change was under way, as younger women began requesting the Pill.

196. Watkins, *On the Pill,* p. 100. See Marks, *Sexual Chemistry,* p. 149, for more on the British report.

197. See S. W. Junod and L. Marks, "Women's Trials: The Approval of the First Oral Contraceptive Pill in the United States and Great Britain," *Journal of the History of Medicine and Allied Sciences,* 57(2002), 117-160. Junod and Marks indicate that this had much to do with early protocols. See also L. Marks, "'Not Just a Statistic': The History of U.S.A. and U.K. Policy Over Thrombotic Disease and the Oral Contraceptive Pill, 1960s to 1970s," *Social Science and Medicine,* 49(1999), 1139-1155.

198. *Time* (Canadian edition), 95(February 9) (1970), 40.

199. D. G. Friend, editor of the *Year Book of Drug Therapy 1970,* Chicago: Year Book Medical Publisher, 1970, p. 164, stated that chlormadinone acetate as an oral

contraceptive looks "promising, but with such a high percentage of breakthrough bleeding most patients would find it unsatisfactory. Whether this agent will be as effective as the dual agent or sequential approach will require much more evaluation. I like the idea of a single agent and hope that further work will support the authors."

200. For comments on doctors in the United States feeling pressured see A. Tone, *Devices and Desires,* pp. 240-241.

201. See Tallin, "The Legal Implications of Non-Therapeutic Practices of Doctors."

202. D. J. Kirby, *The Final Report of Project Outreach: Attitudes Toward and Utilization of Family Planning Services in the City of St. John's,* n.p., 1975.

203. "Oral Contraception and Thromboembolic Disease," *Canadian Medical Association Journal,* 98(1968), 1118.

204. "History of FDA Patient Package Insert Requirements," *American Journal of Hospital Pharmacy,* 37(1980), 1660. See also, A. Tone, *Devices and Desires,* pp. 250-251, and E. S. Watkins, *On the Pill,* pp. 103-131. For a more general account of estrogens, see E. S. Watkins, "'Doctor, Are You Trying to Kill Me?': Ambivalence About the Patient Package Insert for Estrogen," *Bulletin of the History of Medicine,* 76(2002), 84-104.

205. See E. S. Watkins, "'Doctor, Are you Trying to Kill Me?'".

206. "Parliament Hill: Risk from Pill Less than Risk without Pill," *Canadian Medical Association Journal,* 102(1970), 801.

207. "The Canadian Medical Association Comments on the Food and Drug Committee Report, 'Hazards of Oral Contraceptives,'" *Canadian Medical Association Journal,* 103(1970), 1415-1422.

208. "Oral Contraceptives, 1985: A Synopsis," *Canadian Medical Association Journal,* 133(1985), 463-465.

209. For an overview of the ongoing controversy see J. O. Drife, "The Third Generation Pill Controversy (continued). The Risks Are Still Small Compared with Those of Pregnancy," *British Medical Journal,* 323(2001), 119-120.

210. See J. M. Kemmeren, A. Agra, and D. E. Grobee, "Third Generation Oral Contraceptives and Risk of Venous Thrombosis: Meta-Analysis," *British Medical Journal,* 323(2001), 131-134.

211. L. Tyrer, "Introduction of the Pill and Its Impact," *Contraception,* 59(1999), 11S-16S.

212. It is noteworthy that the saga of DES (diethylstilbestrol) could have been sufficient warning for later concerns with estrogens, as indicated by influential activist Barbara Seaman. See B. Seaman and G. Seaman, in *Women and the Crisis in Sex Hormones,* New York: Rawson Associates, 1977, pp. 1-59. Introduced in 1941, DES gained fairly wide usage as a way of reducing the risk of threatened miscarriage (ultimately felt to be of uncertain value), to fatten cattle, and as a morning-after contraceptive. (For the cattle story see A. I. Marcus, *Cancer from Beef: DES Federal Food Regulation and Consumer Confidence,* Baltimore: Johns Hopkins University Press, 1994.) For dilemmas and uncertainties in 1975 see K. Weiss, "Vaginal Cancer: An Iatrogenic 'Disease,'" *International Journal of Health Services,* 5(1975), 235-251. In the mid-1960s, DES daughters—daughters of mothers who had been given DES during pregnancy—began to visit doctors' offices with adenocarcinomas of the vagina or a pre-cancerous condition; a 1971 report found an association, and

in 1973 the FDA issued a warning to physicians not to prescribe DES for pregnant women.

213. For history see E. S. Watkins, "Dispensing with Aging: Changing Rationales for Long-Term Hormone Replacement Therapy, 1960-2000," *Pharmacy in History,* 43(2001), 23-37.

214. I. Palmlund, "The Marketing of Estrogens for Menopausal and Postmenopausal Women," *Journal of Psychosomatic Obstetrics and Gynecology,* 18(1997), 158-164; see also M. N. G. Dukes, "The Menopause and the Pharmaceutical Industry," *Journal of Psychosomatic Obstetrics and Gynecology,* 18(1997), 181-188.

215. See J. L. Lacey, P. J. Mink, J. H. Lukin, M. E. Sherman, T. Troisi, P. Hartge, A. Schatzkin, and C. Schairer, "Menopausal Hormonal Replacement Therapy and Risk of Ovarian Cancer," *Journal of the American Medical Association,* 288(2002), 334-341.

Chapter 6

1. T. R. Harrison, "Severe Angina Pectoris Considerations of Surgical and Medical Management," *Journal of the American Medical Association,* 223(1973), 1022-1026. Found in E. J. Huth and T. J. Murray (eds.), *Medicine in Quotations: Views of Health and Disease Through the Ages,* Philadelphia: American College of Physicians, 2000, p. 362.

2. In 1969, readers of *The Evening Telegram,* August 14, 1969, p. 3 ("Value of Research Stressed at Pharmacists' Convention"), were told, for example, that "the public feels 'drugs are dangerous, and they feel they're overdosed,'" according to a report from the Canadian Pharmaceutical Association.

3. For an informative, detailed analysis of critiques of scientific authority, at least on dietary matters, see S. Hilgartner, *Science on Stage: Expert Advice As Public Drama,* Stanford: Stanford University Press, 2000.

4. I. Illich, *Limits to Medicine—Medical Nemesis: The Expropriation of Health,* Toronto: McClelland and Stewart, 1976. Some sense of the book's resonating influence can be judged from various articles published on "too much medicine" or "medicalization" in a theme issue of the *British Medical Journal,* April 13, 2002.

5. Illich, *Limits to Medicine,* p. 6.

6. For a more general recent account of medicalization, much applauded, see R. Moynihan, *Too Much Medicine? The Business of Health—and Its Risks for You,* Sydney: ABC Books, 1998.

7. Illich, *Limits to Medicine,* pp. 66, 73. For a full discussion of chloramphenicol, see T. Maeder, *Adverse Reactions,* New York: William Morrow, 1994.

8. See L. Lander, *Defective Medicine: Risk, Anger, and the Malpractice Crisis,* New York: Farrar Straus and Giroux, 1978, p. 27. Cf., S. Law and S. Polan, *Pain and Profit: The Politics of Malpractice,* New York: Harper and Row, 1978, who wrote "medical malpractice has come of age." See also, R. M. Patterson (ed.), *Drugs in Litigation: Damage Awards Involving Prescription Drugs,* Charlottesville: The Mitchie Company, 2000.

9. From recollections of M. Schmidt, commissioner of food and drugs 1973-1976, Oral History Project, FDA History, available online at <http://www.fda.gov/oc/history/oralhistories/schmidt/default.htm>, accessed August 2003.

10. For quote see F. J. Ingelfinger, R. V. Ebert, M. Finland, and A. S. Relman, *Controversy in Internal Medicine II,* Philadelphia: W. B. Saunders, 1974, p. 1.

11. P. Talalay (ed.), *Drugs in Our Society,* Baltimore: Johns Hopkins University Press, 1964. See, especially, editor's summary of comments, pp. 269-300.

12. See E. Shorter, "Primary Care" in R. Porter (ed.), *The Cambridge Illustrated History of Medicine,* Cambridge: Cambridge University Press, 1996, p. 143. The phrase was also used specifically as a title of a book: G. C. Robinson, *The Patient As a Person,* New York: Commonwealth Fund, 1939, as noted by R. Porter in *The Greatest Benefit to Mankind: A Medical History of Humanity,* New York: W. W. Norton and Co., 1997, p. 682.

13. Quoted in Porter, *The Greatest Benefit to Mankind,* p. 679.

14. For issues of bedside versus scientific medicine in the first decades of the twentieth century see C. Lawrence, "A Tale of Two Sciences: Bedside and Bench in Twentieth-Century Britain," *Medical History,* 43(1999), 421-449.

15. See S. W. Tracy, "An Evolving Science of Man: The Transformation and Demise of American Constitutional Medicine, 1920-1950," in C. Lawrence and G. Weisz (eds.), *Greater Than the Parts: Holism in Biomedicine, 1920-1950,* New York: Oxford University Press, 1998, pp. 161-188.

16. E. Balint and J. S. Norell, *Six Minutes for the Patient Interactions in General Practice Consultations,* London: Tavistock, 1973. This book was essentially a posthumous tribute. Balint's best-known book was *The Doctor, the Patient, and the Illness,* London: Pitman, 1957.

17. J. T. Hart, "Going to the Doctor," in R. Cooter and J. Pickstone (eds.), *Medicine in the Twentieth Century,* Amsterdam, Netherlands: Harwood, 2000, pp, 543-557, notes that it is hard for later generations to appreciate the hostility of almost all British general practitioners to any psychiatric diagnosis, apart from psychosis. For signs of the movement in the United States, cf., N. Brunori, "General Practitioners and Psychiatry," *American Practitioner,* 2(1951), 138-145. It is impossible to say how widespread the issue was in Newfoundland, but it was the special interest of certain practitioners, notably J. A. Walsh, 1897-1976.

18. This issue is raised in M. Marinker, "'What Is Wrong' and 'How We Know It': Changing Concepts of Illness in General Practice," in I. Loudon, J. Horder, and C. Webster (eds.), *General Practice Under the National Health Service 1948-1997,* London: Clarendon Press, 1998, pp. 65-91.

19. Marinker, "'What is Wrong,'" p. 13.

20. Representative texts include M. Field, *Patients Are People: A Medical-Social Approach to Prolonged Illness,* New York: Columbia University Press, 1967 and E. L. Koos, *The Sociology of the Patient,* New York: McGraw-Hill, 1959. Written for nurses, Koos's book opens with a sense of a movement: "In the past half-century the healing professions have come increasingly to view health and illness in a new light. Instead of placing the sole emphasis upon the disease, the tendency is to recognize that the patient is a person" (p. vii). See also Porter, *The Greatest Benefit to Mankind,* 1997, pp. 668-709.

21. A. P. Cawadias, "Nomen Proprium," *British Medical Journal,* 2(1957), 1547.

22. A review of the literature (1958 onward) through the electronic databases (MEDLINE, OLDMEDLINE, and CINAHL) reveals a continuing rise in the use of the term *patient-centered* to the early 2000s.

23. N. Cousins, *Anatomy of an Illness As Perceived by the Patient: Reflections on Healing and Regeneration*, New York: Norton, 1979.

24. N. Cousins, *The Healing Heart: Antidotes to Panic and Helplessness*, New York: Norton, 1983, pp. 11-12.

25. Women in a southwest coast community in Newfoundland were reported to be "ambivalent in their attitudes toward doctors," especially for treating everyday ailments or more chronic illness. See D. C. Davis, "Medical Misinformation: Communication Between Outport Newfoundland Women and Their Physicians," *Social Science and Medicine*, 18(1984), 273-278. For trust and mistrust see R. R. Andersen, J. K. Crellin, and B. O'Dwyer, *Healthways. Newfoundland Elders: Their Lifestyles and Values*, St. John's: Creative Publishers, 1998, pp. 116-131. This was also a commonplace issue recorded in the Oral History Collection, Medical Communication Group, Department of English, Memorial University of Newfoundland.

26. *Newfoundland Medical Association Journal*, 21(2)(1979), 31-32.

27. *Newfoundland Medical Association Journal*, 22(2)(1980), 18-19.

28. For prompting thoughts about negotiation, along with the emergence of the user movement, see K. Davies, "'Silent and Censured Travellers'? Patients' Narratives and Patients' Voices: Perspectives on the History of Mental Illness Since 1948," *Social History of Medicine*, 14(2001), 267-292.

29. Based on conversations with many Newfoundland physicians, 1997-2002.

30. See Porter, *The Greatest Benefit to Mankind*, pp. 716-717.

31. See also, B. Mintzes and C. Hodgkin, "The Consumer Movements from Single-Issue Campaigns to Long-Term Reform" in P. Davis (ed.), *Contested Ground: Public Purpose and Private Interests—the Regulation of Prescription Drugs*, New York: Oxford University Press, 1996, pp. 76-89.

32. The influence of Social Audit is primarily due to Charles Medawar, who has gained widespread authoritative support as well as detractors. For a list of publications visit the Web at <http://socialaudit.org.uk/121publi.htm>, accessed August 2003.

33. It is appropriate to contrast these with the well-known consumer group Quackwatch in the United States. Founded by physician Stephen Barrett in 1969, this network of volunteers pays particular attention to "health fraud."

34. R. Smith, "The Discomfort of Patient Power," *British Medical Journal*, 324(2002), 497.

35. Differences in mind-set become clear in various sections of this book, but of special interest is a study in 2001 that suggests different mind-sets can begin early in the course of professional education; pharmacy students were shown to be "significantly more likely than engineering, accountancy, social policy and humanities students to believe that medicines in general are beneficial, and were significantly less likely to perceive medicines as potentially harmful" (R. Horne, S. Frost, M. Hankins, and S. Wright, "'In the Eye of the Beholder': Pharmacy Students Have More Positive Perceptions of Medicines Than Students of Other Disciplines," *International Journal of Pharmacy Practice*, 9[2001], 85-89).

36. For recent comments on scare stories see F. Weldon, "Why Scare Stories Are Good for the NHS," *British Medical Journal*, 324(2002), 984. The influence of movies and television is now the subject of a substantial literature with differing interpretations about impact. A further issue is accuracy of information, for example

see A. D. Ross and H. Gibbs, *The Medicine of ER or, How We Almost Die,* New York: Basic Books, 1996.

37. Andersen, Crellin, and O'Dwyer, *Healthways,* pp. 139-140. Such remarks must be put in the context of senior citizens who remember a time when expectations were few, a time when a brain tumor would not be considered for treatment. In those days people "didn't believe in chasing doctors so much" (Ibid., p. 116). Positive benefits are often recognized. As some say: "I think people's got more understanding that doctors are necessary to have good health. I have high blood pressure and I wouldn't be alive today only for my doctor. I have faith in him" (Oral History Collection, Medical Communication Group, file 003). Equally, many "thank God for medication."

38. For examples of such critiques see B. Inglis, *Drugs, Doctors, and Disease,* London: André Deutsch, 1965; A. M. Mintz, *The Therapeutic Nightmare,* Boston: Houghton Mifflin, 1965, and his revised edition, *By Prescription Only,* Boston: Beacon Press, 1967 (a wide-ranging and influential book by a well-respected Washington journalist); G. Johnson, *The Pill Controversy,* Los Angeles: Sherbourne Press, 1967; M. Silverman and P. R. Lee, *Pills, Profits, and Politics,* Berkeley: University of California Press, 1974; A. Melville and C. Johnson, *Cured to Death: The Effects of Prescription Drugs,* New York: Stein and Day, 1982. Most of these books are noted in M. Montagne and B. A. Bleidt, "Social Forces in the Premature Removal of Drug Products from the Market Place," *Clinical Research Practices and Drug Regulatory Affairs,* 5(2-3)(1987), 83-127. M. Weitz, *Health Shock: A Guide to Ineffective and Hazardous Medical Treatment,* Newton Abbott: David and Charles, 1980. An earlier book often noted is H. A. Braille, *The Drug Story,* Washington, DC: Columbia, 1949.

39. For comment on arousal see account by H. F. Dowling, *Medicines for Man: The Development, Regulation, and Use of Prescription Drugs,* New York: Knopf, 1970, p. 198. Dowling's work is of interest as the perspective of a professor of medicine.

40. *Time* (Canadian Edition), 75(April 25) (1960), 56-57.

41. Cf., M. L. Burstall and B. G. Reuben, *Critics of the Pharmaceutical Industry,* London: REMIT Consultants, 1990.

42. "Powell's Pancreas," *The Economist,* 198(1961), 1101.

43. R. A. Fine, *The Great Drug Deception: The Shocking Story of MER/29 and the Folks Who Gave You Thalidomide,* New York: Stein and Day, 1972.

44. Much scientific opinion suggests that the initial review of the literature indicating teratogenicity of Bendectin was incorrect. The legal ramifications of the lawsuits and the nature of scientific evidence raise issues of uncertainty. See J. Sanders, *Bendectin on Trial: A Study of Mass Tort Legislation,* Ann Arbor: University of Michigan Press, 1998.

45. See Maeder, *Adverse Reactions.*

46. O. Hansen, *Inside Ciba-Geigy,* Penang, Malaysia: International Organization of Consumers Unions, 1989. Entero-Vioform caused subacute myelo-optic neuropathy (SMON).

47. J. Gabe and M. Bury, "Halcion Nights: A Sociological Account of a Medical Controversy," *Sociology,* 30(1996), 447-469.

48. J. Abraham, "Bias in Science and Medical Knowledge: The Opren Controversy," *Sociology,* 28(1994), 717-736.

49. See E. Richards, *Vitamin C and Cancer: Medicine or Politics?* New York: St. Martin's Press, 1991.

50. Most analysis has focused on Dalkon Shield. After initial marketing in 1969, the A. H. Robins Company in 1970 acquired the patent and initiated an aggressive sales campaign to promote Dalkon Shield as a safe and reliable alternative to oral contraceptives. However, the company failed to predict side effects and potential health risks, ranging from pelvic inflammatory disease and ectopic pregnancies to birth defects and death. Claims for compensation—worldwide well beyond Britain, Canada, and the United States—against the company started as early as 1974. The relevant literature is vast, but see C. J. Levinson and D. C. Richardson, "The Dalkon Shield Story," *Advances in Planned Parenthood*, 11(1)(1976), 53-63; M. Mintz, *At Any Cost: Corporate Greed, Women, and the Dalkon Shield*, New York: Pantheon Books, 1985; K. M. Hicks, *Surviving the Dalkon Shield IUD: Women v. the Pharmaceutical Industry*, New York: Teachers College Press, 1994.
For a discussion on withholding of information see D. Hailey, "Scientific Harassment by Pharmaceutical Companies: Time to Stop," *Canadian Medical Association Journal*, 162(2000), 212-213.

51. The literature on the tobacco saga is vast, but see S. A. Glantz, J. Slade, L. A. Bero, P. Hanauer, and D. E. Barnes, *The Cigarette Papers*, Berkeley: University of California Press, 1996, for evidence of withholding information about health risks. For Canadian initiatives see R. Cunningham, *Smoke and Mirrors: The Canadian Tobacco War*, Ottawa: International Development Research Centre, 1996.

52. For context see J. Braithwaite, *Corporate Crime in the Pharmaceutical Industry*, London: Routledge and Kegan Paul, 1984.

53. For a 1974 review of the growth and scope of the problem of "adverse reaction," see Silverman and Lee, *Pills, Profits, and Politics*, pp. 258-281. The rise in the number of prescriptions was a significant factor. The authors note that between 1950 and 1972 the average number of prescriptions dispensed by community pharmacies alone to each man, woman, and child in this country has jumped from about 2.4 to 5.5 per year. Hospital prescriptions added to the number.

54. See Talalay (ed.), *Drugs in Our Society*, p. 280.

55. See Silverman and Lee, *Pills, Profits, and Politics*, p. 262; J. N. Hathcock and J. Coon (eds.), *Nutrition and Drug Interrelations*, New York: Academic Press, 1978. See also H. Miller, *Medicine and Society*, London: Oxford University Press, 1973, p. 6.

56. H. Jick, "Drugs—Remarkably Nontoxic," *New England Journal of Medicine*, 291(1974), 824-828. Jick, however, indicated that the effects were minor. Critics felt that Jick's numbers of side effects were too low; see, for example, H. Davies, *Modern Medicine: A Doctor's Dissent*, London: Abelard-Schuman, 1977, p. 37.

57. Jick, "Drugs—Remarkably Nontoxic," p. 825.

58. M. M. Wintrobe, "The Therapeutic Millenium and Its Price: Adverse Reactions to Drugs," in P. Talalay (ed.), *Drugs in Our Society*, pp. 107-114.

59. Burstall and Reuben, *Critics of the Pharmaceutical Industry*, p. 96. Although the general statement comes from discussions with physicians and patients over many years, it needs detailed study, as indicated by the following article, which dealt with blame in managed care: M. Rosenthal and M. Schlesinger, "Not Afraid to

Blame: The Neglected Role of Blame Attribution in Medical Consumerism and Some Implications for Health Policy," *The Milbank Quarterly*, 80(2002), 41-95.

60. See K. E. Laser, P. D. Allen, S. J. Woolhandler, D. U. Himmelstein, S. M. Wolfe, and D. H. Bor, "Timing of New Black Box Warnings and Withdrawals for Prescription Medications," *Journal of the American Medical Association*, 287 (2002), 2215-2220. Not all removals are for safety reasons. For other discussion see H. A. Smith, "A Survey of Drug Products Removed from the Market," *Clinical Research Practices and Drug Regulatory Affairs*, 6(1)(1998), 69-86.

61. R. J. Temple and M. H. Himmel, "Safety of Newly Approved Drugs," *Journal of the American Medical Association*, 287(2002), 2275.

62. Cf., J. Abraham and G. Lewis, "Citizenship, Medical Expertise, and the Capitalist Regulatory State in Europe," *Sociology*, 36(2002), 67-88. See also M. Saks, "Medicine and the Counter Culture," in Cooter and Pickstone (eds.), *Medicine in the Twentieth Century*, pp. 113-123.

63. For discussion see Montagne and Bleidt, "Social Forces in the Premature Removal of Drug Products from the Market Place," 83-127. Critiques of the critics are pervasive. For challenging questions about sociologists' views of medicine see S. J. Williams, "Sociological Imperialism and the Profession of Medicine Revisited: Where Are We Now," *Sociology of Health and Illness*, 23(2001), 135-158.

64. Burstall and Reuben, *Critics of the Pharmaceutical Industry*, pp. 32, 50-53. For more on consumer concerns about safety see Montagne and Bleidt, "Social Forces in the Premature Removal of Drug Products from the Market Place," p. 97.

65. J. Abraham, *Science, Politics, and the Pharmaceutical Industry: Controversy and Bias in Drug Regulation*, New York: St. Martin's Press, 1995, p. 82.

66. Ibid., p. 83 and 80.

67. P. Brown, "Drug Regulation—A Life Sentence on the Industry," *Scrip Magazine* (September 1996), 23. For a consumer perspective see C. Medawar, "Strictly Confidential Transparency," *Scrip Magazine* (May 1994), 18-19, and C. Medawar "Secrecy and Medicines," *International Journal of Risk and Safety in Medicine*, 9(1996), 133-141. See also J. Abraham, J. Sheppard, and T. Reed, "Rethinking Transparency and Accountability in Medicines Regulation in the United Kingdom," *British Medical Journal*, 318(1999), 46-47.

68. J. Lexchin, "Drug Makers and Drug Regulators: Too Close for Comfort. A Study of the Canadian Situation," *Social Science and Medicine*, 31(1990), 1257. For a general discussion on issues in Canada see M. Rachlis and C. Kushner, *Strong Medicine: How to Save Canada's Health Care System*, Toronto: HarperCollins, 1994, pp. 124-151.

69. J. Lexchin, "Drug Makers and Drug Regulators," p. 1250. Lexchin might also have noted thalidomide as discussed in Chapter 5, though contemporaries considered the problem to be with government bureaucracy.

70. J. Lexchin, "Pharmaceuticals: Politics and Policy," in P. Armstrong, H. Armstrong, and D. Coburn (eds.), *Unhealthy Times: Political Economy Perspectives on Health and Care*, Oxford: Oxford University Press, 2001, p. 41.

71. M. D. Rawlins, "Doctors and the Drug Makers," *The Lancet*, 2(1984), 276.

72. Letters in the *British Medical Journal*, 1(1960), 963, 1506.

73. For a note on the British General Medical Council and advice on relationships with the industry see M. D. Rawlins, "Doctors and the Drug Makers."

74. Burstall and Reuben, *Critics of the Pharmaceutical Industry*, p. 62. Pharmacists have long noted that the prescribing patterns of physicians change after a representative visits them.

75. Cf., J. Lexchin, "What Information Do Physicians Receive from Pharmaceutical Representatives?" *Canadian Family Physician*, 43(1997), 941-945.

76. T. J. Wang, J. C. Ausiello, and R. S. Stafford, "Trends in Antihypertensive Drug Advertising, 1985-1996," *Circulation*, 99(1999), 2055-2057.

77. For background on the development of direct-to-consumer advertising see D. A. Kessler and W. L. Pines, "The Federal Regulation of Prescription Drug Advertising and Promotion," *Journal of the American Medical Association*, 264 (1990), 2409-2415, and references in endnotes 72 and 73.

78. B. Mintzes, M. L. Barer, R. L. Kravitz, A. Kazanjian, K. Bassett, J. Lexchin, R. G. Evans, R. Pau, and S. A. Marion, "Influence of Direct to Consumer Pharmaceutical Advertising and Patients' Requests on Prescribing Decisions: Two Site Cross Sectional Study," *British Medical Journal*, 324(2002), 279. A Canadian study that concluded "Concerns about the value of opening up the regulatory environment to permit direct to consumer advertising in the EU and Canada" seem well justified to commentators elsewhere.

79. M. B. Rosenthal, E. R. Berndt, J. M. Donohue, R. G. Frank, and A. M. Epstein, "Promotion of Prescription Drugs to Consumers," *New England Journal of Medicine*, 346(2002), 498-505. See also R. L. Pinkus, "From Lydia Pinkham to Bob Dole: What the Changing Face of Direct-to-Consumer Drug Advertising Reveals About the Professionalism of Medicine," *Kennedy Institute of Ethics Journal*, 12(2002), 141-158.

80. For the concerns of one pressure group, Social Audit, see C. Medawar, "Health, Pharma, and the E.U.: A Briefing to Members of the European Parliament on Direct-To-Consumer Drug Promotion," December 2001. Available online at <http://www.socialaudit.org.uk/5111-005.htm>, accessed September 2002.

81. See C. B. Inlander, L. S. Levin, and E. Weiner, *Medicine on Trial: The Appalling Story of Ineptitude, Malfeasance, Neglect, and Arrogance*, New York: Prentice Hall, 1988, pp. 135-153, for general comments on drugs, including medication errors in the United States. The book, compiled by the directors of the People's Medical Society, "the nation's largest consumer health organization," attracted much interest when published; see also H. Ridley, *Drugs of Choice: A Report on the Drug Formularies Used in NHS Hospitals*, London: Social Audit, 1986, for a British perspective.

82. W. Evans, "Addiction to Medicines," *British Medical Journal*, 2(1962), 722. A useful benchmark is J. P. Martin, *Social Aspects of Prescribing*, London: Heinemann, 1957. Soon after the National Health Service started, physicians whose prescribing costs were above average were having their prescription records examined ("Medical Notes in Parliament. Excessive Prescribing," *British Medical Journal*, 1[1956], 988-989). It is noteworthy that a medical/pharmaceutical textbook published in 1981 stated that medication errors are rarely publicized: N. M. Davis and M. R. Cohen, *Medication Errors: Causes and Prevention*, Philadelphia: Stickley, 1980, preface.

83. I. Tait and S. Graham-Jones, "General Practice, Its Patients, and the Public," in Loudon, Horder, and Webster (eds.), *General Practice Under the National Health Service 1948-1997*, p. 231.

84. See, for example, remarks from a thoughtful British physician, H. Miller, *Medicine and Society,* London: Oxford University Press, 1973, p. 9. Miller added, as would many general practitioners, that the tirades in the main came from physicians not immediately concerned with the personal daily management of distressed patients. Indeed, much of the criticism came from university researchers and from society at large, as reflected in the consumer movement; much attention was given to problems within hospitals, for example see D. W. Bates, N. Spell, D. J. Cullen, E. Burdick, N. Laird, L. A. Petersen, S. D. Small, B. J. Sweitzer, and L. L. Leape, "The Costs of Adverse Drug Events in Hospitalized Patients," *Journal of the American Medical Association,* (1997), 277, 307-311.

85. Report by a Working Party 1975, Council of Europe. European Public Health Community, "Abuse of Medicines, Part Two: Prescription Medicines," *Drug Intelligence and Clinical Pharmacy,* 10(1976), 94-110.

86. The term *victim* is often found in the literature, sometimes used by physicians; see Rachlis and Kushner, *Strong Medicine,* p. 127.

87. D. M. Dunlop, T. L. Henderson, and R. S. Inch, "A Survey of 17,301 Prescriptions on Form E.C. 10," *British Medical Journal,* 1(1952), 294. Another commentator noted that tonics were "demanded" in a South Wales industrial/country practice at the time: J. D. P. Graham, "What Doctors Prescribe," *British Medical Journal,* 1(1952), 435-436.

88. A. Digby, *The Evolution of British General Practice 1850-1948,* Oxford: Oxford University Press, 1999, p. 198.

89. F. Moor, "What Doctors Prescribe," *British Medical Journal,* 1(1952), 436. This was one of many letters following the paper by Dunlop and colleagues that offered insight into prescribing at the time.

90. A. P. Williams, R. Cockerill, and F. H. Lowy, "The Physician As Prescriber: Relations Between Knowledge About Prescription Drugs, Encounters with Patients and the Pharmaceutical Industry, and Prescription Volume," *Health and Canadian Society,* 3(1995), 135.

91. Studies, underway in the 1950s, became more evident from the 1970s onward; representative contributions included K. Dunnell and A. Cartwright, *Medicine Takers, Prescribers, and Hoarders,* London: Routledge and Kegan Paul, 1972, which highlighted many variables (e.g., "Belief in doctors' ability to cure or relieve a number of conditions was not" related to patients' medicine-taking behavior (p. 62); R. Mapes (ed.), *Prescribing Practice and Drug Usage,* London: Croom Helm, 1980; R. Blum with K. Kreitman, "Factors Affecting Individual Use of Medicines," in R. Blum, A. Herxheimer, C. Stenzl, and J. Woodcock (eds.), *Pharmaceuticals and Health Policy,* New York: Holmes and Meier, 1981, pp. 122-185; C. P. Bradley, "Decision Making and Prescribing Patterns—a Literature Review," *Family Practice,* 8(1991), 276-287. Bradley argues that further understanding of prescribing behavior requires a study of the underlying decision-making processes.

On the need to change education, various views recur; e.g., as "little attention has been paid to patients' ideas about medicines [though] such ideas might well have relevance for understanding non-adherence to medication." (N. Britten, "Patients' Ideas About Medicines: A Qualitative Study in a General Practice Population," *British Journal of General Practice,* 44[1994], 465-468). See also K. Pollock, "'I've Not Asked Him, You See, and He's Not Said': Understanding Lay Explanatory Models of Disease Is a Prerequisite for Concordant Consultations," *The International Journal of Pharmacy Practice*, 9(2001), 105-117.

92. See M. Balint, J. Hunt, D. Joyce, M. Marinker, and J. Woodcock, *Treatment or Diagnosis: A Study of Repeat Prescriptions in General Practice*, London: Tavistock/Lippincott, 1970. Blaming patients shifted somewhat in the 1990s to blaming patients for lifestyle-induced illness.

93. N. Britten, "Patients' Demands for Prescriptions in Primary Care," *British Medical Journal*, 310(1995), 1084-1085. Italics added. It should be emphasized that overprescribing is always relative; by the early 1990s, some informants noted that doctors "used to overprescribe" in the past as if to imply that the problem no longer existed, a view in accord with suggestions of increasingly conservative prescribing on the part of British physicians (N. Britten, "Patient Demand for Prescriptions: A View from the Other Side," *Family Practice*, 11[1994], 62-66). Questions are also raised by physicians; see, for example, D. Healy, *The Antidepressant Era*, Cambridge: Harvard University Press, 1997, pp. 226-231.

94. See S. Webb and M. Lloyd, "Prescribing and Referral to General Practice: A Study of Patients' Expectations and Doctors' Actions," *British Journal of General Practice*, 44(1994), 165-169.

95. J. Cockburn and S. Pit, "Prescribing Behaviour in Clinical Practice: Patients' Expectations and Doctors' Perceptions of Patients' Expectations—a Questionnaire Study," *British Medical Journal*, 315(1997), 520-523.

96. E. H. Boath and A. Blankinsopp, "The Rise and Fall of Proton Pump Inhibitor Drugs: Patients' Perspectives," *Social Science and Medicine*, 45(1997), 1571-1579.

97. F. A. Stevenson, C. A. Barry, N. Britten, N. Barber, and C. P. Bradley, "Doctor-Patient Communication About Drugs: The Evidence for Shared Decision Making," *Social Science and Medicine*, 50(2000), 829. See also R. Mahomed, C. Paton, and E. Lee, "Prescribing Hypnotics in a Mental Health Trust: What Consultant Psychiatrists Say and What They Do," *Pharmaceutical Journal*, 268(2002), 657-659.

98. J. Lexchin, "Improving the Appropriateness of Physician Prescribing," *International Journal of Health Services*, 28(1998), 253.

99. For indications of this see P. A. Offit, B. Fass-Offit, and L. M. Bell, *Breaking the Antibiotic Habit: A Parent's Guide to Coughs, Colds, Ear Infections, and Sore Throats*, New York: John Wiley and Sons, 1999, pp. 143-144.

100. For accounts raising the issue of overprescribing J. Whorton, "'Antibiotic Abandon': The Resurgence of Therapeutic Rationalism," in J. Parascandola (ed.), *The History of Antibiotics: A Symposium*, Madison, WI: American Institute of the History of Pharmacy, 1980, pp. 125-136 and D. P. Adams, *"The Greatest Good to the Greatest Number": Penicillin Rationing on the American Home Front, 1940-1945*, New York: Peter Lang, 1991, pp. 153-183; and W. Hewitt, "Penicillin—Historical Impact on Infectious Control," *Annals of the New York Academy of Sciences*, 145 ART. 2(1967), 212-215. Cf., also A. I. Marcus, *Cancer from Beef: DES Federal Food Regulation and Consumer Confidence*, Baltimore: Johns Hopkins University Press, 1994, pp. 68-87. The observations of many druggists that physicians overprescribed ("Too much penicillin given out anyway, especially to children" [Bill O'Mara, personal communication, 2000]) are "anecdotal," but forceful.

101. For more on chloramphenicol see Maeder, *Adverse Reactions*. The author's challenge to readers is to consider the fact that "despite repeated warnings from the FDA and the AMA, three special studies by the National Research Council, two decades of congressional hearings by Estes Kefauver, Hubert Humphrey, Gaylord Nelson, and L. H. Fountain, endless newspaper exposés, professional papers, and journal editorials, and hundreds of lawsuits, doctors continued to prescribe it in enormous quantities for trivial medical conditions" (pp. 8-9).

102. For reference to early recognition of penicillin-resistant strains by A. D. Gardner see L. Bickel, *Rise Up To Life: A Biography of Howard Walter Florey Who Gave Penicillin to the World*, London: Angus and Robertson, 1972, p. 252; see also T. I. Williams, *Howard Florey: Penicillin and After*, Oxford: Oxford University Press, 1984, pp. 166-167.

103. Government spokesperson quoted in "Control of Penicillin," *British Medical Journal*, 2(1946), 71-72.

104. Ibid., p. 71.

105. Second Reading of Penicillin Bill, March 18, 1947, *Hansard's Parliamentary Debates, House of Lords, 1946-1947*, Volume CXLIV (Fifth Series) London: His Majesty's Stationary Office, column 402. Side effects specifically noted were dermatitis and ulcers of the mouth. It is noteworthy that British parliamentarians relied on advice of medical authorities including Sir Alexander Fleming (discoverer of penicillin in 1928), who was always eager to protect his "baby."

106. For social and psychological factors shaping prescribing, see J. G. R. Howie, "Clinical Judgment and Antibiotic Use in General Practice," *British Medical Journal*, 2(1976), 1061-1064.

107. Whitbourne case records. History of Medicine Collection, Faculty of Medicine, Memorial University of Newfoundland.

108. Williams, *Howard Florey*, p. 298.

109. *Newsletter of the Newfoundland Medical Association*, 1(4)(1958), 3-4.

110. P. C. English, *Rheumatic Fever in America and Britain: A Biological, Epidemiological and Medical History*, New Brunswick, NJ: Rutgers University Press, 1999, p. 143. For other discussion see B. F. Massell, *Rheumatic Fever and Streptococcal Infection: Unraveling the Mysteries of a Dread Disease*, Boston: Countway Library of Medicine, 1997.

111. *Time* (Canadian Edition), 75(January 25) (1960), p. 55.

112. E. Chain, "Thirty Years of Penicillin Therapy," *Journal of the Royal College of Physicians of London*, 6(1972), 127-128.

113. S. G. B. Aymes, *Magic Bullets, Lost Horizons: The Rise and Fall of Antibiotics*, London: Taylor and Francis, 2001, p. 204. This was a laboratory demonstration, not a clinical demonstration. See "*Staphylococcus aureus* Resistant to Vancomycin—United States, 2002," *Morbidity and Mortality Weekly Report*, 51 (2002), 565-567, for an account of a vancomycin-resistant organism that was immediately labeled a "superbug" by the press. For rising fears among segments of the population see M. Shnayerson and M. Plotkin, *The Killers Within: The Deadly Rise of Drug-Resistant Bacteria*, New York: Little, Brown and Co., 2002.

114. Select Committee on Science and Technology, *Resistance to Antibiotics and Other Antimicrobial Agents, Session 1997-98, Seventh Report*, London: The Stationary Office, p. 73.

115. *Government Response to the House of Lords Select Committee on Science and Technology Report: Resistance to Antibiotics and Other Antimicrobial Agents,* London: The Stationary Office, 1998.

116. Cf., in the United States, "A Public Health Action Plan to Combat Antimicrobial Resistance" (1999), and the "Antibiotic Resistance Prevention Act" (2001). For World Health Organization activities, see <http://www.who.int/inf-pr-2001/en/pr2001-39.html>, accessed August 15, 2002.

117. Offit, Fass-Offit, and Bell, *Breaking the Antibiotic Habit,* pp. 106, 117.

118. J. M. Hutchinson and R. N. Foley, "Method of Physician Remuneration and Rates of Antibiotic Prescription," *Canadian Medical Association Journal,* 160(1999), 1013-1017. It is hardly surprising that the study was challenged.

119. J. M. Hutchinson, S. Jelinski, D. Hefferton, D. Desaulniers, and P. S. Parfrey, "Role of Diagnostic Labeling in Antibiotic Prescription," *Canadian Family Physician,* 47(2001), 1217-1224.

120. The literature is vast, but see D. Double, "The Limits of Psychiatry," *British Medical Journal,* 324(2002), 900-904, which draws attention to the Critical Psychiatry Network; L. Johnstone, *Users and Abusers of Psychiatry: A Critical Look at Psychiatric Practice,* London: Routledge, 2000; For medicines see C. Medawar, "The Antidepressant Web: Marketing Depression and Making Medicines Work," *International Journal of Risk and Safety in Medicine,* 10(1997), 75-126.

121. "The Barbiturates," *The Lancet,* 253(1947), 583.

122. S. L. Speaker, "'From Happiness Pills' to 'National Nightmare': Changing Cultural Assessment of Minor Tranquilizers in America, 1955-1980," *Journal of the History of Medicine and Allied Sciences,* 52(1997), 338-376.

123. E. Bargmann, S. M. Wolfe, J. Levin, and the Public Citizen Health Research Group, *Stopping Valium,* New York: Warner Books, 1982.

124. Ibid., p. 5.

125. J. Marks, *The Benzodiazepines: Use, Overuse, Misuse, Abuse,* Baltimore: University Park Press, 1978, p. 80; the same message came in the second edition of 1985, perhaps slightly more cautious, but stating: "Therapeutic dependence only very rarely leads on to abuse with dose escalation" (Marks, *The Benzodiazepines: Use, Overuse, Misuse, Abuse,* Second Edition, Lancaster: MTP Press, p. 114).

126. R. Barton and L. Hurst, "Unnecessary Use of Tranquillizers in Elderly Patients," British Journal of Psychiatry, 112(1966), 989-990.

127. For views of dependence and tranquilizer use as a social problem see J. Gabe (ed.), *Understanding Tranquilliser Use: The Role of the Social Sciences,* London: Tavistiock/Routledge, 1991. For an American history of psychological health see E. S. Moskowitz, *In Therapy We Trust: America's Obsession with Self-Fulfillment,* Baltimore: Johns Hopkins University Press, 2001.

128. R. Cooperstock and H. L. Lennard, "Role Strains and Tranquillizer Use" in D. Coburn, C. D'Arcy, and G. Torrance (eds.), *Health and Canadian Society: Sociological Perspectives,* Toronto: University of Toronto Press, 1998, pp. 208, 205, respectively.

129. For advertising changes see M. Smith, *A Social History of the Minor Tranquilizers: The Quest for Small Comfort in the Age of Anxiety,* Binghamton, NY: Pharmaceutical Products Press, 1991, pp. 114-129.

130. *Newfoundland House of Assembly 1st Session, 38th Assembly, 12 July 1979-27 February 1980,* Book 48, p. 4477.

131. A. Melville, "Reducing Whose Anxiety? A Study of the Relationship Between Repeat Prescribing of Minor Tranquillisers and Doctors' Attitudes," in Mapes (ed.), *Prescribing Practice and Drug Usage*, p. 113.

132. See R. Shah, Z. Uren, A. Baker, and A. Majeed, "Deaths from Antidepressants in England and Wales 1993-1997: Analysis of a New National Database," *Psychological Medicine*, 31(2001), 1203-1210; and T. W. Croghan, "The Controversy of Increased Spending for Antidepressants," *Health Affairs*, 20(2)(2001), 129-135. It was more the ascendancy of the antidepressives over the minor tranquilizers in the 1980s, as noted in Chapter 5, that brought change, though the use of minor tranquilizers remained high. For example, in Newfoundland, from February 1999 to January 2000, more benzodiazepines were dispensed than antidepressants, (*PharmaFacts, Newfoundland and Labrador Centre for Health Information*, 1 [1][2001], 1).

133. For specific discussion on the benzodiazepines see J. Gabe and M. Bury, "Anxious Times: The Benzodiazepine Controversy and the Fracturing of Expert Authority," in Davis (ed.), *Contested Ground*, pp. 42-56. For malpractice suits relating to drugs see *Drugs in Litigation: Damage Awards Involving Prescription and Nonprescription Drugs*, Charlottesville,VA: Michie Law Publishers, 2001.

134. One historian concluded that Prozac "produced one massive benefit for the public good: it helped psychiatric conditions begin to seem acceptable in the eyes of the public, although we are still far from speaking of a complete destigmatization of mental illness" (E. Shorter, *A History of Psychiatry*, New York: Wiley, 1997, p. 324). Perhaps the best way to gauge public concerns with Prozac is to conduct an Internet search under "Prozac and safety concerns." In August 2003 the Google search engine listed more than 13,000 hits.

135. N. J. Facchinetti and W. M. Dickson, "Access to Generic Drugs in the 1950s: The Politics of a Social Problem," *American Journal of Public Health*, 72(1982), 468-475. For context in the United States see F. J. Ascione, D. M. Kirking, C. A. Gaither, and L. S. Welage, "Historical Overview of Generic Medication Policy," *Journal of the American Pharmaceutical Association*, 41(2001), 567-577.

136. "Tuppence Coloured," *The Economist*, 206(1963), 448.

137. In Britain, substitution became part of the Labour party's policy in the late 1980s, but it came to naught. For relevant discussion see A. Haynes, "Is Generic Substitution an Option?" *The Pharmaceutical Journal*, 250(1993), 241.

138. For quote see D. G. Hall, "Statement on Generic Prescribing," *Rhode Island Medical Journal*, 50(1967), 693. For some background see Silverman and Lee, *Pills, Profits, and Politics*, pp. 143-145, 166.

139. For a sample of criticism, especially strong from the pharmaceutical industry, see L. C. Hoff, "Repeal of Antisubstitution Laws: Impact on the Consumer," *Medical Marketing and Media*, 11 (December 1976), 20, 22-25. Physicians, on the other hand, were generally split; for one 1970 survey of physicians see C. L. Braucher and A. W. Jowdy, "A Study of Physicians' Attitudes Concerning Generic Prescribing," *Journal of the Medical Association Georgia*, 59(1970), 175-179.

140. For the intensity of debate in the late 1960s in the United States see Silverman and Lee, *Pills, Profits, and Politics*, pp. 147-162.

141. Cf., D. E. Francke, "Bioavailability of Digoxin," *Drug Intelligence and Clinical Pharmacy*, 6(1972), 5.

142. The new discipline can be said to have come of age with the appearance of the *Journal of Pharmacokinetics and Biopharmaceutics* in 1973. For a 1987 review of issues at a significant stage in the development of generics (new legislation had been introduced in 1984) see B. L. Strom, "Generic Drug Substitution Revisited," *New England Journal of Medicine*, 316(1987), 1456-1462. Apart from specific concerns with therapeutic equivalence, concerns existed over good manufacturing practices. For discussion in the 1970s at the height of debate see D. Schwartzman, *Innovation in the Pharmaceutical Industry*, Baltimore: Johns Hopkins University Press, 1976, pp. 212-225.

143. Quote from *Newfoundland House of Assembly, 1st Session, 38th Assembly 12 July 1979—27 February 1980*. Book 48, p. 4471. It was also suggested that it was not government "policy to become involved with private enterprise" (Ibid., p. 4492). The act was implemented in 1981 and was followed by falling provincial drug costs in the mid-1980s.

144. L. A. Klippert and J. G. White, "Generic Substitution for Newfoundland," *Newfoundland Medical Association Journal*, 21(1)(1979), 31-33.

145. This view is not derived from any documentary evidence but from the sentiments of a number of physicians and pharmacists.

146. The revised version was incorporated into the 1994 Pharmaceutical Association Act, "An Act to Continue the Newfoundland Pharmaceutical Association," *Newfoundland Statutes, Chapter P-12* (section 61 [1] for quote). Implicit in this was the pharmacist's role in providing information. Cf., *Newfoundland House of Assembly Proceedings*, 1994, Volume XLII (10) 2622. Another provincial "cost-containment initiative" came in 1998. The initiative set a maximum allowable cost for certain groups of over-the-counter medicines when prescribed by a physician or dentist under the Provincial Drug Plan. Thus druggists could substitute brands of over-the-counter medicines for those under the Senior Citizens' Drug Subsidy Program.

147. See J. Lexchin, "After Compulsory Licensing: Coming Issues in Canadian Pharmaceutical Policy and Politics," *Health Policy*, 40(1997), 69-80. Lexchin outlines issues for debate.

148. M. Anderson and K. Parent, "Timely Access to Generic Drugs: Issues for Health Policy in Canada," available online at <http://www.cdma-acfpp.org/issues/fd_o6.s html>, accessed August 2003.

149. J. R. Graham, "Canada Saves Little with Generic Drugs," available online at <http://www.heartland.org/archives/health/jan02/generic.htm>, accessed August 2003.

150. Relative intensity of interest in generics in the three countries can be judged from citations in online databases such as MEDLINE and IPA. See also reports on class action suits: N. Beavers, "Courts to Decide Whether It's OK to Pay to Delay," *Drug Topics*, 142(November 1998, Supp.) 20S, 22S. For figures see Anonymous, "Consumer Group Touts Generics," *American Journal of Health System Pharmacy*, 56(1999), 2276, 2283, which indicated that 83 percent of those who had taken a generic product believed it was as effective as the brand name.

The 1980s' FDA scandal is discussed in Ascione, Kirking, Gaither, and Welage, "Historical Overview of Generic Medication Policy." For additional insight, a reminder of human resources considerations in policymaking and implementation, see "FDA Oral History Program: Interview with J. Richard Crout available online at <http://www.fda.gov/oc/history/oralhistories/crout/default.htm>, accessed August 2003.

151. J. M. Ganther and D. H. Kreling, "Consumer Perceptions of Risk and Required Cost Savings for Generic Prescription Drugs," *Journal of the American Pharmaceutical Association,* 40(2000), 378-383.

152. For some details on over-the-counter medicine changes see Silverman and Lee, *Pills, Profits, and Politics,* pp. 229-233. For invoking "science": M. C. Gerald, "Judging OTCs Science Narrows the Choices," *American Pharmacy,* NS19(5)(1979), 18-22.

153. The removal of sweet spirits of niter as an over-the-counter remedy was noted in Anonymous, "OTCs Under Review: An Update On What's In and What's Out," *American Pharmacy,* NS20(9)(1980), 11-15.

154. It was reported in 1987 that growth was in the ascendancy, based on safe, effective, and meritorious drugs. See H. I. Silverman, "What Lies Ahead for Rx-to-OTC Switches," *Drug and Cosmetic Industry,* 141(August) (1987), 43-47, 72.

155. By the late 1970s and early 1980s the emphasis on self-care was in full swing on both sides of the Atlantic. For one useful analysis (not a do-it-yourself guide) see J. D. Williamson and K. Dancher, *Self-Care in Health,* London: Croom Helm, 1978. For more on the situation in the 1990s see A. Blankinsopp and C. Bradley, "Patients, Society, and the Increase in Self-Medication," *British Medical Journal,* 312(1996), 629-632, and other articles in the series "OTC," (Ibid., 688-691, 758-760, 835-837).

156. D. M. Vickery, "A Medical Perspective," *Drug Information Journal,* 19(1985), 155-158, points out that physicians' experiences are confined to alarming incidents.

157. Report by a Working Party, 1975, Council of Europe, European Public Health Community, "Abuse of Medicines, Part One: Self-Medication," *Drug Intelligence and Clinical Pharmacy,* 10(January) (1976), 21.

158. Ibid., p. 28.

159. D. Cargill, "Self-Treatment As an Alternative to Rationing of Medical Care," *The Lancet,* 1(1967), 1377-1378.

160. P. V. Rosenau and C. Thoer, "The Liberalization of Access to Medication in the United States and Europe," in Davis (ed.), *Contested Ground: Public Purpose and Private Interest in the Regulation of Prescription Drugs,* pp. 194-206.

161. "FDA Oral History Program. Interview with Alexander M. Schmidt," <http://www.fda.gov/oc/history/oralhistories/Schmidt/default.htm>, accessed August 2003.

162. See G. Rivett, *From Cradle to Grave: Fifty Years of the NHS,* London: King's Fund, 1998, p. 385.

163. M. Berry, *Canadian Pharmacy Law,* Aurora: Aurora Professional Press, 2002, pp. 2-24. In Canada, there is no "pharmacy-only" drug category described in the Food and Drugs Act. However, the National Drug Scheduling System and various provincial schedules describe such categories and even the location of the product for sale, e.g., no public access or on open shelves in pharmacies but not general stores. For the United States: R. R. Abood and D. B. Brushwood, *Pharmacy Practice and the Law,* Gaithersburg, MD: Aspen, 2001, pp. 107-109. The U.S. over-the-counter category is comparable to the General Sales List (GSL) in Britain.

164. B. Berube, "R_x to OTC Bringing in the Switch Hitters," *Canadian Pharmaceutical Journal,* 124(1991), 338-340. Berube cites an industry spokesperson; other factors, such as advertising, could have contributed.

165. Rosenou and Thoer, "The Liberalization of Access to Medication in the United States and Europe," p. 201.

166. Examples include R. Pates, A. J. McBride, S. Li, and R. Ramadan, "Misuse of Over-the-Counter Medicines: A Survey of Community Pharmacies in a South Wales Health Authority," *Pharmaceutical Journal,* 268(2002), 179-182. This study of pharmacists (conducted around 2000) revealed a general awareness of abuse among two-thirds of those surveyed. On the other hand, one-third said they did not consider it a problem in their pharmacies. In the United States the issue was accentuated by direct-to-consumer advertising, e.g., see "Americans at Risk from Self-Medication, Survey Reveals," *American Journal of Health Systems Pharmacy,* 54(1997), 2664, 2666. Yet, in 1992 Canadians were said to appear to have a responsible attitude toward the process of self-medication. See L. G. Suveges, "Surveying the Surveys: An Overview of Four Studies," *Canadian Pharmaceutical Journal,* 125(1992), 380-387, 425.

167. In 2001 over-the-counter sales in Britain grew 10 percent more than in the United States (2 percent) and Europe (4 percent): "Comestic OTC Sales Rise by 10 Percent," *The Pharmaceutical Journal,* 268(2002), 489.

168. For some context to the statement see A. Blenkinsopp and C. Bradley, "Patients, Society, and the Increase in Self-Medication," *British Medical Journal,* 312(1996), 629-632; and M. Ross, "Jumping Over the Counter: Regulators Are Increasingly Taking Drugs Off the Prescription Pad and Letting Them Be Sold Over the Counter. Is This Good for Patients?" *Medical Post,* 36(29)(2000), available online at <http://www.medicalpost.com/mpcontent/article.jsp?content=/content/EXTRACT/RAWART/3629/26A.html>, accessed August 2003. For a sense of expansion of efforts to further shift prescription-only drugs to over-the-counter status or for sale by pharmacists see "Overhaul of POM-P Reclassification Could Mean Big Changes for Pharmacy," *The Pharmaceutical Journal,* 268(2002), 131-132; D. Hibbert, P. Bissell, and P. R. Ward, "Consumerism and Professional Work in the Community Pharmacy," *Sociology of Health and Illness,* 24(2002), 46-65.

169. Nutraceuticals comprise vitamins, minerals, and animal products as well as herbs.

170. R. C. Engs, *Clean Living Movements: American Cycles of Health Reform,* Westport: Praeger, 2000.

171. Cf., M. S. Goldstein, *Alternative Health Care, Medicine, Miracle or Mirage?* Philadelphia: Temple University Press, 1999, pp. 24-39. See also M. Saks, "Medicine and Complementary Medicine: Challenge and Change," in G. Scambler and P. Higgs (eds.), *Modernity, Medicine, and Health,* London: Routledge, 1998, pp. 198-215. Saks discusses the rise of complementary medicine in the context of the characterization of the modern era as postmodern.

172. Herbal practitioners, of course, continue to the present, though very many are formally educated in herbalism or are self-taught from books rather than drawing on family and community knowledge.

173. Advertisement leaflet marketed by entrepreneur Gerald Doyle, Newfoundland Pharmaceutical Association Archives (see Chapter 4).

174. A noteworthy book was B. Inglis', *The Case of Unorthodox Medicine,* New York: Putnam's Sons, 1965 (first American edition; published originally in Britain in 1964).

175. See J. C. Whorton, *Crusaders for Fitness: The History of American Health Reformers,* Princeton: Princeton University Press, 1982, 331-339.

176. Davis's succession of books from the 1950s on "correct" nutrition as the path to health had wide influence. Perhaps her best-known book was *Let's Eat Right to Keep Fit*, First Edition New York: Harcourt Brace, 1954. Davis's writings have been castigated for inaccuracies, see S. Barrett, "Adele Davis's Legacy," <http://www.quackwatch.com/04ConsumerEducation/divis.html>, accessed July 2002.

177. R. Adams and F. Murray, *Megavitamin Therapy*, New York: Larchmont Books, 1973. This book was part of the development of orthomolecular medicine and its popularization.

178. W. Pritzker, *Natural Foods, Eat Better, Live Longer, Improve Your Sex Life*, New York: Defran House, 1971.

179. R. J. Williams, *Nutrition Against Disease: Environmental Prevention*, New York: Bantam, 1981.

180. E.g., G. E. Griffin, *World Without Cancer: The Story of Vitamin B_{17}*, Part 1, Thousand Oaks, CA: American Medica, 1975.

181. H. L. Newhold, *Mega-Nutrients for Your Nerves*, New York: Wyden, 1975.

182. Ibid., p. 132.

183. For example, *The Case for Unorthodox Medicine* was an influential book by British author Brian Inglis. His aim was "to find out why fringe medicine, so long discredited and for a while assumed to be dying out, should have survived and in some cases continued to flourish" (p. 11). One reason he offered was the failure of the medical profession to "provide what the community needs" (p. 64).

184. *Complementary Therapies for Pregnancy and Childbirth*, D. Tiran and S. Mack (eds.), London: Baillière Tindall, 2000, p. 111.

185. Spam e-mail received August 24, 2001.

186. These concepts have a long history, which some see as part of the complementary/alternative medical scene stretching back to 1800s and earlier. Nowadays, this "pedigree" of history is a commonplace sentiment used, generally uncritically, to support both the safety and efficacy of a herb, namely that it has been used for "hundreds," if not "thousands," of years. What is overlooked is the precautions that were believed necessary to be taken before 1950 to deal with side effects of many medicines.

187. See C. A. Karter and J. M. Lee, *Holistic Health Care: Approaches to Health Promotion and Wellbeing*, Monticello, IL: Vance Bibliographies, 1979.

188. The difficulties in defining "holism" are made clear by C. E. Rosenberg, "Holism in Twentieth-Century Medicine," in C. Lawrence and G. Weisz (eds.), *Greater Than the Parts: Holism in Biomedicine, 1920-1950*, New York: Oxford University Press, 1998.

189. The quote is the title of the first chapter in D. A. Tubesing, *Wholistic Health: A Whole-Person Approach in Primary Health Care*, New York: Human Sciences Press, 1979, pp. 19-33. The author, director of the Institute for Whole Person Health Care, Duluth, Minnesota, points out that all over America sick people look for help but often have trouble getting it.

190. J. LaPatra, *Healing the Coming Revolution in Holistic Medicine*, New York: McGraw-Hill, 1978, p. 1.

191. For a recent account see J. K. Crellin and F. Ania, *Professionalism and Ethics in Complementary and Alternative Medicine*, Binghamton, NY: The Haworth Integrative Healing Press, 2002, pp. 20-27.

192. Quote and information on the Wellness Centre from J. K. Crellin and C. Curran, "Contemporary Issues—Health Care in Contemporary Canadian Society: Changing Directions," Course Manual, Philosophy 2807, Distance Education, Memorial University of Newfoundland, 1996, pp. 6-7, transcript of interview with G. Higgins and C. Oliver.

193. *Newfoundland and Labrador Holistic Health Directory 2001 Edition,* St. John's: HealthCare Publications, 2001.

194. For interpretation see J. Vincent, "Self-Help Groups and Health Care in Contemporary Britain," in M. Saks (ed.), *Alternative Medicine in Britain,* Oxford: Clarendon Press, 1992, pp. 137-153.

195. Efforts to harvest the wild herb in Newfoundland encouraged many people to try St. John's wort before the scientific evidence to support its use appeared. Analyses of the Newfoundland supply indicated that concentration of hypericin, then presumed to be the principal active constituent, was especially high; however, new data suggested the hypericin content was not the principal factor contributing to efficacy. For a general review see J. Barnes, "Herbal Therapeutics. 2. Depression," *Pharmaceutical Journal,* 268(2002), 908-910.

196. Clinical trial data on St. John's wort in 2002 still leave much uncertainty. For references, see the constantly updated Cochrane Library Database, <http://cochranelibrary.com>, accessed August 2003.

197. Irish Medicines Board, "Herbal Medicines Project Final Report October 2001," available online at <http://www.dietandbody.com/alternativemedicine/article1029.html>, accessed August 2002.

198. P. Harrison-Read, "Drugs in Psychiatric Practice," in E. M. Tansey, D. A. Christie, and L. A. Reynolds (eds.), *Wellcome Witnesses to Twentieth-Century Medicine,* London: Wellcome Trust, Volume 2, 1998, p. 161.

199. For one example of discussion see E-H. W. Kluge, *Biomedical Ethics in a Canadian Context,* Scarborough, Ontario, Canada: Prentice-Hall, 1992, pp. 77-83.

200. D. T. Steinke, T. M. MacDonald, and P. G. Davy, "Doctor-Patient Relationship and Prescribing Patterns: A View from Primary Care," *PharmacoEconomics,* 16(1999), 599-603.

201. For a general discussion see A. Mitchell and M. Cormack, *The Therapeutic Relationship in Complementary Health Care,* Edinburgh: Churchill Livingstone, 1998.

202. A striking increase in use of the term *quality of life* in medical articles is readily documented by a search in databases such as MEDLINE.

203. Lander, *Defective Medicine: Risk, Anger, and the Malpractice Crisis,* p. 3.

204. C. W. Peck and G. Bryan, "Nomen Proprium," *The Lancet,* 273(1957), 1120 (also published in the *British Medical Journal,* 2[1957], 1366-1367). For analogous cautions from the United States see "Labeling of Prescription Drugs," *Journal of the American Medical Association,* 185(1963), 316.

205. M. Karr, "Complete Labeling of Prescriptions," *New England Journal of Medicine,* 280(1969), 673.

206. S. L. Nightingale, "Written Patient Information on Prescription Drugs: The Evolution of Government and Voluntary Programs in the United States," *International Journal of Technology Assessment in Health Care,* 11(1995), 399-409. See also, L. A. Morris, "The FDA's Approach to Patient Package Inserts: The Four Phases of PPIs" in M. Bogaert, R. Vander Stichele, J.-M. Kaufman, and R. Lefebvre

(eds.), *Patient Package Insert As a Source of Drug Information* (Proceedings of a symposium held in Belgium 1988), Amsterdam: Excerpta Medica, 1989, pp. 59-66. This book provides a general account of international trends up to 1988. It makes clear that the consumer health movement was a strong force in prompting change.

207. R. H. Blum, *The Management of the Doctor-Patient Relationship*, New York: McGraw-Hill, 1960, p. vii.

208. The accuracy of available information has been an issue for consumer groups, especially advertising. Cf., C. Medawar, "Patient Package Inserts, Drug Information and Liability Issues: A Consumer View," Bogaert, Vander Stichele, Kaufman, and LeFebvre, *Patient Package Insert As a Source of Drug Information*, pp. 81-87; and C. Medawar, "Data Sheets: A Consumer Perspective," *The Lancet*, 1(1988), 777-778.

209. Medawar, "Patient Package Inserts Drug Information and Liability Issues: A Consumer View," p. 85.

210. For example, citations in International Pharmaceutical Abstracts (IPA) revealed only thirty-eight citations from 1970 to June 2003 under "illiteracy."

211. M. Kelner, "The Therapeutic Relationship Under Fire," in M. Kelner and B. Wellman (eds.), *Complementary and Alternative Medicine: Challenge and Change*, Amsterdam, Netherlands: Harwood Academic, 2000, p. 94. The data were compiled from *visits* to practitioners. Whether the same distinction would have emerged if the complementary/alternative medicine patients had been recruited into the study when they were visiting a family practitioner is unclear; after all, few people depend on an alternative practitioner alone. Although the differences in practitioner-patient relationships in conventional or complementary/alternative medicine may well reflect the physician's special expert knowledge of drugs (albeit little different from that of homeopathic doctors and their medicines), it has to be recognized that, commonly, the level of trust often fails to lead to "compliance." Discussions on trust commonly suggest that it depends on more than expertise. For concerns about the erosion of trust in the 1990s through managed care in the United States see P. Illingworth, "Trust: The Scarcest of Medical Resources," *Journal of Medicine and Philosophy*, 27(2002), 31-46.

212. S. Anderson, "The Changing Role of the Community Pharmacist in Health Promotion in Great Britain 1930-1985," *Pharmaceutical Historian*, 32(2002), 7-10.

213. Oral History Collection, Newfoundland Pharmaceutical Association, George Young.

214. Ibid.

215. Some multi-ingredient ointments persisted, an indication that many skin problems were relatively untouched by new medications, including the "wonder" preparation hydrocortisone.

216. Some exceptions existed: "Mr. Hutchinson used to make up some fabulous ointments. I used it in my own [St. John's] store. I remember a woman from Botwood came in the 1960s and she had eczema. I made the ointment up for her. It cured her. All [of] Botwood used to come looking for it. A couple of doctors rang me for the formula, but I wouldn't give it to them!" (Oral History Collection, Newfoundland Pharmaceutical Association, James Aylward).

217. Oral History Collection, Newfoundland Pharmaceutical Association, Neil Curtis.

218. Oral History Collection, Newfoundland Pharmaceutical Association, Bill O'Mara.

219. Cf., R. A. Buerki, "The Public Image of the American Pharmacist in the Popular Press," *Pharmacy in History*, 38(1996), 62-78.

220. Oral History Collection, Newfoundland Pharmaceutical Association, Bill O'Mara; *The Evening Telegram*, July 16, 1959, p. 18.

221. Oral History Collection, Newfoundland Pharmaceutical Association, Leo Walsh.

222. It is tempting to see the widening of merchandise as part of an "Americanization" of Newfoundland pharmacy, especially since, as noted in Chapter 4, certain features such as the soda fountain had taken root in the first half of the twentieth century. It can be said that the overt feeling of kinship with British pharmacy was lost after the 1950s. This is seemingly reflected in the changing shop fascias of McMurdo's pharmacy: "T. McMurdo and Co. Chemists, Druggists" (c. 1910); followed by a hanging sign that added "Drugs, Sodas," (c. 1953); finally, in 1963, "McMurdo's Drugs, Soda." Ultimately, the British designations "chemist" or "chemist and druggist" disappeared entirely from all stores in Newfoundland.

223. Oral History Collection, Newfoundland Pharmaceutical Association, Neil Curtis, Bob McCarthy.

224. Oral History Collection, Newfoundland Pharmaceutical Association, Neil Curtis.

225. For representative discussions see J. K. Mount, "Pharmacy's Social Movement at the Turn of the Century: Introduction to Pharmaceutical Care Symposium," *Pharmacy in History*, 43(2001), 66-74; L. J. Muzzin, G. P. Brown, and R. W. Hornosty, "Professional Ideology in Canadian Pharmacy," *Health and Canadian Society*, 1(1993), 319-345; Muzzin, Brown, and Hornosty note Hepler's definition of pharmaceutical care: "the responsible provision of drug therapy for the purpose of achieving definite outcomes that improve a patient's quality of life" (p. 326).

226. *Time* (Canadian edition) 101(March 5, 1973), 73. Oral History Collection, Newfoundland Pharmaceutical Association, Bill Hogan.

227. J. P. Rovers, J. D. Curie, H. P. Hagel, R. P. McDonough, and J. L. Sobotka, *A Practical Guide to Pharmaceutical Care*, Washington, DC: American Pharmaceutical Association, 1998, p. 1. For worldwide trends by 1998 "World-Wide Developments in Pharmaceutical Care," *The Pharmaceutical Journal*, 260(1998), 563-568.

228. Oral History Collection, Newfoundland Pharmaceutical Association, George Hutchins and Bob McCarthy.

229. Oral History Collection, Newfoundland Pharmaceutical Association, Bob McCarthy. For a general discussion on dilemmas in Canada over counseling, Muzzin, Brown, and Hornosty, "Professional Ideology in Canadian Pharmacy."

230. Oral History Collection, Newfoundland Pharmaceutical Association, Cecil Burke.

231. Oral History Collection, Newfoundland Pharmaceutical Association, George Hutchins, who also remembered that when Woolco opened the first discount store in St. John's, "I had to answer to all kinds of people who weren't pharmacists, didn't understand pharmacy, and it was very frustrating at times."

232. See R. Horne, "Representations of Medication and Treatment: Advances in Theory and Measurement," in K. J. Petrie and J. A. Weinman (eds.), *Perceptions of*

Health and Illness: Current Research and Application, Amsterdam, Netherlands: Harwood, pp. 155-188.

233. N. Britten, "Patients' Ideas About Medicines: A Qualitative Study in a General Practice Population," *British Journal of General Practice,* 44(1994), 466. The issue of natural versus synthetic often emerges: "I just don't like artificial things . . . [natural remedies] are not chemically made, like flowers are naturally grown things. I prefer to take those than factory made chemicals" (Ibid., p. 466).

234. See comments by N. Vuckovic and M. Nichter, "Changing Patterns of Pharmaceutical Practice in the United States," *Social Sciences and Medicine,* 44(1997), 1285-1302.

235. Moskowitz, *In Therapy We Trust,* p. 219.

236. The term *commodity* is not widely used in the context of prescription drugs, but it is in line with the growing use of the term *consumer* rather than *patient* (Hibbert, Bissell, and Ward, "Consumerism and Professional Work in the Community Pharmacy"). Commerce of drugs in developing countries has also raised the topic of commodities, e.g., see S. Van Der Geest, "Essential Drugs: Critical Anthropological Note," *Pharmaceutisch Weekblad,* 123(1998), 1101-1104. For challenging comments on "the illness and commodity" see Marinker, "'What is Wrong' and 'How We Know It.'"

237. For quote and other context see M. E. Brown, "Drugs and Desire," *Pharmaceutical Journal,* 268(2002), 374-375.

238. R. Blythe, "Drugs and Medicines Are Not Ordinary Commercial Articles," *Pharmaceutical Journal,* 256(1996), 213.

239. E. Douglas, S. Chapman, S. Hudson, K. Paterson, and C. Duggan, "Patients' Perspectives on Medicines and Pharmacy: Views of Patients with Type 2 Diabetes," *The International Journal of Pharmacy Practice,* 9(suppl.)(2001), R76. Studies that indicate consumers often do not want advice about over-the-counter remedies should be noted, e.g., a Canadian study: J. Taylor, "Reasons Consumers Do Not Ask for Advice on Non-Prescription Medicines in Pharmacies," *The International Journal of Pharmacy Practice,* 2(1994), 209-214.

240. Quoted in F. Smith, S. A. Frank, and E. Rowley, "Group Interviews with People Taking Long-Term Medication: Comparing the Perspectives of People with Arthritis, Respiratory Disease, and Mental Health Problems," *The International Journal of Pharmacy Practice,* 8(June 2000), 90.

241. For example, see R. D. Caplan, E. A. R. Robinson, J. R. P. French Jr., J. R. Caldwell, and M. Shinn, *Adhering to Medical Regimens: Pilot Experiments in Patient Education and Social Support,* Ann Arbor: Institute for Social Research, University of Michigan, 1976. See also A. M. Zifferblatt, "Increasing Patient Compliance Through the Applied Analysis of Behavior," *Preventive Medicine,* 4(1975), 173-182. Zifferblatt indicates a somewhat coercive approach to the problem.

242. R. B. Haynes, D. W. Taylor, and D. L. Sackett (eds.), *Compliance in Health Care,* Baltimore: Johns Hopkins University Press, 1979, p. xv. See also D. L. Sackett and R. B. Haynes (eds.), *Compliance with Therapeutic Regimens,* Baltimore: Johns Hopkins University Press, 1976, p. xi.

243. K. E. Gerber and A. M. Nehemkis, *Compliance: The Dilemma of the Chronically Ill,* New York: Springer Publishing Company, 1986, p. xi. The message of the book is that patients may or may not comply with parts of a regimen.

244. See B. Blackwell, "The Drug Regimen and Treatment Compliance," in Haynes, Taylor, and Sacket (eds.), *Compliance in Health Care,* pp. 144-156.

245. Ibid.

246. For reference to flaws of the human condition with respect to compliance see A. R. Jonsen, "Ethical Issues in Compliance," in Haynes, Taylor, and Sackett (eds.), *Compliance in Health Care,* pp. 113-120.

247. For a telling example of problems see Anonymous, "Living with Warfarin and Diuretics: So Hard to Be Compliant," *Pharmaceutical Journal,* 268(2002), 183.

248. Cf., I. Barofsky, "Compliance, Adherence, and the Therapeutic Alliance: Steps in the Development of Self-Care," *Social Science and Medicine,* 12(1978), 369-376.

249. For a focus on this issue see Royal Pharmaceutical Society of Great Britain, *From Compliance to Concordance: Toward Shared Goals in Medicine Taking,* London: Royal Pharmaceutical Society of Great Britain, 1997.

250. W. W. Weston, "Informed and Shared Decision-Making: The Crux of Patient-Centred Care," *Canadian Medical Association Journal,* 165(2001), 438.

251. The role of hope or hopefulness was often discussed in the same terms as placebo. For James Jackson Putnam's 1895 views on hopefulness see F. G. Gosling, *Before Freud: Neurasthenia and the American Medical Community 1870-1910,* Urbana: University of Illinois Press, 1987, p. 131.

252. See R. R. Parse, *Hope: An International Human Becoming Perspective,* Sudbury, MA: Jones and Bartlett, 1999.

253. J. S. Bradshaw, *Doctors on Trial,* London: Wildwood House, 1978, pp. 312-313.

Epilogue

1. Quote 1: M. B. Strauss (ed.), *Familiar Medical Quotations,* Boston: Little, Brown, 1968, p. 630; quote 2: E. J. Huth and T. J. Murray, *Medicine in Quotations: Views of Health and Disease Through the Ages,* Philadelphia: American College of Physicians, 2000, p. 362; quote 3: R. R. Andersen, J. K. Crellin, and M. Joe, "Spirituality, Values and Boundaries in the Revitalization of a Mi'kmaq Community," in G. Harvey (ed.), *Indigenous Religions: A Companion,* London: Cassell, 2000, p. 251.

2. R. Dunglison, *General Therapeutics and Materia Medica,* Philadelphia: Lea and Blanchard, Volume 1, 1850, p. 17.

3. Even as the second half of the twentieth century opened, the formal teaching of medical students about medicines (as distinct from on the hospital wards) had, for some years, already been in the hands of the basic science of pharmacology, which has always placed much emphasis on mechanisms of action. No longer did textbooks appear with the words "therapeutics" and/or "materia medica" in their titles, except for L. Goodman and A. Gilman's classic textbook *Goodman and Gilman's The Pharmacological Basis of Therapeutics,* first published in 1941. "The primary function of clinical pharmacology in medical education and hospital practice" emerging in the 1950s was stated, in 1972, to provide "a rational basis for drug therapy" (D. E. Hutcheon, "Factors Influencing the Growth of Clinical Pharmacology," *Journal of Clinical Pharmacology and New Drugs,* 12(1972), 365). Totally in-

adequate teaching in U.S. medical schools was also noted, little different from elsewhere. For perspectives on pharmacy see J. Parascandola and J. Swann, "Development of Pharmacology in American Schools of Pharmacy," *Pharmacy in History,* 25(1983), 95-115.

4. I cannot resist reference to a noteworthy conversation (c.1925 or so) between two physicians, albeit fictitious, in Sinclair Lewis, *Arrowsmith,* New York: Harcourt Brace, 1945, p. 183. In response to a question from one doctor to another on treating asthma, the reply mentions that a treatment containing foxes' lungs is fine for asthma. "I told that to a Sioux City pulmonary specialist one time and he laughed at me—said it wasn't scientific—and I said to him, 'Hell!' I said, 'scientific!' I said, 'I don't know if it's the latest fad and wrinkle in science or not,' I said, 'but I get results, and that's what I'm looking for 's results!'" The attitude persists, albeit much less strident.

5. R. S. Downie and J. Macnaughton, *Clinical Judgement: Evidence in Practice,* Oxford: Oxford University Press, 2000. It is of interest to compare this book, with its message of the need to incorporate humane values into clinical judgment, with A. F. Feinstein, *Clinical Judgment,* Baltimore: Williams and Wilkins, 1967, which argues that clinicians should bring science into clinical judgment (e.g., see p. 29).

6. For discussions on Britain that are equally relevant to North America see N. Britten, "Prescribing and the Defense of Clinical Autonomy," *Sociology of Health and Illness,* 23(2001), 478-496; for further developments in prescribing by pharmacists see C. Bellingham, "Space, Time, and Team Working: Issues for Pharmacists Who Wish to Prescribe," *Pharmaceutical Journal,* 268(2001), 562-563.

Index

Note: Page numbers followed by the letter "b" indicate boxed material; those followed by the letter "t" indicate tables.

Printed in the United States
by Baker & Taylor Publisher Services